T0226555

Head and Neck Cancer

Editor

A. DIMITRIOS COLEVAS

HEMATOLOGY/ONCOLOGY CLINICS OF NORTH AMERICA

www.hemonc.theclinics.com

Consulting Editors
GEORGE P. CANELLOS
H. FRANKLIN BUNN

December 2015 • Volume 29 • Number 6

ELSEVIER

1600 John F. Kennedy Boulevard • Suite 1800 • Philadelphia, Pennsylvania, 19103-2899

http://www.theclinics.com

HEMATOLOGY/ONCOLOGY CLINICS OF NORTH AMERICA Volume 29, Number 6
December 2015 ISSN 0889-8588, ISBN 13: 978-0-323-40250-7

Editor: Jennifer Flynn-Briggs
Developmental Editor: Kristen Helm

Hematology/Oncology Clinics (ISSN 0889-8588) is published bimonthly by Elsevier Inc., 360 Park Avenue South, New York, NY 10010-1710. Months of issue are February, April, June, August, October, and December. Business and Editorial Offices: 1600 John F. Kennedy Blvd., Ste. 1800, Philadelphia, PA 19103—2899. Customer Service Office: 3251 Riverport Lane, Maryland Heights, MO 63043. Periodicals postage paid at New York, NY and at additional mailing offices. Subscription prices are $385.00 per year (domestic individuals), $633.00 per year (domestic institutions), $190.00 per year (domestic students/residents), $440.00 per year (Canadian individuals), $783.00 per year (Canadian institutions) $520.00 per year (international individuals), $783.00 per year (international institutions), and $255.00 per year (international and Canadian students/residents). International air speed delivery is included in all *Clinics* subscription prices. All prices are subject to change without notice. **POSTMASTER:** Send address changes to *Hematology/Oncology Clinics of North America*, Elsevier Health Sciences Division, Subscription Customer Service, 3251 Riverport Lane, Maryland Heights, MO 63043. Customer Service (orders, claims, online, change of address): Elsevier Health Sciences Division, Subscription **Customer Service, 3251 Riverport Lane, Maryland Heights, MO 63043. Tel: 1-800-654-2452 (U.S. and Canada); 314-447-8871 (outside U.S. and Canada). Fax: 314-447-8029. E-mail: journalscustomerservice-usa@elsevier.com (for print support); journalsonlinesupport-usa@elsevier.com (for online support)**.

Reprints. For copies of 100 or more, of articles in this publication, please contact the Commercial Reprints Department, Elsevier Inc., 360 Park Avenue South, New York, New York 10010-1710; Tel.: 212-633-3874, Fax: 212-633-3820, E-mail: reprints@elsevier.com.

Hematology/Oncology Clinics of North America is covered in *MEDLINE/PubMed (Index Medicus), EMBASE/ Excerpta Medica, and BIOSIS.*

Contributors

CONSULTING EDITORS

GEORGE P. CANELLOS, MD
William Rosenberg Professor of Medicine, Department of Medical Oncology, Dana-Farber Cancer Institute, Boston, Massachusetts

H. FRANKLIN BUNN, MD
Professor of Medicine, Division of Hematology, Brigham and Women's Hospital, Harvard Medical School, Boston, Massachusetts

EDITOR

A. DIMITRIOS COLEVAS, MD
Division of Medical Oncology, Stanford University, Stanford Cancer Institute, Stanford, California

AUTHORS

PIERRE BLANCHARD, MD, PhD
Consultant, Department of Radiation Oncology, Research in Epidemiology and Population Health, Paris-Saclay University, Gustave-Roussy, Villejuif Cedex, France

MARIA E. CABANILLAS, MD
Department of Endocrine Neoplasia and Hormonal Disorders, The University of Texas MD Anderson Cancer Center, Houston, Texas

GILBERTO CASTRO Jr, MD, PhD
Department of Clinical Oncology, Instituto do Câncer do Estado de São Paulo, Faculdade de Medicina da Universidade de São Paulo, São Paulo, Brazil

NICOLE G. CHAU, MD
Instructor, Center for Head and Neck Oncology, Dana-Farber Cancer Institute, Harvard Medical School; Department of Medical Oncology, Dana-Farber Cancer Institute; Department of Medicine, Brigham and Women's Hospital, Boston, Massachusetts

VERONIQUE WAN FOOK CHEUNG, MD
Fellow, Division of Head and Neck Surgical Oncology, University of Nebraska Medical Center, Omaha, Nebraska

CHRISTINE H. CHUNG, MD
Department of Otolaryngology-Head and Neck Surgery, Sidney Kimmel Comprehensive Cancer Center, The Johns Hopkins University School of Medicine, Johns Hopkins Medical Institutions, Baltimore, Maryland

RAMONA DADU, MD
Department of Endocrine Neoplasia and Hormonal Disorders, The University of Texas MD Anderson Cancer Center, Houston, Texas

MAURA L. GILLISON, MD, PhD
Professor, Cancer Control and Prevention Program, The Ohio State University Comprehensive Cancer Center, The Ohio State University, Columbus, Ohio

ELIZABETH G. GRUBBS, MD
Department of Surgical Oncology, The University of Texas MD Anderson Cancer Center, Houston, Texas

GARY BRANDON GUNN, MD
Department of Radiation Oncology, The University of Texas MD Anderson Cancer Center, Houston, Texas

ROBERT I. HADDAD, MD
Associate Professor, Center for Head and Neck Oncology, Dana-Farber Cancer Institute, Harvard Medical School; Department of Medical Oncology, Dana-Farber Cancer Institute; Department of Medicine, Brigham and Women's Hospital, Boston, Massachusetts

FLOYD CHRISTOPHER HOLSINGER, MD, FACS
Professor and Chief of Head and Neck Surgery, Department of Otolaryngology-Head and Neck Surgery, Stanford University School of Medicine, Palo Alto, California

MIMI I. HU, MD
Department of Endocrine Neoplasia and Hormonal Disorders, The University of Texas MD Anderson Cancer Center, Houston, Texas

PEDRO H. ISAACSSON VELHO, MD
Department of Clinical Oncology, Instituto do Câncer do Estado de São Paulo, Faculdade de Medicina da Universidade de São Paulo, São Paulo, Brazil

STEPHEN Y. LAI, MD, PhD
Departments of Head and Neck Surgery, The University of Texas MD Anderson Cancer Center, Houston, Texas

ANNE W.M. LEE, MD, FRCR
Clinical Professor, Department of Clinical Oncology, Li Ka Shing Faculty of Medicine, The University of Hong Kong, Queen Mary Hospital, Hong Kong; The University of Hong Kong – Shenzhen Hospital, Shenzhen, Guangdong, China

RYAN J. LI, MD
Clinical Instructor, Department of Otolaryngology-Head and Neck Surgery, Stanford University School of Medicine, Palo Alto, California

GIL CHAI LIM, MD
Department of Otolaryngology-Head and Neck Surgery, Jeju National University School of Medicine, Jeju Special Self-Governing Province, Republic of Korea

CHARLES LU, MD
Department of Thoracic/Head and Neck Medical Oncology, The University of Texas MD Anderson Cancer Center, Houston, Texas

WILLIAM M. LYDIATT, MD
Professor and Division Chief, Division of Head and Neck Surgical Oncology, University of Nebraska Medical Center; Head and Neck Surgical Oncology, Nebraska Methodist Hospital, Omaha, Nebraska

JEAN-PASCAL MACHIELS, MD, PhD
Departments of Medical Oncology and Head and Neck Surgery, King Albert II Institute, Cliniques Universitaires Saint-Luc and Institut de Recherche Clinique et Expérimentale (IREC), Université Catholique de Louvain, Brussels, Belgium

DANIELLE N. MARGALIT, MD, MPH
Assistant Professor, Department of Radiation Oncology, Dana-Farber Cancer Institute, Harvard Medical School, Boston, Massachusetts

RENATO G. MARTINS, MD, MPH
Professor, Division of Medical Oncology, Department of Medicine, University of Washington, Seattle, Washington

EDUARDO MÉNDEZ, MD, MS
Associate Professor, Department of Otolaryngology, Head and Neck Surgery, University of Washington; Clinical Research Division, Fred Hutchinson Cancer Research Center, Seattle, Washington

WAI TONG NG, MD, FRCR
Consultant, Department of Clinical Oncology, Pamela Youde Nethersole Eastern Hospital, Chai Wan, Hong Kong, China

ARU PANWAR, MD
Assistant Professor, Division of Head and Neck Surgical Oncology, University of Nebraska Medical Center; Head and Neck Surgical Oncology, Nebraska Methodist Hospital, Omaha, Nebraska

UPENDRA PARVATHANENI, MBBS, FRANZCR
Associate Professor, Division of Radiation Oncology, Department of Medicine, University of Washington, Seattle, Washington

JEAN-PIERRE PIGNON, MD, PhD
Senior Clinical Epidemiologist, Department of Biostatistics and Epidemiology, Ligue National Contre le Cancer Platform of Meta-analyses in Oncology, Research in Epidemiology and Population Health, Paris-Saclay University, Gustave-Roussy, Villejuif Cedex, France

SIDHARTH V. PURAM, MD, PhD
Department of Otolaryngology, Massachusetts Eye and Ear Infirmary; Department of Otology and Laryngology, Harvard Medical School, Boston, Massachusetts

CARLO RESTIGHINI, MD
Medical Oncology, Istituto Nazionale dei Tumori, Milano, Italy

JAMES W. ROCCO, MD, PhD, FACS
Department of Otolaryngology-Head and Neck Surgery, Wexner Medical Center, James Cancer Hospital, Solove Research Institute, The Ohio State University, Columbus, Ohio

CRISTINA P. RODRIGUEZ, MD
Associate Professor, Division of Medical Oncology, Department of Medicine, University of Washington, Seattle, Washington

SANDRA SCHMITZ, MD, PhD
Departments of Medical Oncology and Head and Neck Surgery, King Albert II Institute, Cliniques Universitaires Saint-Luc and Institut de Recherche Clinique et Expérimentale (IREC), Université Catholique de Louvain, Brussels, Belgium

JONATHON D. SCHOENFELD, MD, MPH
Assistant Professor, Department of Radiation Oncology, Dana-Farber Cancer Institute, Harvard Medical School, Boston, Massachusetts

DAVID W. SCHOPPY, MD, PhD
Division of Head and Neck Surgery, Department of Otolaryngology, Stanford University School of Medicine, Stanford, California

JOHN B. SUNWOO, MD
Division of Head and Neck Surgery, Department of Otolaryngology, Stanford University School of Medicine, Stanford, California

HENRY SZE, FRCR
Clinical Assistant Professor, Department of Clinical Oncology, Li Ka Shing Faculty of Medicine, The University of Hong Kong, Queen Mary Hospital, Hong Kong; The University of Hong Kong – Shenzhen Hospital, Shenzhen, Guangdong, China

ROY B. TISHLER, MD, PhD
Director, Head and Neck Radiation Oncology; Associate Professor, Department of Radiation Oncology, Dana-Farber Cancer Institute, Harvard Medical School, Boston, Massachusetts

MICHELLE D. WILLIAMS, MD
Pathology Head and Neck Section, Department of Pathology, The University of Texas MD Anderson Cancer Center, Houston, Texas

Contents

> In spite of a rapidly expanding understanding of head and neck tumor biology and optimization of radiation, chemotherapy, and surgical treatment modalities, head and neck squamous cell carcinoma (HNSCC) remains a major cause of cancer-related morbidity and mortality. Although our biologic understanding of these tumors had largely been limited to pathways driving proliferation, survival, and differentiation, the identification of HPV as a major driver of HNSCC and genomic sequencing analyses has dramatically influenced our understanding of tumor biology and approach to therapy. Here, we summarize molecular aspects of HNSCC biology and identify promising areas for potential diagnostic and therapeutic agents.

> Based on currently available genomic data, most head and neck squamous cell carcinoma have few targetable aberrations and immediate clinical translation is challenging. However, potential therapeutic agents listed in this article need to be thoroughly evaluated because there are compelling scientific rationales supporting their development. Concerted effort is required to identify better predictive biomarkers of clinical benefit and improve the therapeutic index. Clinicians need to better understand resistance mechanisms, generate novel hypotheses for appropriate combination regimens and dosing schedules, develop more accurate model systems, and conduct innovative clinical trials.

> Overexpression of epidermal growth factor receptor (EGFR) is linked with poor prognosis in squamous cell carcinoma of the head and neck (SCCHN). Cetuximab binds specifically to EGFR with high affinity; combined with radiotherapy, it improves locoregional control and survival over radiotherapy alone. Adding cetuximab to platinum-based chemotherapy and 5-fluorouracil improves overall survival in incurable disease. Only a minority of patients benefit from anti-EGFR monoclonal antibodies. A better understanding of the molecular mechanisms involved in treatment resistance and identification of predictive biomarkers are crucial. Potentially more potent anti-EGFR compounds are currently under investigation with the aim of improving treatment efficacy.

> Although head and neck squamous cell carcinoma has traditionally been
> considered to be a very immunosuppressive, or at least nonimmunogenic,
> tumor type, recent results from clinical studies of immune checkpoint
> blockade strategies have led to resurgence in the enthusiasm for immuno-
> therapeutic approaches. Additional strategies for immunotherapy that are
> under active investigation include enhancement of cetuximab-mediated
> antibody-dependent cell-mediated cytotoxicity, tumor vaccines, and engi-
> neered T cells for adoptive therapy. All of these studies have early-phase
> clinical trials under way, and the next several years will be exciting as the
> results of these studies are reported.

> Human papillomavirus (HPV) is the cause of a distinct subset of oropharyn-
> geal cancer rising in incidence in the United States and other developed
> countries. This increased incidence, combined with the strong effect of tu-
> mor HPV status on survival, has had a profound effect on the head and neck
> cancer discipline. The multidisciplinary field of head and neck cancer is in
> the midst of re-evaluating evidence-based algorithms for clinical decision
> making, developed from clinical trials conducted in an era when HPV-
> negative cancer predominated. This article reviews relationships between
> tumor HPV status and gender, cancer incidence trends, overall survival,
> treatment response, racial disparities, tumor staging, risk stratification, sur-
> vival post disease progression, and clinical trial design.

> Most patients diagnosed with head and neck cancer have locally advanced
> disease. Sequential and concurrent chemoradiation are standard, nonsur-
> gical, curative-intent treatment options. Controversy remains regarding the
> superiority of one approach to another. Definitive management strategies
> are evolving with increasing efforts to pursue deintensification of therapy
> for low-risk patients, and to pursue therapeutic intensification for high-
> risk patients. Both sequential therapy and concurrent chemoradiation
> play important roles in shaping treatment paradigms because both ap-
> proaches may be used to investigate deintensification or intensification
> strategies. This article examines the latest evidence and state-of-the-art
> approaches, highlighting ongoing controversies and future directions.

> Traditional open surgical approaches are indicated for treatment of select
> tumor subsites of head and neck cancer, but can also result in major
> cosmetic and functional morbidity. Transoral surgical approaches have
> been used for head and neck cancer since the 1960s, with their application

continuing to evolve with the changing landscape of this disease and recent innovations in surgical instrumentation. The potential to further reduce treatment morbidity with transoral surgery, while optimizing oncologic outcomes, continues to be investigated. This review examines current literature evaluating oncologic and quality-of-life outcomes achieved through transoral head and neck surgery.

The many advances in radiotherapy for squamous cell cancer of the head and neck described in this article will have significant effects on the ultimate outcomes of patients who receive this treatment. The technological and clinical advances should allow one to maintain or improve disease control, while moderating the toxicity associated with head and neck radiation therapy.

Radiotherapy is the primary treatment of nasopharyngeal carcinoma and combination chemotherapy can enhance treatment outcomes for locoregionally advanced disease. The Intergroup 0099 study using concurrent-adjuvant cisplatin-based chemoradiotherapy was the first trial to demonstrate a survival benefit. Since then, there have been attempts to further improve the treatment results by altering the chemotherapy sequence, using different chemotherapeutic agents or schedules, and extending the use of chemotherapy to early-stage disease. This review provides an overview of the data and highlights the current controversies behind international guidelines.

Surgery remains the most important effective treatment for differentiated (DTC) and medullary thyroid cancer (MTC). Radioactive iodine (RAI) is another important treatment but is reserved only for DTC whose disease captures RAI. Once patients fail primary therapy, observation is often recommended, as most DTC and MTC patients will have indolent disease. However, in a fraction of patients, systemic therapy must be considered. In recent decades 4 systemic therapies have been approved by the United States FDA for DTC and MTC. Sorafenib and lenvatinib are approved for DTC and vandetanib and cabozantinib for MTC. Anaplastic thyroid cancer (ATC) is a rare and rapidly progressive form of thyroid cancer with a very high mortality rate. Treatment of ATC remains a challenge. Most patients are not surgical candidates at diagnosis due to advanced disease. External beam radiation and radiosensitizing radiation are the mainstay of therapy at this time. However, exciting new drugs and approaches to therapy are on the horizon but it will take a concerted, worldwide effort to complete clinical trials in order to find effective therapies that will improve the overall survival for this devastating disease.

Cristina P. Rodriguez, Upendra Parvathaneni, Eduardo Méndez, and
Renato G. Martins

> Salivary gland malignant tumors represent a diverse group of neoplasms.
> Their low incidence makes research studies challenging, with most thera-
> peutic recommendations based on case reviews, single-arm trials, or
> small randomized trials. The standard of care for localized disease is sur-
> gical resection. Radiotherapy is the preferred local therapy when surgery is
> not possible or if there is significant morbidity. When symptomatic meta-
> static disease develops, systemic therapy is considered. Recent trial
> accrual success with a cooperative group, treatments based on defined
> molecular targets, and the development of immunotherapies all hold
> promise in improving the care of patients with these tumors.

Aru Panwar, Veronique Wan Fook Cheung, and William M. Lydiatt

> Supportive care and survivorship strategies in the management of head
> and neck squamous cell carcinoma (HNSCC) revolve around continued
> collaborative efforts aimed at early identification and intervention for lo-
> coregional disease recurrence, second primary malignancy, management
> of treatment-related side effects, and provision for psychosocial support.
> Development of evidence-based guidelines and optimization of these
> strategies is increasingly important in the setting of improved survival of
> patients with HNSCC because of a variety of diagnostic and therapeutic
> advances and evolving demographics of HNSCC patient population, spe-
> cifically, p16-associated oropharyngeal squamous cell carcinoma.

HEMATOLOGY/ONCOLOGY CLINICS OF NORTH AMERICA

ISSUE OF RELATED INTEREST

Surgical Oncology Clinics, July 2015 (Vol. 24, Issue 3)
Head and Neck Cancer
John A. Ridge, *Editor*
Available at: http://www.surgonc.theclinics.com/

THE CLINICS ARE AVAILABLE ONLINE!
Access your subscription at:
www.theclinics.com

Preface

New Diseases and New Treatments—Head and Neck Cancer Updates

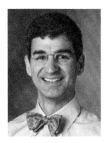

A. Dimitrios Colevas, MD
Editor

It is with great excitement that I introduce this issue of *Hematology/Oncology Clinics of North America*, the focus of which is on head and neck cancers.

Drs Puram and Rocco elegantly update us on what is known about molecular alterations in squamous cell carcinomas of the head and neck. Drs Velho, Castro, and Chung highlight which of these alterations are likely to offer therapeutic fruits in the near future. Subsequent articles on the EGFR receptor, immunotherapy, and HPV-related oropharynx cancers remind us that there are new diseases that must be evaluated and treated differently, and what novel treatment paradigms (immuno-therapy) are emerging. While EGFR-targeted therapies have been around for a while, we are still perfecting how to best use them. One of the most exciting new frontiers in therapeutics is harnessing our own body's immune system from inhibition of immune checkpoints all the way to genetic engineering of autologous T cells to improve outcomes without necessarily intensifying conventional chemotherapy and radiation treatments. This may be particularly relevant for virally induced cancers such as HPV-associated oropharynx cancer and EBV-related nasopharyngeal cancer.

Multimodality therapy is still the primary treatment approach for most patients with localized head and neck cancer, and there have been major leaps forward in both surgical and radiation treatments. Drs Lim, Holsinger, and Li point out that with surgery, less can be more, especially with new technology such as transoral robotics. In the case of radiation, the excitement of new imaging techniques, image-guided adoptive and replaning techniques, as well as the refinement of intensity-modulated radiation therapy and intensity-modified protein therapy are changing what we can offer patients.

Hematol Oncol Clin N Am 29 (2015) xiii–xiv
http://dx.doi.org/10.1016/j.hoc.2015.08.004
0889-8588/15/$ – see front matter © 2015 Published by Elsevier Inc.

Diseases other than the typical squamous cell carcinomas are also noted for exciting developments. In the case of nasopharyngeal cancer, Dr Sze and colleagues point out that some lower-stage patients can be treated with less. In patients with more advanced NPC, we learn more about the use of drugs beyond cisplatin and personalized prognostic markers such as blood EBV DNA levels.

Thyroid carcinoma treatment options have expanded dramatically. Dr Cabanillas and colleagues have elegantly summarized the great leap forward beyond surgery and radioactive iodine with a discussion of the new tyrosine-kinase inhibitors and inhibitors directed against BRAF mutant tumors.

To round out this issue, we have an update on salivary gland cancers, and last, but not least, Drs Panwar, Cheung, and Lydiatt reinforce the importance of paying attention to supportive care and survivorship in our patients, who are living longer and better lives as our treatment modalities improve.

I hope the readers find these articles both useful and stimulating.

A. Dimitrios Colevas, MD
Division of Medical Oncology
Stanford University
Stanford Cancer Institute
875 Blake Wilbur Drive
Stanford, CA 94305-5826, USA

E-mail address:
colevas@stanford.edu

Molecular Aspects of Head and Neck Cancer Therapy

Sidharth V. Puram, MD, PhD[a,b], James W. Rocco, MD, PhD[c,*]

KEYWORDS

- Head and neck cancer • Squamous cell carcinoma • Molecular biology
- Targeted therapy • Synthetic lethality • Genomic sequencing
- Intratumor heterogeneity

KEY POINTS

- Head and neck squamous cell carcinoma (HNSCC) is driven by numerous mutations, with human papilloma virus negative (HPV–) cancers caused by more traditional risk factors (tobacco use/alcohol) tending to harbor more mutations, greater intratumor heterogeneity, and extensive copy number variation.
- Recent genomic insights suggest that targeted therapy of HNSCC will remain a significant challenge. Most mutations identified based on sequencing analyses are loss-of-function mutations in known and putative tumor suppressor genes that may require novel approaches, such as synthetic lethality.
- Oncogenic drivers are few and far between and often are present at low mutant allele frequencies, suggesting they may be poor choices for targeted therapy.
- One exception for targeted therapy may be activating Ras or PI3K mutations that occur at high frequency in HPV+ cancers, offering a potential avenue for therapy that may facilitate deintensification of chemoradiation therapy.
- Identification of genes implicated in tumor-immune interactions as well as loss of function mutations suggest that immunotherapy and modulation of immune surveillance may be a valuable therapeutic approach, supporting ongoing immunotherapy clinical trials.

INTRODUCTION

Despite advances in our understanding of tumor biology, including its evolutionary refinements, as well as radiation, chemotherapy, and surgical treatments,

---

Disclosures/Conflict of Interest: The authors have nothing to disclose.
[a] Department of Otolaryngology, Massachusetts Eye and Ear Infirmary, 243 Charles St., Boston, MA 02114, USA; [b] Department of Otology and Laryngology, Harvard Medical School, 25 Shattuck St., Boston, MA 02115, USA; [c] Department of Otolaryngology-Head and Neck Surgery, Wexner Medical Center, James Cancer Hospital, Solove Research Institute, The Ohio State University, 320 West 10th Avenue, Columbus, OH 43210, USA
* Corresponding author.
E-mail address: james.rocco@osumc.edu

head and neck squamous cell carcinoma (HNSCC) remains the sixth leading cause of cancer-related morbidity and mortality, with 550,000 new cases diagnosed each year.[1,2] These tumors arise from mucosal epithelium in the oral cavity, oropharynx, larynx, and hypopharynx, which together represent 75% of diagnosed cancers.[3]

HNSCC tumors can be broadly divided into those that are human papilloma virus (HPV)-negative (HPV–) and associated with alcohol and tobacco consumption,[4] and those that are HPV-positive (HPV+) and due to HPV infection primarily with serotype 16.[5,6] Although HPV– cancers arise via field cancerization and clonal progression in the setting of repetitive carcinogen application, HPV+ tumors harbor few mutations and are driven by a fundamentally distinct pathophysiologic mechanisms that rely on E6 and E7 viral proteins to inactivate or bypass cellular tumor suppressive responses.[7] Although recent vaccines against HPV (Gardasil, Cervarix) will influence the prevalence of HPV+ HNSCC in the decades to follow, for now, the incidence of HPV+ HNSCC continues to rise. Current estimates suggest that 45% to 90% of oropharyngeal squamous cell carcinomas (OPSCCs) are HPV+ with 90% associated with HPV serotype 16.[8,9] The division of HNSCC into two fundamentally distinct tumor cohorts with widely disparate survival rates based on HPV status represents one of the most significant developments of the past decade in head and neck cancer research and treatment.

Treatment for HNSCC is most often chosen based on the primary tumor subsite, TNM staging, and predicted functional outcomes following different treatment modalities. In general, early-stage (I or II) HNSCC is treated with local therapy, taking advantage of the ability of surgical removal or radiation to offer a curative modality. Advanced disease (stage III or IV) requires multimodality treatment with surgery, radiation, and/or chemotherapy.[10] Although the influence of treatment-related medical complications on mortality has declined,[11] and some improvements in head and neck survival have been documented, these are largely related to the increasing incidence of HPV+ cancers rather than substantive gain in the clinical management of HNSCC. Treatment failure in HNSCC relates to resistance of tumor cells to primary or adjuvant chemoradiation therapy, as well as residual undetectable microscopic disease that remains after surgical resection.

Recent whole-exome sequencing of HNSCC offers several lessons into how these tumors will need to be treated to improve on traditional therapeutic modalities. First, the sequencing of such a large number of tumors from numerous institutions demonstrates the successful endeavor of a multi-institutional collaborative effort to molecularly characterize the biology of head and neck tumors. Second, these analyses have validated that p53 inactivating mutations remain the predominant genetic defect identified, substantiating previous studies and emphasizing the observation that most tumors harbor loss-of-function mutations. Third, sequencing data separates HPV+ and HPV– tumors into distinct groups with completely different mutational profiles. Fourth, we have learned that HNSCC will be challenging to treat: there is no singular target for these tumors. Intratumor heterogeneity will also remain a challenge as we attempt to advance our therapeutic approaches.

In this review, we briefly discuss the molecular pathways driving HNSCC as identified using traditional genetics and biochemistry, but focus primarily on the new and interesting scientific advances in the field. In particular, we emphasize insights from recent whole-exome sequencing analyses of HNSCC, discuss lessons learned from analyses of intratumor heterogeneity, and explore the implications of recent studies on future therapeutic approaches.

TUMOR SUPPRESSORS FREQUENTLY DRIVE HEAD AND NECK SQUAMOUS CELL CARCINOMA BUT ARE DIFFICULT TO TARGET

p53 is a ubiquitous tumor suppressor that is critically altered in a number of human cancers,[12] with up to two-thirds of HNSCCs harboring mutations in exons 5 to 8.[13,14] Mutations in p53 dysregulate the cell cycle and monitoring of genomic integrity, thereby leading to aberrant proliferation, disrupted apoptosis, and defective DNA repair, whereas the HPV viral oncogene E6 targets p53 for degradation (**Fig. 1**). Clinically, alterations in p53 function are associated with resistance to radiation and cisplatin-based chemotherapeutics,[15] emphasizing the importance of this master regulator in HNSCC pathogenesis.

Recent whole exome sequencing analyses have validated these observations in cell lines and in vitro models, confirming that p53 mutations are common in HNSCC with loss-of-function mutations predominating. Stransky and colleagues[16] analyzed 74 tumor-normal pairs with their analysis, suggesting 63% contained mutations or deletions in p53. Analyses from The Cancer Genome Atlas (TCGA) of 279 HNSCCs identified mutations in p53 in 84% of HPV– tumors, with only 3% (1 of 36) of HPV+ tumors containing a p53 mutation (**Fig. 2**).[17] Similarly, inactivating mutations in the cell-cycle regulator CDKN2A were found in 58% of HPV– tumors.[17] Thus, a major conclusion of these whole-exome sequencing analyses has been validating the near-universal loss of function of p53 and CDKN2A inactivation in smoking/alcohol-related HNSCC. The challenge with p53and CDKN2A loss-of-function mutations is reactivation and/or replacing these critical cell-cycle regulators. Adenoviral gene therapy, chemical activators of mutated genes, and antagonists of endogenous p53 inhibitors are all possibilities, but preclinical and clinical trials hold variable promise,[18] and these strategies suffer the inherent limitations of targeting tumor suppressor genes, including efficient delivery, tumor cell target specificity, and public resistance to gene therapy.

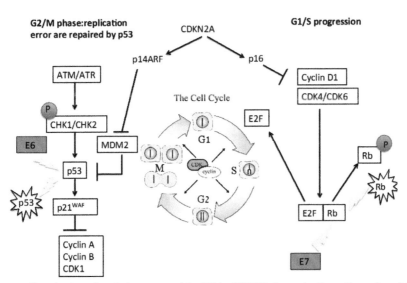

Fig. 1. Cell-cycle signaling is interrupted in HPV+ HNSCC through disruption of multiple cell-cycle checkpoints. (*From* Machiels JP, Lambrecht M, Hanin FX, et al. Advances in the management of squamous cell carcinoma of the head and neck. F1000Prime Rep 2014;6:44.)

A

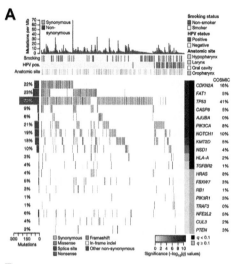

B

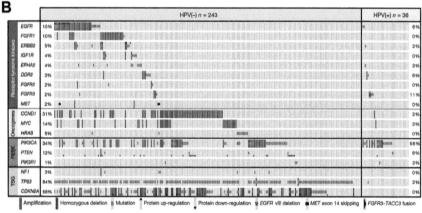

C

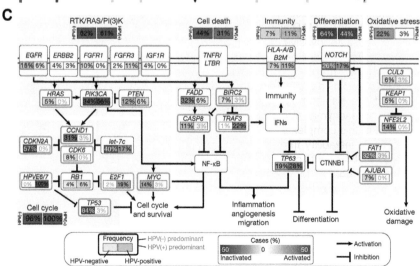

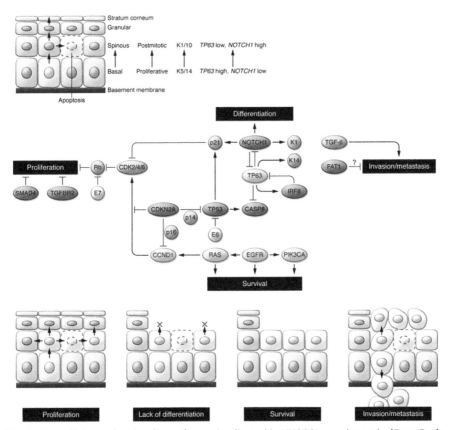

Fig. 3. Key cellular and molecular pathways implicated in HNSCC tumorigenesis. (*From* Rothenberg SM, Ellisen LW. The molecular pathogenesis of head and neck squamous cell carcinoma. J Clin Invest 2012;122(6):1952; with permission.)

Alteration of differentiation pathways through the loss of transforming growth factor β receptor (TGFβR)/SMAD signaling may also promote the transformation of aerodigestive mucosa to invasive SCC by critically altering tumor suppressor pathways (see **Fig. 2**; **Fig. 3**). Loss of function mutations in TGFβR2 as well as in SMAD2 and SMAD4 have been identified.[19,20] Interestingly, data from cutaneous SCC suggest that TGFβ may play a dual role in oncogenesis, initially acting as a tumor suppressor to prevent the transformation to invasive SCC, but subsequently promoting the epithelial-mesenchymal transition and supporting metastasis.[21] Animal data from mice confirm this complex signaling dichotomy: conditional deletion of SMAD4 triggers genomic instability through activation of TGFβ1 and other SMADs,[22] whereas deletion of TGFβR2 acts cooperatively with KRAS (V-Ki-ras2 Kirsten rat sarcoma viral oncogene homolog) to promote metastases.[23] In whole-exome sequencing,

Fig. 2. Whole-exome sequencing of HNSCC reveals novel insights into tumor pathogenesis and mutational profile. (*A*) Significantly mutated genes in HNSCC. (*B*) Candidate therapeutic targets and driver oncogenic events. (*C*) Deregulation of signaling pathways and transcription factors. (*From* Cancer Genome Atlas Network. Comprehensive genomic characterization of head and neck squamous cell carcinomas. Nature 2015;517:576–82; with permission.)

comparison of mutations by subset analyses of anatomic site revealed unique mutations in TGFβR2 in oral cavity tumors, consistent with previously described functions in animal models.[17] Given that TGFβ inhibitors are readily available and already being used in clinical trials for non–small cell lung cancer, colorectal cancer, and prostate cancer,[24] inhibition of these differentiation pathways in HNSCC may be an accessible and exciting avenue for novel therapeutics.

Sequencing data also have provided a rich array of data implicating loss-of-function mutations in additional pathways of differentiation in HNSCC, defining major new potential therapeutic targets. NOTCH1 loss-of-function mutations, for example, were noted in 11% to 19% of tumors, with another 11% to 14% containing NOTCH2 or NOTCH3 mutations (see **Fig. 2A**).[16,17] Interestingly, these same tumors had mutations in gene sets associated with differentiation, such as IRF6 and TP63, implying that these genes may act together with NOTCH1 to ultimately trigger the development of immature, dedifferentiated, highly proliferative basaloid cells. Additional mutations were identified in less well characterized genes such as SYNE1 and 2, which control nuclear polarity, and RIMS2 and piccolo presynaptic cytomatrix protein (PCLO), which regulate calcium sensing during terminal squamous cell differentiation. Thus, dysregulation of programs involving cellular differentiation appears to be a critical component of HNSCC tumor biology. In addition, inhibition of NOTCH activation has been associated with an increased risk of cutaneous SCC, with a recent phase III trial with the gamma-secretase inhibitor semagacestat halted due to an increased rate of cutaneous SCC in the treatment arm compared with placebo.[25] Together, these data suggest that differentiation pathways may be a major regulator of HNSCC tumorigenesis, raising the possibility that dysregulation of differentiation identified in other SCCs of the lung, esophagus, and cervix may be relevant to head and neck biology.

Other tumor suppressor pathways also have been identified using unbiased approaches: FAT1, which has well-described roles in aberrant Wnt signaling, was mutated in 12% to 23% of tumors (see **Fig. 2A**).[16,17] Previous studies have shown that FAT1 encodes a cadherin-related protein that suppresses the nuclear localization of β-catenin and thereby inhibits proliferation.[26] In addition, FAT1 appears to regulate cell migration and invasiveness (see **Fig. 3**),[27] suggesting that there may be multiple effects of FAT1 mutations on HNSCC tumorigenesis. Additional mutations and deletions were identified in apoptosis-related genes (CASP8, DDX3X), histone methyltransferases (PRDM9, EZH2, NSD1), as well as Ajuba, a centrosomal protein that regulates cell division and vertebrate ciliogenesis in an EGFR-RAS-MAPK-dependent manner (see **Fig. 2A, C**)[16,17]; however, further work is required to biologically characterize the mechanism and impact of these mutations on tumorigenesis. Nevertheless, identification of these mutations emphasizes the major role tumor suppressor pathways play in HNSCC pathogenesis.

Targeting tumor suppressor pathways is significantly more challenging than inhibiting oncogenic signaling, as it requires reactivation of tumor suppressor genes or their downstream effectors rather than simple chemical or biological inhibition. In this setting, the concept of synthetic lethality may prove useful for making therapeutic advances. Loss of a tumor suppressor gene may evoke unique susceptibilities to inhibition of a second gene or pathway that is normally not observed. Synthetic lethality leverages this principle that inhibition of two genes is lethal, whereas in contrast, inhibition of either gene alone is not.

There is now great interest in identifying the synthetic lethal partners of inactive genes, such as tumor suppressors, to help identify novel therapeutic targets.[28] A recent data-driven computational approach for genome-wide identification of synthetic lethal interactions has been developed,[28] with the ability to identify synthetic lethal partners of both oncogenes and tumor suppressors. This approach has been used to develop a network analysis of synthetic lethal interactions that predicts which genes are essential and likely to be efficient pharmaceutical targets. Although this analysis has not been completed in HNSCC, it will be critical to move forward swiftly with such an approach, taking advantage of genome-wide short hairpin RNA and small-interfering RNA–mediated drug sensitization and small molecular inhibitor screens.[29] By characterizing the synthetic lethal genes across a broad array of head and neck tumors, one could identify the gene targets worthy of aggressive drug targeting. Such an approach leverages the bioinformatics power of network analyses, rather than trying to simply inhibit or activate a single gene target, an effect that may ultimately be escaped through evolution of the cancer cells themselves.

In more practical terms, McLornan and colleagues[29] broadly characterized the pathways that may be nonoverlapping and unique to cancer cells; thus, targeting these aspects of cell biology may allow for selective targeting of cancer cells through synthetic lethality (**Box 1**). For example, although DNA damage response pathways generally provide a "unified guard" against genomic instability, many malignancies have defects in aspects of DNA repair mechanisms. For example, mutations in the DNA repair gene MSH2 or MLH1 become synthetically lethal when combined with inhibitors of DNA polymerase due to the accumulation of double-strand breaks.[30] Indeed, methotrexate has been shown to induce DNA damage in MSH2-mutant cells compared with wild type, which has been the basis for methotrexate trials in MSH2-deficient colorectal cancer.[31]

Targeting cells with p53 loss of function, which is mutated in 72% of HNSCC,[17] may be one especially important context in which synthetic lethality approaches may prove valuable. In the context of p53 loss of function, cancer cells lose the normal mechanisms of p53-dependent G1-S cell-cycle arrest and become dependent on G2-M checkpoint arrest for DNA repair and survival. Thus, targeting G2-M checkpoint proteins can induce mitotic catastrophe and synthetic lethality in p53 loss-of-function cells. For example, inhibition of stress-activated p38 mitogen-activated protein kinase MAPKAP kinase 2 (MK2), ataxia telangiectasia mutated (ATM), and serum/glucocorticoid regulated kinase 2 (SGK2) or serine/threonine protein kinase 3 (PAK3) may sensitize tumor cells to chemotherapy (MK2, ATM) or induce autophagy (SGK2) or

---

Box 1
Mechanisms for achieving synthetic lethality in cancer cells

Targeting oncogenic drivers

Exploiting DNA-repair or cell-cycle defects

Using new drug combinations derived from screen

Using altered drug timing and sequencing

Exploring the tumor-cell environment

Targeting the stroma

Exploiting the altered metabolome

Targeting the altered proteome

Exploiting nononcogene "addiction"

Adapted from McLornan DP, List A, Mufti GJ. Applying synthetic lethality for the selective targeting of cancer. N Engl J Med 2014;371(18):1725–35.

apoptosis (PAK3).[32–34] Recent computational analyses have identified multiple candidate kinase genes that serve as synthetic lethal partners of p53 mutants, including polo-like kinase 1, cyclin-dependent kinase 1, and aurora kinase A.[35] Within head and neck oncology, this approach has been put into practice with an RNAi kinome viability screen in p53 mutant HNSCC cells to identify oncogenes that may be targeted in this mutational context.[36] Using this method to screen primary human HNSCC tumors, as well as tissue from murine models, several "critical survival kinases" were identified, including the Wee1-like protein kinase (WEE1). Small molecule inhibition of WEE1 using the compound MK-1775 revealed durable effects on HNSCC viability and apoptosis, while also potentiating the efficacy of cisplatin in a mouse xenograft model. This inhibitor is now part of a phase I clinical trial to determine whether it may be useful in combination with neoadjuvant weekly docetaxel and cisplatin before surgery in p53-mutant HNSCC. Exploring these approaches further is likely to yield additional novel therapeutics for loss-of-function mutations that have remained difficult to target.

ONCOGENE MUTATIONS ARE UNCOMMON IN HEAD AND NECK SQUAMOUS CELL CARCINOMA WITH LIMITED POTENTIAL FOR TARGETED THERAPY IN SPECIFIC CONTEXTS

Unlike other malignancies, such as breast cancer or chronic myelogenous leukemia, which stand as examples of cancers driven by oncogenes (epidermal growth factor receptor [EGFR] and BCR-Abl, respectively) which can be inhibited with profound effects on clinical outcomes, HNSCC does not appear to demonstrate significant oncogene addiction. In vitro studies have identified a role for EGFR signaling in HNSCC, but sequencing analyses suggest only 15% of HPV– and 6% of HPV+ tumors contain mutations or amplification of EGFR (see **Fig. 2B**).[17] EGFR is a transmembrane tyrosine kinase receptor in the HER/erbB family of proteins that triggers Ras and PI3K signaling (see **Fig. 2C**). In HNSCC, candidate sequencing studies have shown that EGFR is overexpressed most commonly through gene amplification and increased copy number,[37] rather than activating mutations or truncation mutants such as EGFRvIII.

Based on the limited dependence of HNSCC on EGFR signaling, it is not surprising that inhibitors of EGFR have had variable success. EGFR overexpression appears predictive of poor clinical prognosis and resistance to radiation,[38–40] with data suggesting improved overall survival when cetuximab, a monoclonal antibody against EGFR, is combined with radiation or chemotherapy.[41,42] However, response to cetuximab does not correlate with the degree of overexpression and as a monotherapy, the benefits of cetuximab are limited to a 6% to 13% response rate.[3,41] Similarly, the Radiation Therapy Oncology Group recently completed a Phase III trial exploring the effects of cetuximab in patients with stage III or IV HNSCC who were undergoing concurrent accelerated fractionated radiotherapy and cisplatin treatment.[43] This group found no differences in patient outcomes (mortality, progression-free survival, overall survival, locoregional failure, or distant metastasis) with the addition of cetuximab. These findings suggest that other mechanisms may be activated upon EGFR inhibition or redundant activators of cell survival may limit treatment efficacy, consistent with whole-exome studies suggesting oncogenes have low mutant allele frequencies and rarely drive HNSCC (see **Fig. 2C**).[16,17] Thus, although there has been substantial interest in kinase inhibitors of EGFR in treating HNSCC, these agents have limited clinical impact in a significant portion of HNSCC tumors.

One exception for targeted therapy may be activating Ras or PI3K mutations, which occur at higher frequency in HPV+ cancers, offering a specific context in which targeted therapy may facilitate deintensification of chemoradiation. PI3K signaling is frequently altered in HNSCC through several mechanisms, including loss-of-function mutations in PTEN, which negatively regulates PI3K (40% of HNSCC) and activating mutations in PI3KCA (6%–11% of HNSCC).[44–47] Recent data suggest that the PTEN gene may exhibit a gene dosage effect,[48] with loss of a single allele promoting tumor growth. Interestingly, in the case PI3KCA, mutations may be associated with HPV+ OPSCC,[49] raising the possibility that PI3K acts synergistically with HPV E6 and E7 proteins in this HNSCC subset.

Ras signaling may work in collaboration with PI3K activation or independently to promote HNSCC (see **Fig. 2**C). Although KRAS is frequently mutated in other cancers, HNSCC is associated primarily with HRAS mutations, especially in patients with extensive tobacco exposure.[50,51] Like PI3K, HRAS mutations are also associated with HPV+ tumors.[52] However, Ras family members have proven recalcitrant to inhibition with therapeutic strategies primarily aimed at targeting downstream effectors.

Recent sequencing analyses have validated these in vitro observations identifying amplifications or mutations (specifically the exon 9 helical domain) of PI3K in 56% of HPV+ HNSCC and 34% of HPV– tumors (see **Fig. 2**B).[17] Activating mutations in HRAS were also described in 5% to 8% of HNSCC tumors (see **Fig. 2**A).[16,17] There are numerous ongoing trials evaluating small molecule inhibitors of PI3K.[53] Such molecular inhibitors may be one exception in HNSCC, where oncogene targeting may prove valuable.

HUMAN PAPILLOMA VIRUS INFECTION AND INTEGRATION ALTERS TUMOR BIOLOGY AND TRIGGERS CARCINOGENESIS BY DIVERGENT BIOLOGIC MECHANISMS THAN SMOKING AND ALCOHOL-RELATED HEAD AND NECK SQUAMOUS CELL CARCINOMA

More than a decade of research has made it clear that HPV+ and HPV– HNSCC are distinct entities, with unique etiology, patient demographics, pathophysiology, and clinical outcomes.[7] We now know that HPV– cancers are those that are driven by traditional risk factors, such as smoking and alcohol, with carcinogenesis dependent on the acquisition of multiple epigenetic and genetic alterations yielding a premalignant progenitor that then undergoes additional alterations to become an invasive malignancy. This concept, known as field cancerization, posits that exposure of aerodigestive mucosa to alcohol and tobacco develops genetically distinct fields in which additional mutations may cause transformation. Consistent with this, Slaughter and Southwick[54] made the early observation that 11.2% of HNSCC primaries present with a second primary. Similarly, Sidransky and colleagues examined 87 HNSCCs including analysis of preinvasive lesions using microsatellite analyses for loss of heterozygosity at 10 distinct loci. These analyses revealed progressive chromosomal loss when comparing benign hyperplasia to dysplasia to carcinoma in situ to invasive cancer, suggesting a common clonal progenitor and clonal expansion.[55]

In contrast, HPV+ tumors are driven by HPV infection, usually by serotype16, with the integration of viral DNA into the host genome and the activation of specific and consistent molecular regulators, including p16 (INK4A) and viral proteins E6 and E7 (see **Fig. 1**). Cell lines transfected with p16 and the alternate transcript p14arf displayed markedly inhibited growth,[56] arresting in G1consistent with a role for p16 in blocking the G1-S transition. Indeed, transfection of p16-INK4A adenovirus demonstrated a 96% reduction in proliferation of HNSCC cell lines and in vivo studies in nude mice showed a significant decline in xenograft tumor growth.[57] More recent studies have linked p16-positive IHC (best defined as ≥70% cytoplasmic and nuclear staining) with HPV+ tumors[58] and suggested that p16 overexpression be used as an independent factor to risk stratify OPSCC.[59] Interestingly, epigenetic regulation of p16 through hypermethylation may also play an important role in predicting clinical prognosis and outcomes.[60,61]

The biologic mechanisms explaining differences in clinical outcomes with HPV status are likely multifactorial. The absence of field cancerization certainly reduces the incidence of locoregional recurrence and second primaries, whereas the persistence of functional p53 may explain the improved response to chemotherapy and radiation.[62,63] There is also growing evidence that tumor-immune interactions may explain the improved response of HPV+ tumors: HPV positivity is associated with a more substantial lymphocyte response[64–66] and animal models suggest that immunocompetence is essential for complete tumor eradication.[67]

More recent genome-wide studies of HPV+ and HPV− tumors reveal a clear divergence of these tumors at the genomic level. Compared with HPV− tumors, HPV+ HNSCC has lower rates of mutations and less frequent copy number alterations, indicating that there is less genomic instability in this cohort.[16,17] In a recent study, Akagi and colleagues[68] subsequently demonstrated that HPV integrants flank extensive regions of the host genome, resulting in amplifications and rearrangement. In addition, looping of HPV integrant-mediated replication leads to viral-host concatemers, thereby triggering oncogenesis. However, by DNA analysis there is no consistency in the site of HPV integration: interrogation of RNA transcripts demonstrated transcription across the viral-human integration locus with no recurrent genes identified, suggesting there are diverse mechanisms related to HPV integration, adding another potential source of intratumor and intertumor heterogeneity.[17]

At the level of individual genes, recent whole-exome sequencing studies suggest that HPV+ tumors have infrequent mutations in p53 and CDKN2A in stark contrast to HPV− tumors where these genes are commonly altered.[16,17] Interestingly, HPV+ tumors are distinguished by recurrent deletions and truncation mutations in tumor necrosis factor receptor–associated factor 3 (TRAF3),[17] which has been implicated in innate and acquired viral response to Epstein-Barr virus, HPV, and human immunodeficiency virus. Loss of TRAF3 promotes aberrant nuclear factor kappa B (NFκB) signaling with diverse downstream effects on cytokine signaling and cell death.[69] Thus, there is now unequivocal evidence that mechanistically separates HPV+ and HPV− HNSCC, clarifying the biological basis for the distinct clinical behavior of these distinct head and neck tumors.

INTRATUMOR HETEROGENEITY POSES UNIQUE THERAPEUTIC CHALLENGES AND OPPORTUNITIES IN HEAD AND NECK SQUAMOUS CELL CARCINOMA

Although many tumors are fairly homogeneous, HNSCC is characterized by tremendous intratumor diversity and heterogeneity. Early studies characterizing intratumor heterogeneity used microsatellite marker testing of distinct areas of tumor to demonstrate intratumor heterogeneity at the molecular level.[70] These findings were validated with dual-fluorescence in situ hybridization studies, which demonstrated changes in DNA ploidy and intrasample heterogeneity in 68 of 89 tumors.[71] Interestingly, heterogeneity was more substantial in primary tumors compared with metastatic samples. These early efforts established the presence of intratumor heterogeneity at the genetic level.

To determine the impact of intratumor genetic heterogeneity on clinical outcomes, more recent studies have introduced novel measures of genetic heterogeneity and correlated these findings with primary patient data. For example, we have defined a mutant allele tumor heterogeneity (MATH) score, which is defined as the ratio of the width to the center of the distribution of mutant-allele fractions at tumor-specific mutated loci (**Fig. 4**A).[72] MATH scores were calculated for 74 HNSCCs with publicly available next-generation sequencing data, revealing higher scores in 3 well-established patient cohorts with poor outcomes, namely tumors with inactivating mutations in TP53 (compared with wild-type or nondisruptive mutations), HPV– tumors (compared with HPV+ tumors), and HPV– tumors from smokers with higher pack-years of smoking. Additional analyses demonstrated that higher MATH scores corresponded with shorter overall survival as well as adverse treatment outcomes in clinically high-risk patients (see **Fig. 4**B).[73] Together, these findings serve as the first clinical correlation of genetic intratumor heterogeneity to poor patient outcomes, providing an ideal biomarker that could be used to quantify intratumor genetic heterogeneity.

More recently, we have applied this analysis of intratumor heterogeneity to the TCGA database of 305 patients with HNSCC.[74] Tumor MATH scores were calculated based on whole-exome sequencing data, revealing a substantiating association between high MATH scores and decreased overall survival (hazard ratio of 2.2 for high vs low heterogeneity). This difference was independent of other clinical or biologic differences, such as patient age, HPV status, tumor grade, TP53 mutations, and nodal disease. Based on analyses using MATH, a substantial improvement in overall prognostication compared with traditional staging analyses was demonstrated using

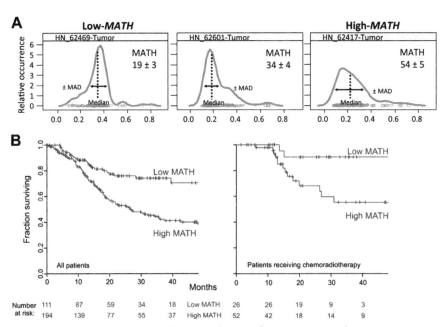

Fig. 4. (*A*) Representative mutant allele distributions from 3 HNSCCs. A heterogenous tumor with a high MATH score will have a broader distribution, shorter peak, and lower median mutant allele fraction compared with a more homogeneous, low MATH score tumor. (*B*) Relationship of intratumor heterogeneity as captured by MATH score with overall survival in HNSCC. (*From* [A] Rocco JW. Mutant allele tumor heterogeneity (MATH) and head and neck squamous cell carcinoma. Head Neck Pathol 2015;9(1):3, with permission; and [B] Mroz EA, Tward AM, Hammon RJ, et al. Intra-tumor genetic heterogeneity and mortality in head and neck cancer: analysis of data from the Cancer Genome Atlas. PLoS Med 2015;12(2):e10001786.)

multivariate analyses, establishing MATH as a useful predictor of tumor behavior and patient outcomes. Collectively, these studies emphasize the importance of intratumor heterogeneity as a major influence on tumor progression, treatment resistance, and metastatic potential, with implications for patient care and prognosis.

Unfortunately, our previous studies do not pinpoint a biological explanation for why intratumor heterogeneity and higher MATH scores correlate with poorer clinical outcomes. Detailing the genetic and biochemical basis of intratumor heterogeneity in HNSCC remains one of the major challenges and opportunities within head and neck oncology. New sequencing technology may enable high-fidelity studies of HNSCC and allow the identification of distinct cellular subpopulation and cancer cell subcohorts. For example, a recent study demonstrated that single-cell RNA sequencing of human tumors can be leveraged to identify distinct intratumor subpopulations and characterize the gene expression profile of these differing cohorts.[75]

A similar analysis in HNSCC would be informative: not only would it allow a detailed characterization of the subpopulations present and their gene expression profiles, it would provide insight into the distinct contributions of each of these populations to tumor pathogenesis. For example, a uniquely expressed gene among the tumor stroma might be predictive of patient outcomes or serve as a novel therapeutic target following tumor resection. Similarly, if matched lymph nodes also could be sequenced, then theoretically one might identify differences in cellular subpopulations as well as unique genetic programs upregulated within the context of regional metastases. Clearly, single-cell analyses of HNSCC hold great promise in improving diagnosis, prognosis, and treatment approaches; this work should proceed expeditiously, as it will have important implications for clinical management of HNSCC.

ADDITIONAL FRONTIERS IN HEAD AND NECK SQUAMOUS CELL CARCINOMA DIAGNOSTICS AND THERAPEUTICS

Despite advances in our understanding of HNSCC, the challenges discussed previously have restricted the management of HNSCC to the same tools used decades ago, namely surgery, radiation therapy, and chemotherapy. However, there is growing interest into several areas of promise with ongoing clinical trials that may yield new biologic agents and therapeutics.

Biomarkers Remain Elusive but Are Worthy of Pursuit

The difficulty of HNSCC surveillance due to limited recurrent tumor size, occult growth and progression, and localization in a variety of anatomic subsites emphasizes the need for reliable biomarkers so as to improve clinical management. This is especially critical considering the importance of early detection before the development of locoregional or distant metastases. To date, there is no usable serum or tissue biomarker that can be used for diagnosis of HNSCC. Hypermethylated circulating tumor DNA has been proposed as one potential candidate: a recent study examined serum from 100 patients with HNSCC and 50 healthy controls to evaluate methylation status of endothelin receptor type B (EDNRB), p16, and deleted in colorectal carcinoma (DCC) using quantitative methylation-specific polymerase chain reaction methods.[76] EDNRB hypermethylation was found in 10% of patients with HNSCC (compared with 0% in controls), whereas DCC hypermethylation and p16 hypermethylation were rarely detected. Thus, EDNRB hypermethylation may be a highly specific, albeit insensitive, biomarker for HNSCC. Nevertheless, this approach may be used to identify a methylation profile for multiple genes, which could improve the sensitivity of testing and aid in the diagnosis and early detection of HNSCC.[77]

To date, HPV is the only example of a biomarker in HNSCC that is used to predict prognosis. However, there is a still a real need to further stratify HPV+ patients given that a portion of these patients still have locoregional recurrences. Kumar and colleagues[78] suggested that HPV status be combined with measures of EGFR, p16, p53, and Bcl-XL expression to predict prognosis. Based on their analyses, patients with low EGFR, high HPV/p16, or low p53 with low Bcl-XL have improved overall survival and disease-free survival. Similar work has shown that increased Bcl-2 expression is an independent predictor of overall and disease-free survival in OPSCC.[79] Interestingly, Bcl-2 expression was specifically associated with distant metastases rather than locoregional recurrences.

Genetic intratumor heterogeneity based on next-generation sequencing may also serve as a potential biomarker. In the validating the TCGA HNSCC data set, both MATH and HPV status were significantly related to overall survival in bivariate Cox proportional hazards analysis, and a substantial portion of the relationship of MATH with outcome was independent of its relationship with HPV status.[74] Importantly, MATH analysis improved HNSCC patient outcome prognostication beyond what was provided by HPV status alone. Ongoing prospective analysis in an oropharyngeal cohort will ultimately determine the role of MATH as a biomarker. Thus, additional biomarkers may help to further stratify HPV+ patients and provide insight into prognosis, thereby guiding the aggressiveness of clinical therapy a priori and facilitating deintensification of chemoradiation therapy.

MicroRNAs in Head and Neck Squamous Cell Carcinoma Offer an Additional, Poorly Understood Layer of Regulation in Tumor Biology

Although microRNAs (miRNAs) have been well studied within the context of developmental biology and other tumor sites, within head and neck oncology, a role for miRNAs has been poorly characterized. The miRNAs are short, 18-bp to 25-bp noncoding RNAs that modulate gene expression by binding to messenger RNA (mRNA) after transcription. miRNAs bind to the 3′ untranslated region (UTR), coding sequences, or the 5′ UTR of mRNA to inhibit translation or silence target transcripts by binding to the RNA-induced silencing complex (**Fig. 5**). There is now growing evidence that dysregulation of miRNAs through direct genetic mutation, epigenetic changes, modifications in biogenesis, altered transcription factor expression, or changes in target sites may contribute to tumor progression.[80] Several studies have cataloged the miRNAs present in HNSCC, identifying both oncogenic and

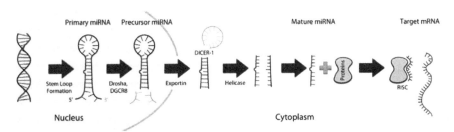

Fig. 5. Schematic demonstrating the mechanism for miRNA based mRNA silencing. (*From* Sethi N, Wright A, Wood H, et al. MicroRNAs and head and neck cancer: reviewing the first decade of research. Eur J Cancer 2014;50(15):2619–35; with permission.)

tumor suppressor transcripts.[81] For example, miR-130b is upregulated in HNSCC, with a presumed role in regulating the epithelial-mesenchymal transition.[80,82] In contrast, miR-99 dysregulation and downregulation promotes oral squamous cell carcinoma survival through likely regulation of mTOR signaling, consistent with a tumor suppressor function.[83] The Let-7 family of miRNAs, which is the largest family of miRNAs, is also downregulated in HNSCC.[84–87]

Recent genome-wide analyses of HNSCC have focused attention on miRNAs and convey the importance of miRNA-mRNA networks in HNSCC.[17] These analyses identified decreased expression of Let-7c-5p and miR-100-5p in tumors compared with normal tissue, with a corresponding association with increased target gene expression of the cell-cycle protein CDK6, transcription elongation factor E2F1, mitosis protein PLK1, and transcription factor HMGA2.[17] These critical observations raise the possibility of potentially novel therapeutics for HNSCC. Because miRNAs can be easily expressed through genetic constructs, an understanding of the role of miRNAs may allow for unique treatments or serum/tissue biomarkers. In addition, because many miRNAs have a more global regulatory role whereby they influence the activity of multiple signaling cascades, modulation of miRNAs offers the possibility of more extensive inhibition or activation of relevant pathways than may be possible with small molecule agents.

Networking Analyses Can Identify Transcriptional and Regulatory Cassettes

Based on recent whole-exome sequencing analyses, there are cohorts of tumor with characteristic signaling pathways, beginning the difficult task of capturing signaling networks within HNSCC. TCGA has used their whole-exome sequencing data to define 4 molecular subtypes of HNSCC (atypical, mesenchymal, basal, and classical). These subtypes are defined by characteristic signaling cassettes and mutations. For example, p53 mutations, CDKN2A loss-of-function mutations, chromosome (chr) 3q amplification, changes in oxidative stress genes, and heavy smoking were associated with the classical subtype, whereas NOTCH1 mutations and HRAS-CASP8 comutations were associated with the basal subtype, suggesting that disrupted cell death is a common finding in this latter subtype.[17] The atypical subtype lacked chr 7 amplifications, and the mesenchymal subtype had mutations in genes involved in innate immunity, such as CD56.[17]

In addition, TCGA has also leveraged unsupervised clustering analysis of copy number alterations (CNAs) to delineate additional HNSCC cohorts. For example, this group describes an "M" class of tumors, which is driven primarily by mutations rather than CNAs.[17] This cohort consists of a subset of oral cavity tumors with a characteristic 3-gene pattern of HRAS activating mutations, inactivating CASP8 mutations, and wild-type p53. This cohort had a more favorable clinical outcome with what appears to be an alternative tumorigenesis pathway involving Ras and alterations in cell death/NFκB.

Recent work has focused on the biologic importance of NFκB in HNSCC by exploring the utility of bortezomib, a proteasome inhibitor that inactivates NFκB, in patients receiving concurrent chemoradiation therapy for recurrent or metastatic HNSCC.[88] Preliminary data reveal a reduction of greater than 50% tumor size in 2 of 6 treated patients. NFκB-regulated cytokines were decreased in patients with clinical responses, and bortezomib was shown to induce apoptotic effects based on terminal deoxynucleotidyl transferase dUTP nick end labeling analyses. This same group is now completing a phase I clinical trial investigating the safety profile of bortezomib when combined with cetuximab with or without cisplatin in patients with stage IV head and neck cancer undergoing radiation therapy.[89]

In the future, further bioinformatic analyses of existing larger tumor data sets (eg, TCGA) will allow additional transcriptional and regulatory cassettes to be identified, perhaps setting up additional opportunities for translational therapeutics. Single-cell analyses of HNSCC will be of great help in this regard, allowing similar analyses to be completed for tumor subpopulations and enabling a comprehensive characterization of tumor-stroma interactions and the signaling pathways governing cellular cross-talk.

Epigenetic Changes and Histone Modification May Enable Tumor Resistance

There has been recent interest in epigenetic changes, including histone modification, as a driver of tumorigenesis. Epigenetic changes have been touted as a major method for tumor resistance to chemotherapy, with cancer stem cells serving as a depot of self-renewing and self-propagating cells that may underlie treatment resistance. Epigenetic modifications may allow these cells to adapt to treatment regimens without requiring the acquisition of new mutations.[90] For example, NFκB has been shown to localize to the nucleus in HNSCC, where it modifies chromatin organization by influencing histone 3 acetylation and thereby condenses chromatin and desensitizes tumor cells to chemotherapy.[91] Accordingly, treatment of cells with a histone deacetylase (HDAC) inhibitor mimics the effect of NFκB inhibition, providing a potential avenue for sensitizing tumor cells to chemotherapy.[90] Interestingly, the same HDAC inhibitors appear to be required for the maintenance of cancer stem cells based on tumor sphere assays,[92] suggesting that HNSCC progression and growth may critically depend on dynamic changes in chromatic organization through histone acetylation. Unfortunately, early trials with HDAC inhibitors have been disappointing: a phase II trial with romidepsin, a potent HDAC inhibitor derived from *Chromobacterium violaceum*, effectively inhibited HDAC in vivo but yielded no objective clinical response.[93] However, there are additional ongoing trials exploring other promising HDAC inhibitors. For example, Ohio State University has an ongoing clinical trial exploring the role of the HDAC inhibitor vorinostat in combination with chemoradiation for the treatment of stage III and IVA oropharyngeal SCC[94] based on promising preclinical data in cell line and animal models of HNSCC.[95,96] These additional studies should help clarify if HDAC inhibitors hold therapeutic promise.

Tumor-Immune Interactions and Immunotherapy Offer Novel Methods for Cancer Surveillance

There has been substantial interest in the interaction between immune infiltrates and tumor cells (see Head and Neck immuno-oncology section).[97] Briefly, these immune cells, known as tumor-infiltrating lymphocytes (TILs), have been characterized in several solid malignancies, including HNSCC.[98] Most studies in HNSCC have focused on the prognostic impact of TILs. For example, Rajjoub and colleagues[99] used tissue microarrays to catalog 48 OPSCCs and determined the CD3+ T cells that were present. They found that tumors with more CD3 cells tended to have decreased rates of metastasis; however, multivariate analyses suggested that the difference was only statistically significant for HPV+ tumors. Similar analyses of CD8+ T cells have yielded mixed conclusions.[98] Unfortunately, a detailed study of the biologic characteristics of HNSCC TILs has been lacking. Single-cell sequencing of HNSCC, including the CD45+ immune infiltrate, may be one method of accomplishing this goal.

If these cells can be better characterized, then it may be possible to develop immunomodulatory therapies that can harness a patient's own immune surveillance mechanisms to target HNSCC. In addition, it may be possible to manipulate patient immune responses through ex vivo alterations in immune cells followed by reimplantation.

Although there is significant progress to be made, biologic agents leveraging TILs may be a useful adjunct to current therapies, providing a method for cellular surveillance of cancer cells that escape traditional treatment modalities.

There are several ongoing clinical trials related to immunotherapy in HNSCC. For example, Merck has sponsored an open phase II trial investigating the role of MK-3475 (Pembrolizumab), a potent inhibitor of PD-1 receptor, in recurrent or metastatic HNSCC after treatment with platinum-based and cetuximab therapy.[100] It would be informative to biologically characterize these tumors before and after treatment with pembrolizumab to better understand how molecular signaling is altered with immunotherapy.

A Darwinian View of Head and Neck Oncology Offers Creative Perspectives into Cancer Biology and Treatment

The past decade of research has seen an explosion of interest in the in situ evolution of tumorigenesis and the adaptation of cancer cells to their environment, not unlike Darwin's theory of evolution as it applies to species fitness.[101] In the case of HNSCC, a Darwinian perspective emphasizes new angles of basic research that remain poorly characterized: What is the role of the "environment" (ie, tumor niche) in carcinogenesis? What are the environmental "perturbations" (ie, therapeutic silver bullets), if any, that might yield clonal extinction and eliminate the cancer so swiftly that none of its constituent members (individual cells) may adapt and survive? Is there a role for metronomic therapy in yielding better long-term control on HNSCC?[102] How can we slow clonal evolution to advance the efficacy of therapy? Although abstract, this new understanding and perspective has begun to trickle down and influence how HNSCC may ultimately be successfully targeted. Certainly, collaboration with developmental and systems biologists is likely to maximize strides in HNSCC, providing new insight ranging from phylogenetic analysis of tumor clones to novel methods of targeting tumor resistance.

SUMMARY

Our molecular understanding of HNSCC has undergone tremendous growth and evolution over the past several decades. We now know there are two clear cohorts of HNSCC: HPV+, which is caused by HPV infection and viral integration, and HPV−, which is driven by acquired mutations and alterations from environmental exposures, such as tobacco and alcohol. Recent whole-exome sequencing studies of HNSCC have provided dramatic insights into HNSCC tumor biology, demonstrating that tumor suppressors are the primary regulators of HNSCC, with oncogenes rarely driving tumorigenesis.

In parallel, a host of new observations have demonstrated the challenge and complexity of developing targeted therapies for HNSCC. Intratumor heterogeneity poses a major challenge to a "silver bullet" for HNSCC, providing genetic diversity that may allow clonal escape and tumor resistance. In addition, new insights from epigenetic studies, the identification of novel miRNA regulators, and tumor-immune system interactions suggest additional layers of regulation and control. Future work should leverage single-cell sequencing and transcriptional network analyses to better characterized molecular cross-talk and cellular interactions, thereby providing a more complete and comprehensive view of HNSCC signaling.

Although we have much to learn about HNSCC, we must not limit the lesson learned to those obtained directly from studying this tumor. Sequencing analyses have conveyed the point, more than ever, that dysregulation of differentiation is a major contribution to head and neck oncology. It has not gone unnoticed that similar pathways are aberrantly regulated in other SCCs of the cervix, skin, lung, and esophagus. In the end, we may find that the biology of these tumors is more of a reflection of their underlying tissue of origin than their anatomic subsite. By combining findings from HNSCC with these other tumors, we may be able to identify more dramatic insights that synergistically improve the treatment of other SCCs as well.

Although numerous clinical trials are ongoing, there is a necessity for greater translation research into areas of promise, such as synthetic lethality and immunotherapy. Although the mainstays of head and neck cancer treatment, including surgery, radiation, and chemotherapy, are likely to persist, the development of useful biological adjuncts could dramatically influence the way conventional therapy is used, offering the possibility of deescalation and deintensification of treatment, while simultaneously improving patient outcomes and quality of life.

REFERENCES

1. International Agency for Research on Cancer. World Health Organisation. Estimated cancer incidence, mortality and prevalence worldwide in 2012. Globocan 2014; http://globoscan.iarc.fr.
2. Rothenberg SM, Ellisen LW. The molecular pathogenesis of head and neck squamous cell carcinoma. J Clin Invest 2012;122(6):1951–7.
3. Machiels JP, Lambrecht M, Hanin FX, et al. Advances in the management of squamous cell carcinoma of the head and neck. F1000Prime Rep 2014;6:44. eCollection.
4. Curado MP, Hashibe M. Recent changes in the epidemiology of head and neck cancer. Curr Opin Oncol 2009;21(3):194–200.
5. Gillison ML. Human papillomavirus-associated head and neck cancer is a distinct epidemiologic, clinical, and molecular entity. Semin Oncol 2004;31:744–54.
6. Chaturvedi AK, Anderson WF, Lortet-Tieulent J, et al. Worldwide trends in incidence rates for oral cavity and oropharyngeal cancers. J Clin Oncol 2013;31: 4550–9.
7. Bonilla-Velez J, Mroz EA, Hammon RJ, et al. Impact of human papillomavirus on oropharyngeal cancer biology and response to therapy: implications for treatment. Otolaryngol Clin North Am 2013;46(4):521–43.
8. Joseph AW, D'Souza G. Epidemiology of human papillomavirus-related head and neck cancer. Otolaryngol Clin North Am 2012;45(4):739–64.
9. Marur S, D'Souza G, Westra WH, et al. HPV-associated head and neck cancer: a virus-related cancer epidemic. Lancet Oncol 2010;11(8):781–9.
10. National Cancer Institute. Head and Neck Cancer. 2014. Available at: http://www.cancer.gov/cancertopics/types/head-and-neck. Accessed May 1, 2015.
11. Lin HW, Bhattacharyya N. Contemporary assessment of medical morbidity and mortality in head and neck surgery. Otolaryngol Head Neck Surg 2012;146(3):385–9.
12. Nigro JM, Baker SJ, Preisinger AC, et al. Mutations in the p53 gene occur in diverse human tumour types. Nature 1989;342(6250):705–8.
13. Gasco M, Crook T. The p53 network in head and neck cancer. Oral Oncol 2003; 39(3):222–31.
14. Somers KD, Merrick MA, Lopez ME, et al. Frequent p53 mutations in head and neck cancer. Cancer Res 1992;52(21):5997–6000.
15. Ohnishi K, Ota I, Takahashi A, et al. Transfection of mutant p53 gene depresses X-ray- or CDDP-induced apoptosis in a human squamous cell carcinoma of the head and neck. Apoptosis 2002;7(4):367–72.

16. Stransky N, Egloff AM, Tward AD, et al. The mutational landscape of head and neck squamous cell carcinoma. Science 2011;333(6046):1157–60.
17. Cancer Genome Atlas Network. Comprehensive genomic characterization of head and neck squamous cell carcinomas. Nature 2015;517:576–82.
18. Tassone P, Old M, Teknos TN, et al. p53-based therapeutics for head and neck squamous cell carcinoma. Oral Oncol 2013;49(8):733–7.
19. Wang D, Song H, Evans JA, et al. Mutation and downregulation of the transforming growth factor beta type II receptor gene in primary squamous cell carcinomas of the head and neck. Carcinogenesis 1997;18(11):2285–90.
20. Qiu W, Schonleben F, Li X, et al. Disruption of transforming growth factor beta–Smad signaling pathway in head and neck squamous cell carcinoma as evidenced by mutations of SMAD2 and SMAD4. Cancer Lett 2007;245(1–2):163–70.
21. Han G, Lu SL, Li AG, et al. Distinct mechanisms of TGF-beta1-mediated epithelial-to-mesenchymal transition and metastasis during skin carcinogenesis. J Clin Invest 2005;115(7):1714–23.
22. Bornstein S, White R, Malkoski S, et al. Smad4 loss in mice causes spontaneous head and neck cancer with increased genomic instability and inflammation. J Clin Invest 2009;119(11):3408–19.
23. Lu SL, Herrington H, Reh D, et al. Loss of transforming growth factor beta type II receptor promotes metastatic head and-neck squamous cell carcinoma. Genes Dev 2006;20(10):1331–42.
24. Nagaraj NS, Datta PK. Targeting the transforming growth factor-beta signaling pathway in human cancer. Expert Opin Investig Drugs 2010;19(1):77–91.
25. Doody RS, Raman R, Farlow M, et al. A phase 3 trial of semagacestat for treatment of Alzheimer's disease. N Engl J Med 2013;369(4):341–50.
26. Morris LG, Kaufman AM, Gong Y, et al. Recurrent somatic mutation of FAT1 in multiple human cancers leads to aberrant Wnt activation. Nat Genet 2013; 45(3):253–61.
27. Nishikawa Y, Miyazaki T, Nakashiro K, et al. Human FAT1 cadherin controls cell migration and invasion of oral squamous cell carcinoma through the localization of β-catenin. Oncol Rep 2011;26(3):587–92.
28. Jerby-Arnon L, Pfetzer N, Waldman YY, et al. Predicting cancer-specific vulnerability via data-driven detection of synthetic lethality. Cell 2014;158(5): 1199–209.
29. McLornan DP, List A, Mufti GJ. Applying synthetic lethality for the selective targeting of cancer. N Engl J Med 2014;371(18):1725–35.
30. Martin SA, McCabe N, Mullarkey M, et al. DNA polymerases as potential therapeutic targets for cancers deficient in the DNA mismatch repair proteins MSH or MLH1. Cancer Cell 2010;17:235–48.
31. Martin SA, McCarthy A, Barber LJ, et al. Methotrexate induces oxidative DNA damage and is selectively lethal to tumour cells with defects in the DNA mismatch repair gene MSH2. EMBO Mol Med 2009;1:323–37.
32. Morandell S, Reinhardt HC, Cannell IG, et al. A reversible gene-targeting strategy identifies synthetic lethal interactions between MK2 and p53 in the DNA damage response in vivo. Cell Rep 2013;5:868–77.
33. Jiang H, Reinhardt HC, Bartkova J, et al. The combined status of ATM and p53 link tumor development with therapeutic response. Genes Dev 2009;23: 1895–909.
34. Baldwin A, Grueneberg DA, Hellner K, et al. Kinase requirements in human cells: V. Synthetic lethal interactions between p53 and the protein kinases SGK2 and PAK3. Proc Natl Acad Sci U S A 2010;107:12463–8.

35. Wang X, Simon R. Identification of potential synthetic lethal genes to p53 using a computational biology approach. BMC Med Genomics 2013;6:30.
36. Moser R, Xu C, Kao M, et al. Functional kinomics identifies candidate therapeutic targets in head and neck cancer. Clin Cancer Res 2014;20(16):4274–88.
37. Kalyankrishna S, Grandis JR. Epidermal growth factor biology in head and neck cancer. J Clin Oncol 2006;24:2666–72.
38. Temam S, Kawaguchi H, El-Naggar AK, et al. Epidermal growth factor receptor copy number alterations correlate with poor clinical outcome in patients with head and neck squamous cancer. J Clin Oncol 2007;25:2164–70.
39. Chung CH, Ely K, McGavran L, et al. Increased epidermal growth factor receptor gene copy number is associated with poor prognosis in head and neck squamous cell carcinomas. J Clin Oncol 2006;24:4170–6.
40. Chiang WF, Liu SY, Yen CY, et al. Association of epidermal growth factor receptor (EGFR) gene copy number amplification with neck lymph node metastasis in areca-associated oral carcinoma. Oral Oncol 2008;44:270–6.
41. Vermorken J, Mesia R, Rivera F, et al. Platinum-based chemotherapy plus cetuximab in head and neck cancer. N Engl J Med 2008;11:1116–27.
42. Bonner JA, Harari PM, Giralt J, et al. Radiotherapy plus cetuximab for locoregionally advanced head and neck cancer: 5-year survival data from a phase 3 randomised trial, and relation between cetuximab-induced rash and survival. Lancet Oncol 2010;11:21–8.
43. Ang KK, Zhang Q, Rosenthal DI, et al. Randomized phase III trial of concurrent accelerated radiation plus cisplatin with or without cetuximab for stage III to IV head and neck carcinoma: RTOG 0522. J Clin Oncol 2014;32(27):2940–50.
44. Okami K, Wu L, Riggins G, et al. Analysis of PTEN/MMAC1 alterations in aerodigestive tract tumors. Cancer Res 1998;58(3):509–11.
45. Shao X, Tandon R, Samara G, et al. Mutational analysis of the PTEN gene in head and neck squamous cell carcinoma. Int J Cancer 1998;77(5):684–8.
46. Qiu W, Schönleben F, Li X, et al. PIK3CA mutations in head and neck squamous cell carcinoma. Clin Cancer Res 2006;12(5):1441–6.
47. Qiu W, Tong GX, Manolidis S, et al. Novel mutant-enriched sequencing identified high frequency of PIK3CA mutations in pharyngeal cancer. Int J Cancer 2008;122(5):1189–94.
48. Berger AH, Knudson AG, Pandolfi PP. A continuum model for tumour suppression. Nature 2011;476(7359):163–9.
49. Henken FE, Banerjee NS, Snijders PJ, et al. PIK3CA-mediated PI3-kinase signalling is essential for HPV-induced transformation in vitro. Mol Cancer 2011;10:71.
50. Saranath D, Chang SE, Bhoite LT, et al. High frequency mutation in codons 12 and 61 of H-ras oncogene in chewing tobacco-related human oral carcinoma in India. Br J Cancer 1991;63(4):573–8.
51. Anderson JA, Irish JC, Ngan BY. Prevalence of RAS oncogene mutation in head and neck carcinomas. J Otolaryngol 1992;21(5):321–6.
52. Anderson JA, Irish JC, McLachlin CM, et al. H-ras oncogene mutation and human papillomavirus infection in oral carcinomas. Arch Otolaryngol Head Neck Surg 1994;120(7):755–60.
53. Engelman JA. Targeting PI3K signalling in cancer: opportunities, challenges and limitations. Nat Rev Cancer 2009;9(8):550–62.
54. Slaughter DP, Southwick HW. 'Field cancerization' in oral stratified squamous epithelium. Clinical implications of multicentric origin. Cancer 1953;6:963–8.

55. Califano J, van der Riet P, Westra W, et al. Genetic progression model for head and neck cancer: implications for field cancerization. Cancer Res 1996;56(11): 2488–92.

56. Liggett WH Jr, Sewell DA, Rocco J, et al. p16 and p16 beta are potent growth suppressors of head and neck squamous carcinoma cells in vitro. Cancer Res 1996;56(18):4119–23.

57. Rocco JW, Li D, Liggett WH Jr, et al. p16INK4A adenovirus-mediated gene therapy for human head and neck squamous cell cancer. Clin Cancer Res 1998; 4(7):1697–704.

58. Grønhøj Larsen C, Gyldenløve M, Jensen DH, et al. Correlation between human papillomavirus and p16 overexpression in oropharyngeal tumours: a systematic review. Br J Cancer 2014;110(6):1587–94.

59. Lewis JS Jr. p16 Immunohistochemistry as a standalone test for risk stratification in oropharyngeal squamous cell carcinoma. Head Neck Pathol 2012; 6:S75–82.

60. Sailasree R, Abhilash A, Sathyan KM, et al. Differential roles of p16INK4A and p14ARF genes in prognosis of oral carcinoma. Cancer Epidemiol Biomarkers Prev 2008;17(2):414–20.

61. Ogi K, Toyota M, Ohe-Toyota M, et al. Aberrant methylation of multiple genes and clinicopathological features in oral squamous cell carcinoma. Clin Cancer Res 2002;8(10):3164–71.

62. Licitra L, Perrone F, Bossi P, et al. High-risk human papillomavirus affects prognosis in patients with surgically treated oropharyngeal squamous cell carcinoma. J Clin Oncol 2006;24(36):5630–6.

63. Butz K, Geisen C, Ullmann A, et al. Cellular responses of HPV-positive cancer cells to genotoxic anti-cancer agents: repression of E6/E7-oncogene expression and induction of apoptosis. Int J Cancer 1996;68(4):506–13.

64. Vu HL, Sikora AG, Fu S, et al. HPV-induced oropharyngeal cancer, immune response and response to therapy. Cancer Lett 2010;288(2):149–55.

65. Wansom D, Light E, Worden F, et al. Correlation of cellular immunity with human papillomavirus 16 status and outcome in patients with advanced oropharyngeal cancer. Arch Otolaryngol Head Neck Surg 2010;136(12):1267–73.

66. Wansom D, Light E, Thomas D, et al. Infiltrating lymphocytes and human papillomavirus-16–associated oropharyngeal cancer. Laryngoscope 2012;122(1):121–7.

67. Spanos WC, Nowicki P, Lee DW, et al. Immune response during therapy with cisplatin or radiation for human papillomavirus-related head and neck cancer. Arch Otolaryngol Head Neck Surg 2009;135(11):1137–46.

68. Akagi K, Li J, Broutian TR, et al. Genome-wide analysis of HPV integration in human cancers reveals recurrent, focal genomic instability. Genome Res 2014; 24(2):185–99.

69. Ni CZ, Welsh K, Leo E, et al. Molecular basis for CD40 signaling mediated by TRAF3. Proc Natl Acad Sci U S A 2000;97(19):10395–9.

70. el-Naggar AK, Hurr K, Luna MA, et al. Intratumoral genetic heterogeneity in primary head and neck squamous carcinoma using microsatellite markers. Diagn Mol Pathol 1997;6(6):305–8.

71. Götte K, Schäfer C, Riedel F, et al. Intratumoral genomic heterogeneity in primary head and neck cancer and corresponding metastases detected by dual-FISH. Oncol Rep 2004;11(1):17–23.

72. Mroz EA, Rocco JW. MATH, a novel measure of intratumor genetic heterogeneity, is high in poor-outcome classes of head and neck squamous cell carcinoma. Oral Oncol 2013;49(3):211–5.

73. Mroz EA, Tward AD, Pickering CR, et al. High intratumor genetic heterogeneity is related to worse outcome in patients with head and neck squamous cell carcinoma. Cancer 2013;119(16):3034–42.

74. Mroz EA, Tward AM, Hammon RJ, et al. Intra-tumor genetic heterogeneity and mortality in head and neck cancer: analysis of data from the Cancer Genome Atlas. PLoS Med 2015;12(2):e1001786. eCollection.

75. Patel AP, Tirosh I, Trombetta JJ, et al. Single-cell RNA-seq highlights intratumoral heterogeneity in primary glioblastoma. Science 2014;344(6190): 1396–401.

76. Mydlarz WK, Hennessey PT, Wang H, et al. Serum biomarkers for detection of head and neck squamous cell carcinoma. Head Neck 2014. [Epub ahead of print].

77. Arantes LM, de Carvalho AC, Melendez ME, et al. Methylation as a biomarker for head and neck cancer. Oral Oncol 2014;50(6):587–92.

78. Kumar B, Cordell KG, Lee JS, et al. EGFR, p16, HPV Titer, Bcl-xL and p53, sex, and smoking as indicators of response to therapy and survival in oropharyngeal cancer. J Clin Oncol 2008;26(19):3128–37.

79. Nichols AC, Finkelstein DM, Faquin WC, et al. Bcl2 and human papilloma virus 16 as predictors of outcome following concurrent chemoradiation for advanced oropharyngeal cancer. Clin Cancer Res 2010;16(7):2138–46.

80. Cao P, Zhou L, Zhang J, et al. Comprehensive expression profiling of microRNAs in laryngeal squamous cell carcinoma. Head Neck 2013;35:720–8.

81. Sethi N, Wright A, Wood H, et al. MicroRNAs and head and neck cancer: reviewing the first decade of research. Eur J Cancer 2014;50(15):2619–35.

82. Avissar M, Christensen BC, Kelsey KT, et al. MicroRNA expression ratio is predictive of head and neck squamous cell carcinoma. Clin Cancer Res 2009;15: 2850–5.

83. Yan B, Fu Q, Lai L, et al. Downregulation of microRNA 99a in oral squamous cell carcinomas contributes to the growth and survival of oral cancer cells. Mol Med Rep 2012;6:675–81.

84. Hui AB, Lenarduzzi M, Krushel T, et al. Comprehensive microRNA profiling for head and neck squamous cell carcinomas. Clin Cancer Res 2010;16:1129–39.

85. Childs G, Fazzari M, Kung G, et al. Low-level expression of microRNAs let-7d and miR-205 are prognostic markers of head and neck squamous cell carcinoma. Am J Pathol 2009;174:736–45.

86. Maclellan SA, Lawson J, Baik J, et al. Differential expression of miRNAs in the serum of patients with high-risk oral lesions. Cancer Med 2012;1:268–74.

87. Yang WH, Lan HY, Tai SK, et al. Repression of bone morphogenetic protein 4 by let-7i attenuates mesenchymal migration of head and neck cancer cells. Biochem Biophys Res Commun 2013;433:24–30.

88. Chang AA, Conley BA, Lebowitz PF, et al. Bortezomib with concurrent radiation therapy in head and neck squamous cell carcinoma. Otolaryngol Head Neck Surg 2004;131(2):117.

89. National Cancer Institute. Radiation therapy and bortezomib and cetuximab with or without cisplatin to treat head and neck cancer. Clinicaltrials.gov; 2013. Available at: https://clinicaltrials.gov/ct2/show/NCT01445405.

90. Le JM, Squarize CH, Castilho RM. Histone modifications: targeting head and neck cancer stem cells. World J Stem Cells 2014;6(5):511–25.

91. Almeida LO, Abrahao AC, Rosselli-Murai LK, et al. NFκB mediates cisplatin resistance through histone modifications in head and neck squamous cell carcinoma (HNSCC). FEBS Open Bio 2014;4:96–104.

92. Giudice FS, Pinto DS Jr, Nör JE, et al. Inhibition of histone deacetylase impacts cancer stem cells and induces epithelial-mesenchyme transition of head and neck cancer. PLoS One 2013;8(3):e58672.

93. Haigentz M Jr, Kim M, Sarta C, et al. Phase II trial of the histone deacetylase inhibitor romidepsin in patients with recurrent/metastatic head and neck cancer. Oral Oncol 2012;48(12):1281–8.

94. Ohio State University Comprehensive Cancer Center. Ph I vorinostat in the treatment of advanced staged oropharyngeal squamous cell carcinoma. Clinicaltrials.gov; 2015. Available at: https://www.clinicaltrials.gov/ct2/show/NCT01064921.

95. Erlich RB, Kherrouche Z, Rickwood D, et al. Preclinical evaluation of dual PI3K-mTOR inhibitors and histone deacetylase inhibitors in head and neck squamous cell carcinoma. Br J Cancer 2012;106(1):107–15.

96. Zhang Y, Jung M, Dritschilo A, et al. Enhancement of radiation sensitivity of human squamous carcinoma cells by histone deacetylase inhibitors. Radiat Res 2004;161(6):667–74.

97. Schoppy DW, Sunwoo JB. Immunotherapy for head and neck squamous cell carcinoma. Hematol Oncol Clin N Am 2015, in press.

98. Uppaluri R, Dunn GP, Lewis JS Jr. Focus on TILs: prognostic significance of tumor infiltrating lymphocytes in head and neck cancers. Cancer Immun 2008;8:16.

99. Rajjoub S, Basha SR, Einhorn E, et al. Prognostic significance of tumor-infiltrating lymphocytes in oropharyngeal cancer. Ear Nose Throat J 2007;86(8):506–11.

100. Merck Sharpe and Dohme Corpo. Study of MK-3475 (Pembrolizumab) in recurrent or metastatic head and neck squamous cell carcinoma after treatment with platinum-based and cetuximab therapy (MK-3475–055/KEYNOTE-055). Clinicaltrials.gov; 2015. Available at: https://clinicaltrials.gov/ct2/show/NCT02255097.

101. Greaves M, Maley CC. Clonal evolution in cancer. Nature 2012;481(7381):306–13.

102. Scharovsky OG, Mainetti LE, Rozados VR. Metronomic chemotherapy: changing the paradigm that more is better. Curr Oncol 2009;16(2):7–15.

Novel Targeted Agents in Head and Neck Squamous Cell Carcinoma

Pedro H. Isaacsson Velho, MD[a], Gilberto Castro Jr, MD, PhD[a], Christine H. Chung, MD[b,c],*

KEYWORDS

- DNA damage response • Cell cycle regulation • PI3K/mTOR • NOTCH • c-MET
- FGFR • Axl • Angiogenesis

KEY POINTS

- Based on current genome-wide sequencing and copy number data, there are only a few oncogenes in HNSCC that can be immediately exploited with novel targeted agents.
- Novel approaches targeting key pathways including DNA damage response and cell cycle regulation, PI3K/mTOR, NOTCH, transmembrane growth factor receptors (c-MET, FGFR, and Axl), and angiogenesis are discussed.
- Moving forward, concerted effort is required to identify better predictive biomarkers of clinical benefits and improve the therapeutic index of targeted agents.

INTRODUCTION

Recent genomic findings in head and neck squamous cell carcinoma (HNSCC) reveal a wide spectrum of genomic alterations.[1–5] A heterogeneous disease by nature, HNSCC encompasses a disparate collection of anatomic sites with complex tumor biology. One of the most distinguishing features of HNSCC is the human papillomavirus (HPV) status of the tumor, HPV-positive HNSCC having more favorable

[a] Department of Clinical Oncology, Instituto do Câncer do Estado de São Paulo, Faculdade de Medicina da Universidade de São Paulo, São Paulo, Brazil; [b] Department of Oncology, Sidney Kimmel Comprehensive Cancer Center, The Johns Hopkins University School of Medicine, Johns Hopkins Medical Institutions, 1550 Orleans Street CRB-2 Room 546, Baltimore, MD 21287-0014, USA; [c] Department of Otolaryngology-Head and Neck Surgery, Sidney Kimmel Comprehensive Cancer Center, The Johns Hopkins University School of Medicine, Johns Hopkins Medical Institutions, 1550 Orleans Street CRB-2 Room 546, Baltimore, MD 21287-0014, USA
* Corresponding author. Department of Otolaryngology-Head and Neck Surgery, Sidney Kimmel Comprehensive Cancer Center, The Johns Hopkins University School of Medicine, Johns Hopkins Medical Institutions, 1550 Orleans Street CRB-2 Room 546, Baltimore, MD 21287-0014.
E-mail address: cchung11@jhmi.edu

Hematol Oncol Clin N Am 29 (2015) 993–1009
http://dx.doi.org/10.1016/j.hoc.2015.07.006
0889-8588/15/$ – see front matter © 2015 Elsevier Inc. All rights reserved.

hemonc.theclinics.com

outcomes compared with HPV-negative HNSCC.[6,7] This genomic heterogeneity of HNSCC tumors creates an obstacle for the identification of an effective targeting agent likely to benefit most patients with HNSCC. The most successful implementation of the genomic alterations in recent years has been based on functionally activating gene mutations (eg, c-KIT activating mutations in gastrointestinal stromal tumor[8]) and copy number gain in oncogenes (eg, ERBB2/HER2 amplification in breast cancer[9]).

However, based on current genome-wide sequencing and copy number data, there are only a few oncogenes in HNSCC that can be immediately exploited with novel targeted agents. This article focuses on novel approaches targeting potentially critical pathways that are frequently altered in HNSCC, including DNA damage response and cell cycle regulation, PI3K/mTOR, NOTCH, transmembrane growth factor receptors (c-MET, FGFR, and Axl), and angiogenesis. The established therapeutic target inhibitors including epidermal growth factor receptor (EGFR) and immune check point proteins (eg, PD1 and PD-L1) are discussed elsewhere in this issue.

DNA DAMAGE RESPONSE AND CELL CYCLE REGULATION TARGETED AGENTS
Targeting Dysfunctional p53

The gene *TP53* (tumor protein p53, *p53*, or *Trp53*), was in 1979 the first tumor-suppressor gene to be identified, and the protein product of this gene, p53, is one of the most important molecules in biology, integrating numerous signals that control cell cycling and apoptosis.[10,11] The p53 network is normally inactive and responds to stimuli, such as cellular damage or stress, to perform its tumor-suppressing function.[12] There are many ways in which p53 protein malfunctions in human cancers, and at least six different mechanisms are cited: (1) amino-acid-changing mutation in the DNA binding domain; (2) deletion of the carboxy-terminal domain; (3) multiplication of the MDM2 gene in the genome; (4) viral infection; (5) deletion of the p14ARF gene; and (6) mislocalization of p53 to the cytoplasm, outside the nucleus.[12]

In HNSCC, the cause of p53 dysfunction differs between HPV-positive and HPV-negative tumors. The HPV-positive HNSCC lacks functional p53 because ubiquitination of p53 by an ubiquitin ligase, E6AP, and a viral oncoprotein, E6, leads to rapid degradation of p53, whereas *TP53* mutation is very rare.[1–4,13,14] However, *TP53* is the most frequently mutated gene in HPV-negative HNSCC, with an incidence of 47% to 87%.[1–4] These mutations can occur throughout the entire gene and typically involve missense mutations, which alter protein conformation or affect how p53 binds its DNA targets. It is also known that any *TP53* mutations in tumor DNA are associated with reduced survival after surgical treatment of HNSCC.[15–17]

Given the biologic importance of p53, there has been a significant effort to identify effective therapeutic approaches for HNSCC with p53 dysfunction. However, direct targeting of a tumor suppressor, such as p53, is currently not feasible because restoration of a lost protein function in the appropriate cellular regulatory context is difficult compared with the inhibition of overly active proteins, such as deregulated oncoproteins.[12,18] One of the ways to circumvent this problem is to find a synthetic lethal partner for dysfunctional p53. The synthetic lethality therapeutic approaches consist of a combination of two or more separate genes/proteins' functional loss leading to cell death, whereas functional loss of only one of the genes/proteins does not reduce cell viability.[19]

Moser and colleagues[20] applied a functional kinomic approach using a high-throughput RNA interference platform to identify new targets exploiting dependence on G2-M cell cycle regulators of *TP53*-mutant tumors for their viability (**Fig. 1**A and

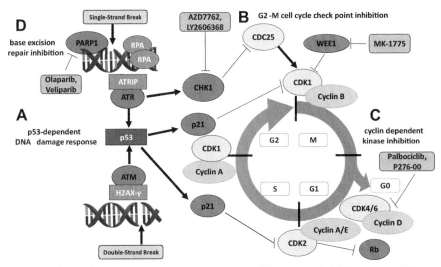

Fig. 1. (*A, B*) p53-dependent DNA damage response. When there is DNA damage, ATR and ATM initiate p53-dependent cell cycle arrest. In p53 mutant tumors, there is increased dependence on the G2-M cell cycle check point regulation; therefore, CHK1 inhibitors (AZD7762 and LY2606368) and a Wee inhibitor (MK-1775 or AZD-1775) are thought to be more effective in p53 mutant tumors. (*C*) Palbociclib is a selective CDK4 and CDK6 inhibitor and P276-00 inhibits CDK1, CDK4, and CDK9. (*D*) Olaparib and veliparib inhibits poly-ADP ribose polymerase (PARP) 1, which is a key driver of base excision repair on a single-strand break. CDK, cyclin-dependent kinase.

B). WEE1 (a G2-M cell cycle regulator), CAM2KB, and NEK4 were identified as the most promising candidate target kinases. MK-1775 (AZD1775), the WEE1 kinase inhibitor, had the broadest and most significant effect on cell viability and apoptosis in primary and recurrent/metastatic HNSCC-derived cells. Sensitivity to MK-1775 depended on several factors including the mutational status of *TP53*, HPV status, and concomitant cisplatin use. *TP53*-mutant cell lines were more sensitive to MK-1775 than *TP53* wild-type cell lines, and the use of MK-1775 combined with cisplatin enhanced the response when compared with cisplatin alone. Based on these preclinical results, several clinical trials are evaluating an MK-1775 monotherapy or a combination of MK-1775 and platinum chemotherapy (NCT02196168, NCT01748825, and NCT02341456).

Targeting Cyclin-Dependent Kinases

There are four distinct phases in the cell cycle (G1, S, G2, and M) and G0 for when the cells are resting or in a quiescent state (see **Fig. 1**).[21] The cyclin-dependent kinases (CDKs) are enzymes that control transition through the cell cycle by forming a complex with cyclins.[21] The functions of several CDKs are well characterized. For example, CDK1 (cell division cycle 2, G1 to S and G2 to M or CDC2) is a key determinant for mitotic progression, CDK2 is relevant for DNA replication, and CDK4 and CDK6 are responsible for numerous growth regulatory signals and cell cycle progression.[22]

In HNSCC, comprehensive gene expression analyses suggest that there is a fundamental difference in the cell cycle regulation depending on the HPV status. In HPV-positive HNSCC, cyclin B, cyclin E, CDK1, and CDK2 are upregulated, whereas cyclin D, CDK4, and CDK6 are upregulated in HPV-negative HNSCC.[23] The prognostic role of cyclins in HNSCC has been evaluated. The gene encoding cyclin D1, *CCND1*, is frequently amplified and an established poor prognostic marker in HNSCC.[3,24–26] A recent meta-analysis evaluated the prognostic role of cyclin D1 in HNSCC and again demonstrated that cyclin D1 overexpression, determined by immunohistochemistry, was associated with lymph node metastasis and worse disease-free survival.[27] Currently, direct inhibition of cyclin D1 is not feasible; therefore, the therapeutic focus is on inhibition of the CDKs (**Fig. 1**C).[21]

For example, an oral inhibitor of CDK4 and CDK6, palbociclib, has been approved for hormone-positive metastatic breast cancer and is being evaluated in HNSCC.[28,29] A phase I trial to evaluate the maximum tolerated dose and to assess the response rate of the combination of cetuximab and palbociclib in patients with incurable HNSCC is ongoing.[30] Of the nine patients enrolled, two patients achieved a partial response, five patients achieved stable disease, one patient progressed, and one patient was not yet evaluable. The maximum tolerated dose was never reached during this trial because there were no dose-limiting toxicities or adverse event-related treatment discontinuation. Several clinical trials are currently evaluating CDK inhibitors in HNSCC in combination with radiation, chemotherapy, or cetuximab (NCT00899054, NCT00824343, and NCT02101034).

Targeting Poly-ADP Ribose Polymerase

Human DNA is repetitively exposed to insults that have the ability to cause a range of damage, such as single-strand breaks; double-strand breaks; bulky adduct formation; and base mismatches, insertions, deletions, and alkylation.[31] Different DNA repair pathways repair the damage to preserve genomic stability and integrity.[31,32] Single-strand breaks are repaired by a base excision repair mechanism and poly-ADP ribose polymerase (PARP) is a key protein involved in this process (**Fig. 1**D). The PARP inhibitors have been developed in *BRCA1* mutant tumors because of the evidence of synthetic lethality.[19] Olaparib has been approved to treat women with advanced ovarian cancer associated with a defective *BRCA1*.[33,34]

The great interest in developing PARP inhibitors in HNSCC comes from the preclinical data showing PARP inhibition is associated with enhanced tumor sensitivity to radiation in lung cancer cell lines.[35] One potential mechanism for the increased response to combination therapy of radiation and PARP inhibitors is that cells are unable to repair radiation-induced single-strand breaks.[36] Moreover, evaluation of HNSCC cell lines demonstrated a potent radiosensitization effect with PARP inhibitors, particularly in HPV/p16-positive HNSCC cell lines.[36,37]

In the clinical context of a deintensified treatment of HPV-positive HNSCC with a favorable prognosis, the PARP inhibitors may provide an alternative to cisplatin and radiotherapy. Based on the synthetic lethality approach, the combination of DNA-damaging chemotherapy agents (eg, platinum agents, topoisomerase-I inhibitors, and alkylating agents) and PARP inhibitors are being evaluated in clinical trials. There are four ongoing trials evaluating the use of PARP inhibitors as a radiosensitizer and in combination with chemotherapy in HNSCC (NCT02308072, NCT01711541, NCT02229656, and NCT01366144).

PI3K-mTOR TARGETED AGENTS

The PI3K-mTOR pathway regulates numerous cellular functions including cell cycle, survival, metabolism, motility, genomic instability, angiogenesis, and inflammatory cell recruitment.[38,39] The PI3K-mTOR pathway is the most frequently altered pathway in human tumors, with *PIK3CA* and *PTEN* being the most frequently altered genes in the pathway; therefore, enumerable therapeutic agents targeting this pathway are being developed.[40] In HNSCC, approximately 30% of both HPV-positive and -negative tumors have genomic alterations in the pathway.[41] Current data suggest that deregulation of this pathway plays an important role in development of HNSCC and response to PI3K-mTOR inhibitors.[41–43]

Because of the prodigious preclinical evidence that PI3K-mTOR signaling represents an integral component of HNSCC signal transduction, several clinical trials are currently underway to evaluate the efficacy of small molecules that inhibit key points of this pathway (**Table 1**). For example, PI3K inhibitors (BYL-719 and buparlisib) and mTOR inhibitors (everolimus, temsirolimus, sirolimus, and ridaforolimus) are actively being investigated in phase II trials as a single agent or in combination with previously established radiation and chemotherapy regimens in HNSCC.[44] Because PI3K and mTOR share several structural similarities, some compounds have been developed to inhibit the class I PI3K isoforms and mTORC1/2,[45] and several of these dual PI3K/mTOR inhibitors are in clinical development including NVP-BEZ235 and LY3023414. Metformin, a biguanide commonly used to manage type II diabetes, is also being investigated as a chemotherapeutic in HNSCC. Although it is not a direct mTOR inhibitor, metformin indirectly inhibits mTORC1 by increasing intracellular AMP levels mediated by AMPK-dependent and independent mechanisms.[46,47]

Contrary to the perception that the presence of *PIK3CA* mutations would highly correlate with response to PI3K inhibitors, the trial evaluating cetuximab or cetuximab and PX-866 combination showed that the *PIK3CA* mutations were not associated with response in both arms.[48] In addition, a recent study revealed that HNSCC cell lines with *PIK3CA* mutations or amplification were initially more sensitive to a PI3Kα isoform-specific inhibitor, BYL719, compared with the cell lines with wild-type *PIK3CA*. Acquired resistance, however, emerged through an interaction among the EGFR, Axl, and PI3K pathway and subsequent downstream activation of mTOR.[49] The addition of mTOR inhibitor (RAD001 and AZD8055) resensitized the BYL719-resistant cells, confirming that the acquired resistance to the PI3K inhibition was mediated through maintained activity of mTOR. Furthermore, the combined inhibition of PI3Kα and either EGFR or Axl reversed the resistance, thereby showing that the maintained mTOR activity was through the interaction between EGFR and Axl and downstream activation of PKC. This study provided the scientific rationale to combine PI3K inhibitors with EGFR, Axl, or PKC inhibitors. The next step in the development of PI3K-mTOR inhibitors is to identify better predictive biomarkers of clinical benefits and to further understand the resistance mechanisms to improve the therapeutic index through appropriate combination regimens.

NOTCH PATHWAY TARGETED AGENTS

The NOTCH pathway comprises of four receptors (NOTCH 1–4) and two families of ligands: JAG1/2 (Jagged 1 and 2) and DLL1/3/4 (Delta-like 1, 3, and 4).[50] The pathway is initiated when one cell expressing the appropriate ligand (Jagged or Delta-like) interacts with another cell expressing a NOTCH receptor. These cell surface receptors are expressed by various cell types and are generally involved in multiple biologic functions including differentiation, regulation of self-renewal capacity, cell-cycle exit, proliferation, angiogenesis, and survival.[50–52] The importance of this pathway in HNSCC was demonstrated by whole-exome sequencing studies that reported 10% to 15% of HNSCC harbor *NOTCH1* mutations.[1–3] A prognostic significance of the mutation was reported by Song and colleagues[53] that patients with *NOTCH1* mutations had a significantly shorter overall and disease-free survival compared with those whose

Table 1
Active clinical trials evaluating PI3K/AKT/mTOR targeted agents for locally advanced and recurrent and/or metastatic HNSCC patients

Targeted Agent	Additional Targeted Agent	Additional Therapy	Inclusion Criteria	Phase	Clinical Trial Identifier
mTOR inhibitor					
Everolimus	—	—	Advanced HNSCC	II	NCT01111058
	—	—	Advanced/recurrent HNSCC	II	NCT01051791
	—	IMRT, cisplatin	Advanced HNSCC	I	NCT00858663
	—	Docetaxel, cisplatin	Advanced HNSCC	I	NCT00935961
	—	Carboplatin, paclitaxel	Advanced HNSCC	I/II	NCT01333085
	Cetuximab	Carboplatin, paclitaxel	Recurrent HNSCC	I/II	NCT01283334
	Cetuximab	Cisplatin, paclitaxel	Advanced HNSC	II	NCT01133678
	Erlotinib	—	Recurrent HNSCC	II	NCT00942734
Temsirolimus	—	—	Recurrent HNSCC	II	NCT01172769
	—	Carboplatin, paclitaxel	Advanced/recurrent HNSCC	I/II	NCT01016769
	Cetuximab	—	Recurrent HNSCC	II	NCT01256385
	Cetuximab	Cisplatin	Advanced/recurrent HNSCC	I/II	NCT01015664
	Erlotinib	—	Platinum-refractory HNSCC	II	NCT01009203
Sirolimus	—	—	Advanced HNSCC	I/II	NCT01195922
Ridaforolimus	Cetuximab	—	Advanced HNSCC/NSCLC/CRC	I	NCT01212627
Metformin	—	Paclitaxel	Recurrent/metastatic HNSCC	II	NCT01333852
PI3K inhibitor					
Buparlisib	—	—	Metastatic head and neck cancer recurrent or progressive under platin and cetuximab-based chemotherapy	I	NCT01737450
Buparlisib	Cetuximab	—	Advanced/recurrent HNSCC	I/II	NCT01816984
Buparlisib	—	Cisplatin, radiotherapy	Locally advanced HNSCC	Ib	NCT02113878
Buparlisib	—	Paclitaxel	Metastatic head and neck cancer previously pretreated with a platinum therapy	II	NCT01852292
BYL719	Cetuximab	—	Recurrent/metastatic HNSCC	Ib/II	NCT01602315
BYL719	—	Paclitaxel, cisplatin	Stage III-IVa, HPV-associated oropharyngeal squamous cell carcinoma	I/II	NCT02298595
BYL719	—	Paclitaxel	Recurrent/metastatic HNSCC	Ib	NCT02051751
PX-866	—	Docetaxel	Advanced HNSCC/NSCLC	I/II	NCT01204099
PX-866	Cetuximab	—	Advanced HNSCC/CRC	I/II	NCT01252628

Abbreviations: CRC, colorectal cancer; IMRT, intensity-modulated radiation therapy; NSCLC, non-small cell lung cancer.
Data from All trial data available at www.clinicaltrials.gov. Accessed March 02, 2015.

tumors carried no *NOTCH1* mutation in a sequencing study of 51 oral squamous cell carcinomas. In addition, all 15 patients with lymph node metastasis and *NOTCH1* mutations had tumor relapse or metastasis after attempted curative treatment, and 14 (93%) of the patients died during the follow-up period compared with only 2 (15%) of the 13 patients with no lymph node metastasis and no *NOTCH1* mutation.

Another study examined the comprehensive genetic, epigenetic, and transcriptional alterations of NOTCH signaling in a cohort of HNSCC patients.[54] Overexpression of downstream Notch effectors was seen in 32% of HNSCC (44 HNSCC tumors and 25 normal mucosal samples). When DNA copy number, methylation, and gene expression of the 47 NOTCH signaling pathway genes were evaluated, a bimodal pattern of NOTCH pathway alterations emerged. A small subset exhibited inactivating *NOTCH1* mutations, but a larger subset exhibited other NOTCH1 pathway alterations including increased gene copy number of the receptors or ligands, increased gene expression, and downstream pathway activation. These findings suggested that the NOTCH pathway is a potential therapeutic target in a subset of HNSCC. As seen in these studies, NOTCH pathway is either tumor suppressive or oncogenic in HNSCC depending on the genetic context; therefore, development of biomarkers will enable the appropriate subset of patients to be treated with NOTCH inhibitors in clinical development.

TRANSMEMBRANE GROWTH FACTOR RECEPTOR TARGETED AGENTS
c-MET Receptor

The hepatocyte growth factor (HGF) receptor, also known as c-Met, is a transmembrane tyrosine kinase receptor associated with migration, invasion, and angiogenesis when overexpressed in cancer.[55] Both c-MET and HGF are deregulated in HNSCC resulting in aberrant activation of the pathway.[56] The prevalence of mutations in or amplification of *MET* or its ligand *HGF* is relatively low, reported in 6% or 2% to 13% of HNSCC, respectively, but overexpression of the MET receptor protein has been frequently shown in HNSCC.[56] MET overexpression in HNSCC is associated with advanced clinical stage, worse survival rate, and inferior response to radiotherapy and chemotherapy.[57–63] In addition, acquired *MET* amplification or upregulation is a well-established mechanism of EGFR inhibitor resistance by compensating for the EGFR signaling inhibition at the PI3K and MAPK nodes.[56,64,65]

Foretinib (GSK1363089 or XL880) is an oral multikinase inhibitor that primarily targets signaling of HGF/MET and vascular endothelial growth factor (VEGF) receptor-2 (VEGFR2) pathways.[66–68] It has demonstrated antitumor activity in human HNSCC cell lines.[68] Foretinib was tested in a single-arm, open, multicenter, nonrandomized phase II trial in patients with recurrent or metastatic HNSCC with a primary end point of response rate.[69] Foretinib was administered at doses of 240 mg orally for 5 consecutive days of a 14-day treatment cycle to 14 unselected patients. Moderate activity was observed with 50% (7 of 14) stable disease, 43% (6 of 14) tumor shrinkage but less than partial response, and 14% (2 of 14) prolonged disease stabilization for more than 13 months. Fatigue, constipation, and hypertension were the most common adverse effects, but it was well tolerated. Despite the lack of objective responses to treatment, there was evidence of modest activity and it may warrant further development with combination approaches in a carefully selected patient population.

Fibroblast Growth Factor Receptors

The fibroblast growth factor receptor (FGFR) signaling pathway is involved in numerous fundamental biologic processes including tissue development, angiogenesis, and tissue regeneration.[70] There are five FGFR members in the receptor family, and FGFR1 has emerged as a therapeutic target in several human solid cancers including HNSCC.[71,72] Recently, Göke and colleagues[72] evaluated *FGFR1* amplification and its mRNA and protein expression levels in association with FGFR inhibitor sensitivity. In this study, HNSCC cell lines were assessed for FGFR1-3 and their ligand FGF2 for their gene copy number, mRNA, and protein expression, and patient tumor-derived xenografts were evaluated for FGFR1 expression. The cell lines and patient tumor-derived xenografts were subsequently treated with an FGFR inhibitor, BGJ398, and their response was correlated with the expression levels of FGFR1. They found that only the FGFR1 mRNA and protein expression levels were associated with response ($P = .04$ and $P = .0002$, respectively) rather than increased *FGFR1* copy number, FGFR2/3 expression, or FGF2 expression. In addition, 452 primary HNSCC were evaluated of which 353 tumors had measurable *FGFR1* copy number by fluorescent *in situ* hydridization (FISH) and mRNA levels by *n situ* hydridization (ISH). They found that 31% and 18% of the primary HNSCC had FGFR1 mRNA expression and *FGFR1* copy number gain, respectively; however, only 35% of the tumors with *FGFR1* copy number gain expressed mRNA suggesting the gene copy number is a poor predictor of the FGFR inhibitor response. There are no clinical studies with FGFR inhibitors in HNSCC with mature data; however, there are a few ongoing early studies (NCT01976741, NCT01831726, and NCT01703481).

Axl

In the 1990s, O'Bryan and colleagues[73] described a new subclass of tyrosine kinase receptors, Axl, which belongs to the TAM (Tyro3, Axl, and Mertk) family of receptor tyrosine kinases. Gas6 (growth-arrest-specific protein 6) is a ligand for Axl. Activation of Axl inhibits apoptosis, and also increases migration, aggregation, and growth through multiple downstream pathways.[74] Axl is overexpressed in many human cancers including HNSCC.[75,76] Axl expression is associated with poor survival[77] and resistance to EGFR inhibitors in HNSCC.[75,76] The disruption of Axl signaling using a small-molecule inhibitor or a monoclonal antibody is known to affect the tumor and stromal cell compartments, further supporting it as a potential therapeutic target. To date, Axl has been mostly studied as a resistance mechanism of EGFR inhibitors through a receptor crosstalk. Giles and colleagues[75] evaluated a small-molecule Axl inhibitor (R428) in HNSCC cell lines with acquired resistance to erlotinib. The results showed that the Axl inhibition reduced the resistant cell viability and completely blocked the resistant cell migration. In addition, *Axl* mRNA expression was evaluated in 334 HNSCCs. Fifty percent of the tumors overexpressed Axl and the overexpression was associated with poor survival in the HNSCC patients.

ANGIOGENESIS TARGETED AGENTS

Angiogenesis is one of the hallmarks of cancer.[78] The neovascularization promoted by angiogenesis is required for tumor progression, invasion, and metastasis. A monoclonal antibody against VEGF and several anti-VEGF receptor small-molecule tyrosine kinase inhibitors are approved for cancer treatments.[79–82] Angiogenesis plays an important role in HNSCC.[83] Overexpression of VEGF, detected by immunohistochemistry, is associated with disease aggressiveness and worse overall survival.[84,85] Based on this, VEGF and its receptors, VEGFRs, emerged as a therapeutic target in HNSCC.

Among the antiangiogenic agents, bevacizumab, a recombinant humanized monoclonal antibody targeting VEGF-A isoform, has been the most extensively studied. Several clinical trials have been conducted evaluating the combination of bevacizumab and other targeted agents, chemotherapy, or radiotherapy in HNSCC (**Table 2**).

Table 2
Completed trials with antiangiogenic agents in head and neck cancer

Trial Reference	Phase of Trial	Targeted Agent	Other Modalities and Agents in the Regimen	Inclusion Criteria	Results
Salama et al,[92] 2011	II	Bevacizumab	RT/5-FU/hydroxyurea/bevacizumab (BFHX) vs RT/5-FU/hydroxyurea (FHX)	Stage II–III (T1-3, N0-1) and T4, N0-1 HNSCC	2-y survival: 68% (58% with bevacizumab; 89% without bevacizumab) 2-y disease-free survival: 75% (59% with bevacizumab; 89% without bevacizumab)
Fury et al,[93] 2012	II	Bevacizumab	RT/cisplatin/bevacizumab	Stage III-IVB HNSCC	2-y survival: 88% 2-y disease-free survival: 75.9%
Yao et al,[94] 2014	II	Bevacizumab	RT/docetaxel/bevacizumab	Stage III-IVB HNSCC	3-y progression-free survival: 68.2% 3-y disease-free survival: 61.7%
Hainsworth et al,[95] 2011	II	Bevacizumab and erlotinib	Induction chemotherapy (paclitaxel, carboplatin, 5-FU and bevacizumab) followed by RT, paclitaxel, bevacizumab, and erlotinib	Stage III-IVB HNSCC	3-y disease-free survival: 71% 3-y overall survival: 82%
Yoo et al,[96] 2012	II	Bevacizumab and erlotinib	RT/cisplatin/erlotinib/bevacizumab	Stage III-IVB HNSCC	3-y overall survival: 86% 3-y progression-free survival: 82%
Argiris et al,[97] 2011	II	Bevacizumab	Bevacizumab/pemetrexed	Previously untreated recurrent/metastatic HNSCC	Time to progression: 5 mo Median overall survival: 11.3 mo
Cohen et al,[86] 2009	I/II	Bevacizumab and erlotinib	Bevacizumab/erlotinib	Recurrent/metastatic HNSCC	Median overall survival: 7.1 mo Progression-free survival: 4.1 mo Best response rate: 15%
Argiris et al,[98] 2013	II	Bevacizumab and cetuximab	Bevacizumab/cetuximab	Recurrent/metastatic HNSCC	Median overall survival: 7.5 mo Progression-free survival: 2.8 mo Best response rate: 16%

(continued on next page)

Table 2
(continued)

Trial Reference	Phase of Trial	Targeted Agent	Other Modalities and Agents in the Regimen	Inclusion Criteria	Results
Elser et al,[87] 2007	II	Sorafenib	Sorafenib	Recurrent/metastatic HNSCC	Time to progression: 1.8 mo Median overall survival: 4.2 mo Objective response rate: 3.7%
Williamson et al,[88] 2010	II	Sorafenib	Sorafenib	Recurrent/metastatic HNSCC	Median progression-free survival: 4.0 mo Median overall survival: 9.0 mo
Choong et al,[89] 2010	II	Sunitinib	Sunitinib	Recurrent/metastatic HNSCC	Time to progression: 8.4 wk and 10.5 wk (for PS 0–1 and PS 2, respectively) Median overall survival: 21 wk and 19 wk (for PS 0–1 and PS 2, respectively)
Fountzilas et al,[90] 2010	II	Sunitinib	Sunitinib	Recurrent/metastatic HNSCC	Time to progression: 2.3 mo Median overall survival: 4.0 mo
Machiels et al,[91] 2010	II	Sunitinib	Sunitinib	Recurrent/metastatic HNSCC	Median progression-free survival: 2 mo Median overall survival: 3.4 mo

Abbreviation: RT, radiotherapy.
Data from Refs.[86–98]

Table 3
Ongoing trials with angiogenesis targeting agents in HNSCC

Antiangiogenic Agent	Phase	Regimen	Inclusion Criteria	Sample Size/Primary End Point	NCT
Bevacizumab	II	Cisplatin/bevacizumab and concurrent IMRT	Stage III/IV HNSCC	42 patients/2-y PFS	NCT00423930
Bevacizumab	III	Chemotherapy (cisplatin/docetaxel, carboplatin/docetaxel, cisplatin/5-FU, carboplatin/5- FU) ± bevacizumab	Recurrent/metastatic HNSCC	400 patients/overall survival	NCT00588770 ECOG1305
Bevacizumab	II	Induction docetaxel, cisplatin, cetuximab, and bevacizumab followed by concurrent radiation, cisplatin, cetuximab, and bevacizumab	Stage III/IV HNSCC	33 patients/rate of complete response	NCT01588431
Bevacizumab	II	Bevacizumab, cetuximab, cisplatin, and concurrent IMRT	Stage III/IV HNSCC	30 patients/2-y PFS	NCT00968435
Sorafenib	I–II	Cisplatin, docetaxel, sorafenib	Recurrent/metastatic HNSCC	41 patients/PFS	NCT02035527
Sorafenib	II	Carboplatin, paclitaxel, sorafenib	Recurrent/metastatic HNSCC	40 patients/PFS	NCT00494182
Axitinib	II	Axitinib (single agent)	Recurrent/metastatic HNSCC	40 patients/PFS	NCT1469546
Pazopanib	II	Pazopanib (single agent)	Recurrent/metastatic HNSCC, refractory to platinum-based therapy	45 patients/response rate	NCT1377298
Pazopanib	I	Pazopanib, cetuximab	Recurrent/metastatic HNSCC	33 patients/maximum tolerated dose	NCT0176416
Vandetanib	II	Vandetanib (single agent)	Preventing head and neck cancer in patients with precancerous head and neck lesions	54 patients/MVD (mutations and microvessel density)	NCT01414426

Abbreviations: MVD, microvessel density; PFS, progression-free survival.

Unfortunately, the results have been quite disappointing. Initial trials of anti-VEGFR small-molecule tyrosine kinase inhibitors, such as sorafenib and sunitinib, demonstrated a promising antitumor effect; however, subsequent studies showed no clinical benefit in recurrent and/or metastatic HNSCC.[86–91] The results from currently ongoing trials with newer agents and a phase III study with a larger sample size are highly anticipated (**Table 3**).

SUMMARY

Based on currently available genomic data, most HNSCCs have only few targetable aberrations and immediate clinical translation is challenging. It is also apparent that a targeted agent monotherapy is not clinically beneficial in most of the patients, considering numerous trials are negative. However, potential therapeutic agents listed in this article need to be thoroughly evaluated because there are compelling scientific rationales supporting their development. Moving forward, concerted effort is required to identify better predictive biomarkers of clinical benefit and improve the therapeutic index. Clinicians need to better understand resistance mechanisms, generate novel hypotheses for appropriate combination regimens and dosing schedules, develop more accurate model systems, and conduct innovative clinical trials.

REFERENCES

1. Stransky N, Egloff AM, Twatd AD, et al. The mutational landscape of head and neck squamous cell carcinoma. Science 2011;333:1157–60.
2. Agrawal N, Frederick MJ, Pickering CR, et al. Exome sequencing of head and neck squamous cell carcinoma reveals inactivating mutations in NOTCH1. Science 2011;333:1154–7.
3. Cancer Genome Atlas Network. Comprehensive genomic characterization of head and neck squamous cell carcinomas. Nature 2015;517:576–82.
4. Chung CH, Guthrie VB, Masica DL, et al. Genomic alterations in head and neck squamous cell carcinoma determined by cancer gene-targeted sequencing. Ann Oncol 2015;26:1216–23.
5. Seiwert TY, Zuo Z, Keck MK, et al. Integrative and comparative genomic analysis of HPV-positive and HPV-negative head and neck squamous cell carcinomas. Clin Cancer Res 2015;21(3):632–41.
6. Fakhry C, Westra WH, Li S, et al. Improved survival of patients with human papillomavirus-positive head and neck squamous cell carcinoma in a prospective clinical trial. J Natl Cancer Inst 2008;100:261–9.
7. Ang KK, Harris J, Wheeler R, et al. Human papillomavirus and survival of patients with oropharyngeal cancer. N Engl J Med 2010;363:24–35.
8. Heinrich MC, Corless CL, Demetri GD, et al. Kinase mutations and imatinib response in patients with metastatic gastrointestinal stromal tumor. J Clin Oncol 2003;21:4342–9.
9. Slamon DJ, Leyland-Jones B, Shak S, et al. Use of chemotherapy plus a monoclonal antibody against HER2 for metastatic breast cancer that overexpresses HER2. N Engl J Med 2001;344:783–92.
10. Lane DP, Crawford LV. T antigen is bound to a host protein in SV40-transformed cells. Nature 1979;278:261–3.
11. Foulkes WD. p53–master and commander. N Engl J Med 2007;357:2539–41.
12. Vogelstein B, Lane D, Levine AJ. Surfing the p53 network. Nature 2000;408: 307–10.

13. Scheffner M, Huibregtse JM, Vierstra RD, et al. The HPV-16 E6 and E6-AP complex functions as a ubiquitin-protein ligase in the ubiquitination of p53. Cell 1993; 75:495–505.
14. Scheffner M, Werness BA, Huibregtse JM, et al. The E6 oncoprotein encoded by human papillomavirus types 16 and 18 promotes the degradation of p53. Cell 1990;63:1129–36.
15. Poeta ML, Manola J, Goldwasser MA, et al. TP53 mutations and survival in squamous-cell carcinoma of the head and neck. N Engl J Med 2007;357: 2552–61.
16. Lindenbergh-van der Plas M, Brakenhoff RH, Kuik DJ, et al. Prognostic significance of truncating TP53 mutations in head and neck squamous cell carcinoma. Clin Cancer Res 2011;17:3733–41.
17. Licitra L, Perrone F, Bossi P, et al. High-risk human papillomavirus affects prognosis in patients with surgically treated oropharyngeal squamous cell carcinoma. J Clin Oncol 2006;24:5630–6.
18. Vogelstein B, Kinzler KW. The genetic basis of human cancer. New York: McGraw-Hill Health Professions Division; 1998.
19. McLornan DP, List A, Mufti GJ. Applying synthetic lethality for the selective targeting of cancer. N Engl J Med 2014;371:1725–35.
20. Moser R, Xu C, Kao M, et al. Functional kinomics identifies candidate therapeutic targets in head and neck cancer. Clin Cancer Res 2014;20(16):4274–88.
21. Asghar U, Witkiewicz AK, Turner NC, et al. The history and future of targeting cyclin-dependent kinases in cancer therapy. Nat Rev Drug Discov 2015;14: 130–46.
22. Drapkin R, Le Roy G, Cho H, et al. Human cyclin-dependent kinase-activating kinase exists in three distinct complexes. Proc Natl Acad Sci U S A 1996;93: 6488–93.
23. Pyeon D, Newton MA, Lambert PF, et al. Fundamental differences in cell cycle deregulation in human papillomavirus-positive and human papillomavirus-negative head/neck and cervical cancers. Cancer Res 2007;67:4605–19.
24. Fujii M, Ishiguro R, Yamashita T, et al. Cyclin D1 amplification correlates with early recurrence of squamous cell carcinoma of the tongue. Cancer Lett 2001;172: 187–92.
25. Walter V, Yin X, Wilkerson MD, et al. Molecular subtypes in head and neck cancer exhibit distinct patterns of chromosomal gain and loss of canonical cancer genes. PLoS One 2013;8:e56823.
26. Khan H, Gupta S, Husain N, et al. Prognostics of cyclin-D1 expression with chemoradiation response in patients of locally advanced oral squamous cell carcinoma. J Cancer Res Ther 2014;10:258–64.
27. Gioacchini FM, Alicandri-Ciufelli M, Kaleci S, et al. The prognostic value of cyclin D1 expression in head and neck squamous cell carcinoma. Eur Arch Otorhinolaryngol 2014. [Epub ahead of print].
28. Finn RS, Crown JP, Lang I, et al. The cyclin-dependent kinase 4/6 inhibitor palbociclib in combination with letrozole versus letrozole alone as first-line treatment of oestrogen receptor-positive, HER2-negative, advanced breast cancer (PALOMA-1/TRIO-18): a randomised phase 2 study. Lancet Oncol 2015;16:25–35.
29. Turner NC, Ro J, Andre F, et al. Palbociclib in hormone-receptor-positive advanced breast cancer. N Engl J Med 2015;373(3):209–19.
30. Michel LS, Ley JC, Wildes TM, et al. Phase I trial of the addition of the CDK 4/6 inhibitor palbociclib to cetuximab in patients with incurable head and neck squamous cell carcinoma (HNSCC). J Clin Oncol 2015;33 [Abstr: 6063].

31. Lord CJ, Ashworth A. The DNA damage response and cancer therapy. Nature 2012;481:287–94.
32. Ashworth A. A synthetic lethal therapeutic approach: poly(ADP) ribose polymerase inhibitors for the treatment of cancers deficient in DNA double-strand break repair. J Clin Oncol 2008;26:3785–90.
33. Fong PC, Boss DS, Yap TA, et al. Inhibition of poly(ADP-ribose) polymerase in tumors from BRCA mutation carriers. N Engl J Med 2009;361:123–34.
34. Ledermann J, Harter P, Gourley C, et al. Olaparib maintenance therapy in platinum-sensitive relapsed ovarian cancer. N Engl J Med 2012;366:1382–92.
35. Albert JM, Cao C, Kim KW, et al. Inhibition of poly(ADP-ribose) polymerase enhances cell death and improves tumor growth delay in irradiated lung cancer models. Clin Cancer Res 2007;13:3033–42.
36. Rieckmann T, Tribius S, Grob TJ, et al. HNSCC cell lines positive for HPV and p16 possess higher cellular radiosensitivity due to an impaired DSB repair capacity. Radiother Oncol 2013;107:242–6.
37. Guster JD, Weissleder SV, Busch CJ, et al. The inhibition of PARP but not EGFR results in the radiosensitization of HPV/p16-positive HNSCC cell lines. Radiother Oncol 2014;113:345–51.
38. Engelman JA, Luo J, Cantley LC. The evolution of phosphatidylinositol 3-kinases as regulators of growth and metabolism. Nat Rev Genet 2006;7:606–19.
39. Thorpe LM, Yuzugullu H, Zhao JJ. PI3K in cancer: divergent roles of isoforms, modes of activation and therapeutic targeting. Nat Rev Cancer 2015;15:7–24.
40. Kandoth C, McLellan MD, Vandin F, et al. Mutational landscape and significance across 12 major cancer types. Nature 2013;502:333–9.
41. Lui VW, Hedberg ML, Li H, et al. Frequent mutation of the PI3K pathway in head and neck cancer defines predictive biomarkers. Cancer Discov 2013;3:761–9.
42. Fenic I, Steger K, Gruber C, et al. Analysis of PIK3CA and Akt/protein kinase B in head and neck squamous cell carcinoma. Oncol Rep 2007;18:253–9.
43. Suda T, Hama T, Kondo S, et al. Copy number amplification of the PIK3CA gene is associated with poor prognosis in non-lymph node metastatic head and neck squamous cell carcinoma. BMC Cancer 2012;12:416.
44. Isaacsson Velho PH, Castro G Jr, Chung CH. Targeting the PI3K pathway in head and neck squamous cell carcinoma. Am Soc Clin Oncol Educ Book 2015;35:123–8.
45. Sturgill TW, Hall MN. Activating mutations in TOR are in similar structures as oncogenic mutations in PI3KCalpha. ACS Chem Biol 2009;4:999–1015.
46. Dowling RJ, Zakikhani M, Fantus IG, et al. Metformin inhibits mammalian target of rapamycin-dependent translation initiation in breast cancer cells. Cancer Res 2007;67:10804–12.
47. Kalender A, Selvaraj A, Kim SY, et al. Metformin, independent of AMPK, inhibits mTORC1 in a rag GTPase-dependent manner. Cell Metab 2010;11:390–401.
48. Jimeno A, Shirai K, Choi M, et al. A randomized, phase II trial of cetuximab with or without PX-866, an irreversible oral phosphatidylinositol 3-kinase inhibitor, in patients with relapsed or metastatic head and neck squamous cell cancer. Ann Oncol 2015;26(3):556–61.
49. Elkabets M, Pazarentzos E, Juric D, et al. AXL mediates resistance to PI3Kalpha inhibition by activating the EGFR/PKC/mTOR axis in head and neck and esophageal squamous cell carcinomas. Cancer Cell 2015;27:533–46.
50. Hori K, Sen A, Artavanis-Tsakonas S. Notch signaling at a glance. J Cell Sci 2013;126:2135–40.
51. Kerbel RS. Tumor angiogenesis. N Engl J Med 2008;358:2039–49.

52. Kang H, Kiess A, Chung CH. Emerging biomarkers in head and neck cancer in the era of genomics. Nat Rev Clin Oncol 2015;12(1):11–26.
53. Song X, Xia R, Li J, et al. Common and complex notch1 mutations in Chinese oral squamous cell carcinoma. Clin Cancer Res 2014;20:701–10.
54. Sun W, Gaykalova DA, Ochs MF, et al. Activation of the NOTCH pathway in head and neck cancer. Cancer Res 2014;74:1091–104.
55. Peruzzi B, Bottaro DP. Targeting the c-Met signaling pathway in cancer. Clin Cancer Res 2006;12:3657–60.
56. Seiwert TY, Jagadeeswaran R, Faoro L, et al. The MET receptor tyrosine kinase is a potential novel therapeutic target for head and neck squamous cell carcinoma. Cancer Res 2009;69:3021–31.
57. Marshall DD, Kornberg LJ. Overexpression of scatter factor and its receptor (c-met) in oral squamous cell carcinoma. Laryngoscope 1998;108:1413–7.
58. Chen YS, Wang JT, Chang YF, et al. Expression of hepatocyte growth factor and c-met protein is significantly associated with the progression of oral squamous cell carcinoma in Taiwan. J Oral Pathol Med 2004;33:209–17.
59. Kim CH, Moon SK, Bae JH, et al. Expression of hepatocyte growth factor and c-Met in hypopharyngeal squamous cell carcinoma. Acta Otolaryngol 2006;126:88–94.
60. Sawatsubashi M, Sasatomi E, Mizokami H, et al. Expression of c-Met in laryngeal carcinoma. Virchows Arch 1998;432:331–5.
61. Lo Muzio L, Farina A, Rubini C, et al. Effect of c-Met expression on survival in head and neck squamous cell carcinoma. Tumour Biol 2006;27:115–21.
62. Aebersold DM, Kollar A, Beer KT, et al. Involvement of the hepatocyte growth factor/scatter factor receptor c-met and of Bcl-xL in the resistance of oropharyngeal cancer to ionizing radiation. Int J Cancer 2001;96:41–54.
63. Akervall J, Guo X, Qian CN, et al. Genetic and expression profiles of squamous cell carcinoma of the head and neck correlate with cisplatin sensitivity and resistance in cell lines and patients. Clin Cancer Res 2004;10:8204–13.
64. Engelman JA, Zejnullahu K, Mitsudomi T, et al. MET amplification leads to gefitinib resistance in lung cancer by activating ERBB3 signaling. Science 2007;316:1039–43.
65. Chau NG, Perez-Ordonez B, Zhang K, et al. The association between EGFR variant III, HPV, p16, c-MET, EGFR gene copy number and response to EGFR inhibitors in patients with recurrent or metastatic squamous cell carcinoma of the head and neck. Head Neck Oncol 2011;3:11.
66. Qian F, Engst S, Yamaguchi K, et al. Inhibition of tumor cell growth, invasion, and metastasis by EXEL-2880 (XL880, GSK1363089), a novel inhibitor of HGF and VEGF receptor tyrosine kinases. Cancer Res 2009;69:8009–16.
67. Knowles LM, Stabile LP, Egloff AM, et al. HGF and c-Met participate in paracrine tumorigenic pathways in head and neck squamous cell cancer. Clin Cancer Res 2009;15:3740–50.
68. Liu L, Shi H, Liu Y, et al. Synergistic effects of foretinib with HER-targeted agents in MET and HER1- or HER2-coactivated tumor cells. Mol Cancer Ther 2011;10:518–30.
69. Seiwert T, Sarantopoulos J, Kallender H, et al. Phase II trial of single-agent foretinib (GSK1363089) in patients with recurrent or metastatic squamous cell carcinoma of the head and neck. Invest New Drugs 2013;31:417–24.
70. Touat M, Ileana E, Postel-Vinay S, et al. Targeting FGFR signaling in cancer. Clin Cancer Res 2015;21:2684–94.
71. Marshall ME, Hinz TK, Kono SA, et al. Fibroblast growth factor receptors are components of autocrine signaling networks in head and neck squamous cell carcinoma cells. Clin Cancer Res 2011;17:5016–25.

72. Goke F, Franzen A, Hinz TK, et al. FGFR1 expression levels predict BGJ398-sensitivity of FGFR1-dependent head and neck squamous cell cancers. Clin Cancer Res 2015. [Epub ahead of print].

73. O'Bryan JP, Frye RA, Cogswell PC, et al. Axl, a transforming gene isolated from primary human myeloid leukemia cells, encodes a novel receptor tyrosine kinase. Mol Cell Biol 1991;11:5016–31.

74. Holland SJ, Powell MJ, Franci C, et al. Multiple roles for the receptor tyrosine kinase axl in tumor formation. Cancer Res 2005;65:9294–303.

75. Giles KM, Kalinowski FC, Candy PA, et al. Axl mediates acquired resistance of head and neck cancer cells to the epidermal growth factor receptor inhibitor erlotinib. Mol Cancer Ther 2013;12:2541–58.

76. Byers LA, Diao L, Wang J, et al. An epithelial-mesenchymal transition gene signature predicts resistance to EGFR and PI3K inhibitors and identifies Axl as a therapeutic target for overcoming EGFR inhibitor resistance. Clin Cancer Res 2013; 19:279–90.

77. Lee CH, Yen CY, Liu SY, et al. Axl is a prognostic marker in oral squamous cell carcinoma. Ann Surg Oncol 2012;19(Suppl 3):S500–8.

78. Hanahan D, Weinberg RA. Hallmarks of cancer: the next generation. Cell 2011; 144:646–74.

79. Saltz LB, Clarke S, Diaz-Rubio E, et al. Bevacizumab in combination with oxaliplatin-based chemotherapy as first-line therapy in metastatic colorectal cancer: a randomized phase III study. J Clin Oncol 2008;26:2013–9.

80. Sandler A, Gray R, Perry MC, et al. Paclitaxel-carboplatin alone or with bevacizumab for non-small-cell lung cancer. N Engl J Med 2006;355:2542–50.

81. Tewari KS, Sill MW, Long HJ III, et al. Improved survival with bevacizumab in advanced cervical cancer. N Engl J Med 2014;370:734–43.

82. Motzer RJ, Hutson TE, McCann L, et al. Overall survival in renal-cell carcinoma with pazopanib versus sunitinib. N Engl J Med 2014;370:1769–70.

83. Vassilakopoulou M, Psyrri A, Argiris A. Targeting angiogenesis in head and neck cancer. Oral Oncol 2015;51:409–15.

84. Kyzas PA, Cunha IW, Ioannidis JP. Prognostic significance of vascular endothelial growth factor immunohistochemical expression in head and neck squamous cell carcinoma: a meta-analysis. Clin Cancer Res 2005;11:1434–40.

85. Kyzas PA, Stefanou D, Batistatou A, et al. Prognostic significance of VEGF immunohistochemical expression and tumor angiogenesis in head and neck squamous cell carcinoma. J Cancer Res Clin Oncol 2005;131:624–30.

86. Cohen EE, Davis DW, Karrison TG, et al. Erlotinib and bevacizumab in patients with recurrent or metastatic squamous-cell carcinoma of the head and neck: a phase I/II study. Lancet Oncol 2009;10:247–57.

87. Elser C, Siu LL, Winquist E, et al. Phase II trial of sorafenib in patients with recurrent or metastatic squamous cell carcinoma of the head and neck or nasopharyngeal carcinoma. J Clin Oncol 2007;25:3766–73.

88. Williamson SK, Moon J, Huang CH, et al. Phase II evaluation of sorafenib in advanced and metastatic squamous cell carcinoma of the head and neck: Southwest Oncology Group Study S0420. J Clin Oncol 2010;28:3330–5.

89. Choong NW, Kozloff M, Taber D, et al. Phase II study of sunitinib malate in head and neck squamous cell carcinoma. Invest New Drugs 2010;28:677–83.

90. Fountzilas G, Fragkoulidi A, Kalogera-Fountzila A, et al. A phase II study of sunitinib in patients with recurrent and/or metastatic non-nasopharyngeal head and neck cancer. Cancer Chemother Pharmacol 2010;65:649–60.

91. Machiels JP, Henry S, Zanetta S, et al. Phase II study of sunitinib in recurrent or metastatic squamous cell carcinoma of the head and neck: GORTEC 2006-01. J Clin Oncol 2010;28:21–8.
92. Salama JK, Haraf DJ, Stenson KM, et al. A randomized phase II study of 5-fluorouracil, hydroxyurea, and twice-daily radiotherapy compared with bevacizumab plus 5-fluorouracil, hydroxyurea, and twice-daily radiotherapy for intermediate-stage and T4N0-1 head and neck cancers. Ann Oncol 2011;22:2304–9.
93. Fury MG, Lee NY, Sherman E, et al. A phase 2 study of bevacizumab with cisplatin plus intensity-modulated radiation therapy for stage III/IVB head and neck squamous cell cancer. Cancer 2012;118:5008–14.
94. Yao M, Galanopoulos N, Lavertu P, et al. Phase II study of bevacizumab in combination with docetaxel and radiation in locally advanced squamous cell carcinoma of the head and neck. Head Neck 2014. [Epub ahead of print].
95. Hainsworth JD, Spigel DR, Greco FA, et al. Combined modality treatment with chemotherapy, radiation therapy, bevacizumab, and erlotinib in patients with locally advanced squamous carcinoma of the head and neck: a phase II trial of the Sarah Cannon oncology research consortium. Cancer J 2011;17:267–72.
96. Yoo DS, Kirkpatrick JP, Craciunescu O, et al. Prospective trial of synchronous bevacizumab, erlotinib, and concurrent chemoradiation in locally advanced head and neck cancer. Clin Cancer Res 2012;18:1404–14.
97. Argiris A, Karamouzis MV, Gooding WE, et al. Phase II trial of pemetrexed and bevacizumab in patients with recurrent or metastatic head and neck cancer. J Clin Oncol 2011;29:1140–5.
98. Argiris A, Kotsakis AP, Hoang T, et al. Cetuximab and bevacizumab: preclinical data and phase II trial in recurrent or metastatic squamous cell carcinoma of the head and neck. Ann Oncol 2013;24:220–5.

Epidermal Growth Factor Receptor Inhibition in Squamous Cell Carcinoma of the Head and Neck

Jean-Pascal Machiels, MD, PhD*, Sandra Schmitz, MD, PhD

KEYWORDS

- Epidermal growth factor receptor • Head and neck cancer
- Anti-EGFR monoclonal antibodies • Tyrosine kinase inhibitors • Pan-HER inhibitors

KEY POINTS

- Up to 90% of squamous cell carcinomas of the head and neck express high levels of epidermal growth factor receptor (EGFR).
- Overexpression and high *EGFR* gene copy number are associated with poor prognosis.
- Cetuximab improves overall survival either as curative treatment in combination with radiation therapy or as palliative treatment in combination with chemotherapy.
- A minority of patients derive long-term benefit of anti-EGFR treatment, outlining the importance of developing novel treatment strategies.
- Potentially more potent anti-EGFR compounds as well as combination strategies are under investigation to improve treatment efficacy.

THE EPIDERMAL GROWTH FACTOR RECEPTOR

The epidermal growth factor receptor (EGFR) is a transmembrane glycoprotein commonly expressed in many normal tissues. It is a member of the human epidermal receptor (HER) tyrosine kinase receptor family composed of 4 different receptors (EGFR/c-erbB-1, c-erbB-2/HER-2/neu, c-erbB-3/HER-3 and c-erbB4/HER-4), all of which are transmembrane proteins with tyrosine kinase activity (**Fig. 1**).

Conflicts of Interest: Dr J.P. Machiels is a member of the advisory board of Boerhinger-Ingelheim (without financial compensation).
Departments of Medical Oncology and Head and Neck Surgery, King Albert II Institute, Cliniques universitaires Saint-Luc and Institut de Recherche Clinique et Expérimentale (IREC), Université catholique de Louvain, 10 avenue Hippocrate, Brussels 1200, Belgium
* Corresponding author. Service d'oncologie médicale, Cliniques universitaires Saint-Luc, Université catholique de Louvain, 10 Avenue Hippocrate, Brussels 1200, Belgium.
E-mail address: jean-pascal.machiels@uclouvain.be

Hematol Oncol Clin N Am 29 (2015) 1011–1032
http://dx.doi.org/10.1016/j.hoc.2015.07.007
0889-8588/15/$ – see front matter © 2015 Elsevier Inc. All rights reserved.

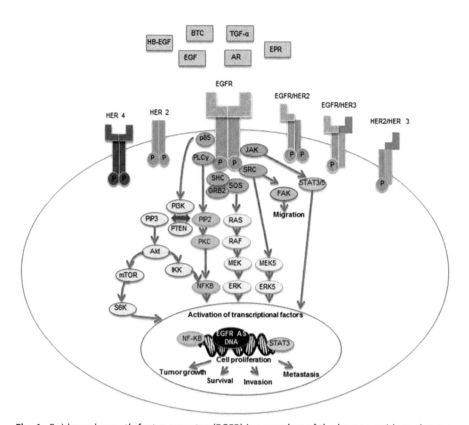

Fig. 1. Epidermal growth factor receptor (EGFR) is a member of the human epidermal receptor (HER) tyrosine kinase receptor family composed of 4 different receptors (EGFR/c-erbB-1, c-erbB-2/HER-2/neu, c-erbB-3/HER-3 and c-erbB4/HER-4), all of which are transmembrane proteins with tyrosine kinase activity. The EGFR has an extracellular domain, which provides a ligand-binding site for multiple ligands. Epidermal growth factor (EGF), transforming growth factor alpha (TGF-α) and amphiregulin (AR) are specific ligands of the EGFR, while β-cellulin (BTC), heparin-binding EGF (HB-EGF), and epiregulin (EPR) are less specific ligands that bind EGFR and ErbB4. Upon ligand fixation, EGFR homodimerization or heterodimerization with another HER receptor occurs, leading to the activation of the intracellular tyrosine kinase. This stimulates kinase signal transduction pathways involved in tumor proliferation, apoptosis, angiogenesis and cell migration/invasion. Downstream signaling through the Ras/Raf/Mek/Erk pathway controls gene transcription, cell proliferation, and cell-cycle progression, whereas the phosphatidylinositol-3-kinase (PI3K)/protein kinase B (PI3K/Akt) pathway stimulates numerous antiapoptotic signals in the cell. Src tyrosine kinase, phospholipase-Cγ, protein kinase C (PKC), and signal transducer and activator of transcription (STAT) activation have also been documented.

The EGFR has an extracellular domain, which provides a ligand-binding site for multiple ligands. Upon ligand fixation, EGFR homodimerization or heterodimerization with another HER receptor occurs, leading to the activation of the intracellular tyrosine kinase. This leads to activation of molecular pathways involved in tumor proliferation, apoptosis, angiogenesis, and cell migration/invasion.[1] Downstream signaling through the Ras/ Raf/Mek/Erk pathway controls gene transcription, cell proliferation, and cell-cycle progression, whereas the phosphatidylinositol-3-kinase/protein kinase B (PI3K/Akt) pathway stimulates numerous antiapoptotic signals. Other proteins activated by EGFR include the Src tyrosine kinase, the phospholipase-C gamma, the protein kinase C, and the signal transducer and activator of transcription.[2]

Up to 90% of squamous cell carcinoma of the head and neck (SCCHN) express high levels of EGFR[2] and overexpression of EGFR and transforming growth factor-α are associated with poor prognosis[3–6] and radioresistance.[3,6,7] Increased *EGFR* gene copy number has been reported in 10% to 58% of patients with SCCHN and has also been described as an indicator of poor survival, locoregional failure, and radioresistance.[8–11]

In non–small cell lung cancer, *EGFR* mutations (especially in exons 19 and 20) are correlated with better treatment response to EGFR tyrosine kinase inhibitors.[12] These mutations are, however, rarely found in SCCHN. EGFRvIII is the result of an in-frame deletion of exons 2 through 7 (deletion of amino acids 30–297, involving 801 base pairs), resulting in a truncated extracellular EGF-binding domain that is constitutively activated.[13] Although earlier reports documented EGFRvIII in about 40% of SCCHN, EGFRvIII variant was identified in less than 0.5% of the samples analyzed by the Cancer Genome Atlas project.[14–16] The reasons for this discrepancy are unknown and require further investigation (methodologic issues, difference between early stage and recurrent SCCHN, etc).

INHIBITION OF EPIDERMAL GROWTH FACTOR RECEPTOR

There are 2 ways to inhibit EGFR signaling (**Fig. 2**). First, monoclonal antibodies (mAbs) administered intravenously can bind specifically to the EGFR with high affinity and thereby block ligand-binding–induced receptor activation. Second, oral tyrosine kinase competitive inhibitors can reversibly or irreversibly inhibit the binding of adenosine 5'-triphosphate to the phosphate-binding loop of the adenosine 5'-triphosphate binding site in the intracellular domain of EGFR, thereby abrogate downstream signaling.

Anti-Epidermal Growth Factor Receptor Monoclonal Antibodies

In SCCHN, cetuximab, panitumumab, and zalutumumab are the most investigated mAbs that specifically bind to EGFR with high affinity. Cetuximab is a chimeric human/murine immunoglobulin (Ig)G1 mAb, whereas zalutumumab (IgG1) and panitumumab (IgG2) are fully human mAbs. In addition to this direct effect on the EGFR, cetuximab and zalutumumab could also activate antibody-dependent cellular cytotoxicity through the binding of their Fc tail to Fc gamma receptors on natural killer cells, monocytes, dendritic cells, and other granulocytes.[17,18] EGFR blockade is also thought to possibly act via inhibition of DNA double-strand break repair that contributes to resistance to radiotherapy and DNA damage induced by chemotherapeutic agents by preventing nuclear import of EGFR.[19] The main trials investigating anti-EGFR mAbs in SCCHN are summarized in **Table 1**.

The role of anti-epidermal growth factor receptor monoclonal antibodies in the multimodal curative treatment

Radiotherapy plus anti-epidermal growth factor receptor monoclonal antibodies versus radiotherapy Bonner and colleagues[20,21] compared radiotherapy alone with radiotherapy plus cetuximab in stage III/IV SCCHN. They found that the addition of cetuximab improved median overall survival (OS) from 29.3 to 49.0 months (*P* = .03) and locoregional control (LCR) from 14.9 to 24.4 months (*P* = .005). Because the patients with oropharynx cancer seemed to be the subgroup that benefitted the most from cetuximab, the human papilloma virus (HPV) status using

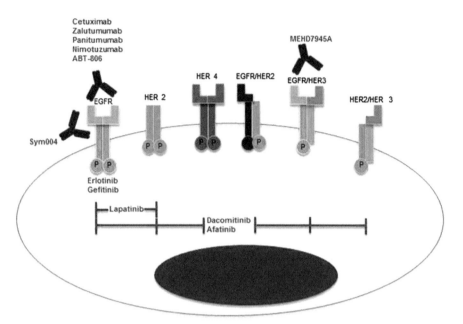

Fig. 2. There are 2 ways to inhibit epidermal growth factor receptor (EGFR) signaling. First, several monoclonal antibodies (mAbs) administered intravenously can specifically bind to the EGFR with high affinity and thereby block ligand-binding–induced receptor activation. Second, oral tyrosine kinase competitive inhibitors can reversibly or irreversibly inhibit the binding of adenosine 5′-triphosphate (ATP) to the phosphate-binding loop of the ATP binding site in the intracellular domain of EGFR and thereby abrogate downstream signaling.

tumor p16 as a surrogate marker was assessed retrospectively. The univariate analysis showed a more pronounced treatment effect of radiotherapy and cetuximab versus radiotherapy in patients with p16-positive tumors. However, interaction tests in p16-positive and -negative populations did not demonstrate a significant interaction between p16 status and treatment effect.[22] Therefore, we cannot conclude definitively from this trial that p16 positivity is a predictive biomarker for cetuximab activity in this setting.

Radiotherapy plus anti-epidermal growth factor receptor monoclonal antibodies versus chemoradiation The GSTTC Italian Study Group randomized patients with unresectable stage III/IV SCCHN according to a 2 × 2 factorial design: 2 cycles of cisplatin/5-fluorouracil concomitant to radiotherapy (arm A1), cetuximab concomitant to radiotherapy (arm A2), 3 cycles of induction cisplatin, docetaxel, and 5-fluorouracil (TPF) followed by concurrent platinum-based chemoradiation (arm B1) and 3 cycles of TPF followed by cetuximab and radiotherapy (arm B2).[23] Interestingly, no differences for grades 3 and 4 in-field skin and mucositis toxicities were observed, challenging the concept that cetuximab added to radiation therapy is less toxic than cisplatin-based chemoradiation. Both regimens showed similar efficacy: median progression-free survival (PFS) and OS were 21.6 months and 44.7 months for the chemoradiation arm and 20.7 months and 44.7 months for the cetuximab and radiotherapy arm. However, this study was not adequately powered to demonstrate that cetuximab plus radiation therapy is equivalent to cisplatin-based chemoradiation.

Table 1
Selected trials with anti-EGFR monoclonal antibodies

Trial	Regimens	N	Disease Stage	Locoregional Control	Progression-Free Survival	Overall Survival
Radiotherapy vs radiotherapy plus an anti-EGFR mAb						
Bonner (phase III)[20,21]	Radiotherapy + cetuximab versus	213	Stage III or IV squamous cell carcinoma of the head and neck	24.4 mo[a] (median)	17.1 mo[a] (median)	49 mo[a] (median)
	Radiotherapy	211		14.9 mo (median)	12.4 mo (median)	29 mo (median)
Chemoradiation vs radiotherapy plus an anti-EGFR mAb						
GSTTC Italian study group (phase III)[23,28]	Radiotherapy + cetuximab versus	161	Stage III or IV squamous cell carcinoma of the head and neck	NA	20.7 mo (median)	44.7 mo (median)
	Chemoradiation (2 cycles of cisplatin/5-fluorouracil)	260			21.6 mo (median)	44.7 mo (median)
CONCERT-2 (phase II)[24]	Radiotherapy + panitumumab versus	90	Stage III or IV squamous cell carcinoma of the head and neck	61% (rate at 2 y)	41% (rate at 2 y)	63% (rate at 2 y)
	Chemoradiation (2 cycles of high-dose cisplatin)	61		51% (rate at 2 y)	62% (rate at 2 y)	71% (rate at 2 y)
NCIC clinical trial group HN.6 trial (phase III)[25]	Radiation therapy (70 Gy) + cisplatin 100 mg/m² d 1, 22, 43 versus	156	Stage III or IV squamous cell carcinoma of the head and neck	—	73% (rate at 2 y)	85% (rate at 2 y)
	Accelerated radiotherapy + panitumumab day –7, 15, 36	159			76% (rate at 2 y)	88% (rate at 2 y)
Induction chemotherapy followed by radiotherapy plus an anti-EGFR mAb						
TREMPLIN (phase II)[27]	TPF followed by chemoradiation (3 cycles of high-dose cisplatin) versus	60	Resectable squamous cell carcinoma of the larynx and hypopharynx	NA	NA	75% (rate at 3 y)
	TPF followed by cetuximab plus radiation	56				73% (rate at 3 y)

(continued on next page)

Table 1
(continued)

Trial	Regimens	N	Disease Stage	Locoregional Control	Progression-Free Survival	Overall Survival
Chemoradiation vs chemoradiation plus an anti-EGFR mAb						
RTOG 0522 (phase III)[29]	Chemoradiation (2 cycles of high-dose cisplatin) versus	447	Stage III or IV squamous cell carcinoma of the head and neck	NA	61% (rate at 3 y)	73% (rate at 3 y)
	Chemoradiation plus cetuximab	444			59% (rate at 3 y)	76% (rate at 3 y)
CONCERT-1 (phase II)[30,31]	Chemoradiation (3 cycles of high-dose cisplatin) versus	63	Stage III or IV squamous cell carcinoma of the head and neck	68% (rate at 2 y)	65% (rate at 2 y)	78% (rate at 2 y)
	Chemoradiation plus panitumumab	87		61% (rate at 2 y)	61% (rate at 2 y)	69% (rate at 2 y)
DAHANCA 19 (phase III)[32]	(Chemo)radiation plus nimorazole versus	309	Squamous cell carcinoma of the head and neck (89% were stage III and IV; 70% received chemoradiation)	73% (rate at 4 y)	NA	Hazard ratio: 1.22
	(Chemo)radiation plus nimorazole and zalutumumab	310		71% (rate at 4 y)		
Anti-EGFR mAbs as adjuvant therapy						
Mesia (phase II)[34]	Radiotherapy plus concomitant cetuximab versus	46	Stage III/IV oropharyngeal cancer	44% (rate at 2 y)	35.3 mo (median)	33.6 mo (median)
	Radiotherapy plus concomitant and adjuvant cetuximab (12 wk)	45		44% (rate at 2 y)	41 mo (median)	39.9 mo (median)
Anti-EGFR mAbs in recurrent and/or metastatic (R/M) disease						
ECOG E5397 (phase III)[36]	Cisplatin versus	60	R/M squamous cell carcinoma: first-line	NA	2.7 mo (median)	8 mo (median)
	Cisplatin and cetuximab	57			4.2 mo (median)	9.2 mo (median)
EXTREME (phase III)[37]	Platin/5-fluorouracil versus	220	R/M squamous cell carcinoma: first-line	NA	3.3 mo[a] (median)	7.4 mo[a] (median)
	Cisplatin/5-fluorouracil/cetuximab	222			5.6 mo[a] (median)	10.1 mo[a] (median)

Study	Treatment	N	Population			
SPECTRUM (phase III)[39]	Cisplatin/5-fluorouracil versus	330	R/M squamous cell carcinoma: first-line	NA	4.6 mo[a] (median)	9 mo (median)
	Cisplatin/5-fluorouracil/panitumumab	327			5.8 mo[a] (median)	11.1 mo (median)
PARTNER (randomized phase II)[40]	Cisplatin/docetaxel versus	51	R/M squamous cell carcinoma: first-line	NA	5.5 mo (median)	13.8 mo (median)
	Cisplatin/docetaxel/panitumumab	52			6.9 mo (median)	12.9 mo (median)
ZALUTE (phase III)[46]	Best supportive care or methotrexate versus	95	R/M squamous cell carcinoma: second-line (platinum failure)	NA	8.4 wk[a] (median)	5.2 mo (median)
	Zalutumumab	191			9.9 wk[a] (median)	6.7 mo (median)

Abbreviations: EGFR, epidermal growth factor receptor; mAb, monoclonal antibody; NA, nonapplicable or not available; R/M, recurrent and/or metastatic; TPF, induction chemotherapy with cisplatin, 5-fluorouracil, and docetaxel.

[a] *P*<.05.

Data from Refs.[20,21,23–25,27–32,34,36,37,39,40,46]

In the CONCERT-2 trial, the investigators compared the safety and efficacy of radiation therapy combined with panitumumab versus concurrent chemoradiation. The investigators reported a trend in favor of concurrent chemoradiation for LCR at 2 years (the primary endpoint): 51% with irradiation plus panitumumab compared with 61% with concurrent chemoradiation. Both PFS ($P = .03$) and OS ($P = .10$) outcomes favored the concurrent chemoradiation arm.[24]

The NCI Canadian group randomized 320 stage 3 and 4 SCCHN patients between standard fractionated radiotherapy (70 Gy over 7 weeks) plus cisplatin (100 mg/m^2, 3 cycles) versus accelerated radiotherapy (70 Gy over 6 weeks) plus panitumumab (9 mg/kg for 3 doses). The 2-year PFS was 73% and 76%, respectively. In addition, noninferiority of bioradiotherapy was not proven in this study.[25]

Therefore, so far, in locally advanced (LA) SCCHN, the combination of radiation therapy and anti-EGFR mAb has not been proven to be equivalent to platinum-based chemoradiation. The results of the RTOG 1016 study that randomized p16-positive oropharyngeal cancer patients between accelerated chemoradiation (high-dose cisplatin) and accelerated radiotherapy plus cetuximab are pending. Outside clinical trials, platinum-based chemoradiation remains the standard of care for fit patients.[26] Cetuximab plus radiotherapy should be only considered for patients with stage 3 and 4 SCCHN and when contraindications to cisplatin such as kidney dysfunction, hearing loss, or cardiovascular insufficiency are present.

Anti-epidermal growth factor receptor monoclonal antibodies and concurrent radiotherapy after induction chemotherapy Lefebvre and colleagues[27] reported the results of a phase II trial comparing the efficacy and safety of induction chemotherapy (TPF) followed by concurrent regimens for larynx preservation (TREMPLIN). Poor responders to induction chemotherapy (<50% response) underwent salvage surgery. Responders were assigned randomly to conventional radiotherapy plus either cisplatin or cetuximab. The primary end point was 3-month larynx preservation. In an intent-to-treat analysis, there was no difference between the arms in the rates of larynx preservation at 3 months and OS at 18 months, but this study was not powered adequately to address these questions. Treatment compliance was higher in the cetuximab plus radiation therapy arm.

In the GSTTC Italian Study Group described, an analysis that compared the induction versus noninduction arms was reported recently. The authors found that induction TPF followed by chemoradiation or concurrent cetuximab plus radiotherapy significantly improved PFS and OS (53 vs 30 months ($P = .015$); independent from the type of concomitant strategy).[28] The benefit of induction chemotherapy seemed to be greater in the cetuximab arm and for patients with non-oropharyngeal cancer. However, the 2×2 factorial design decreases the number of patients in each arm, precluding definitive conclusions owing to a lack of statistical power. With the data we have available presently, TPF followed by concurrent cetuximab and radiotherapy cannot be considered as a standard of care.

Chemoradiation versus chemoradiation plus anti-epidermal growth factor receptor monoclonal antibodies The RTOG 0522 trial investigated the addition of cetuximab to platinum-based chemoradiation in patients with stage III/IV SCCHN.[29] No difference was observed between the 2 groups. The 3-year PFS in the chemoradiation group was 61%, whereas in the chemoradiation group plus cetuximab it was 59%. The 3-year OS was 73% and 76%, respectively. However, local toxicity was higher in the cetuximab-containing arm, with grade 3 and 4 stomatitis being observed in 43% versus 33% and in-field dermatitis in 25% versus 15%.

The phase II CONCERT-1 study showed that the addition of panitumumab to cisplatin-based chemoradiation resulted in increased toxicity with no improvement in response rate or survival. LCR at 2 years was 68% in the chemoradiation group and 61% in the panitumumab group.[30,31]

The DAHANCA 19[32] trial randomized 619 patients between accelerated radiotherapy plus nimorazole and, in case of stage 3 and 4 disease, weekly cisplatin versus the same regimens plus zalutumumab. Seventy percent of the patients received cisplatin. The 4-year LCR rate was 71% in the zalutumumab arm and 73% in the control arm. Survival was similar between the 2 arms.

A randomized, phase II trial (RTOG-0234) investigated concurrent chemoradiotherapy and cetuximab in the postoperative treatment of patients with SCCHN with high-risk pathologic features.[33] Patients were randomly assigned to 60 Gy radiation with cetuximab once per week plus either cisplatin 30 mg/m^2 or docetaxel 15 mg/m^2 once per week. The 2-year OS was 69% for the cisplatin arm and 79% for the docetaxel arm; the 2-year disease-free survival was 57% and 66%, respectively. Although these results look promising, they need to be validated or not in a larger trial (RTOG 1216).

Consequently, chemoradiation without anti-EGFR mAb remains the standard of care in LA SCCHN. Most of these trials adding an anti-EGFR mAb to standard (chemo)radiation have been conducted before HPV-induced oropharyngeal cancer was recognized as a different molecular and clinical disease compared with tobacco and alcohol-induced SCCHN. Therefore, it is possible that we have diluted the effect of anti-EGFR mAb in 1 of these subgroups.

Anti-epidermal growth factor receptor monoclonal antibodies as adjuvant therapy Adjuvant therapy consists of starting or continuing a targeted agent after definitive treatment. A randomized, phase II trial investigated the efficacy and safety of cetuximab maintenance therapy given for 12 weeks after radiotherapy in patients with stage III/IV oropharyngeal cancer.[34] LCR at 1 year was superior among patients treated with cetuximab maintenance (59% vs 47%). However, LCR was similar between both arms after 2 years of follow-up. In another phase II trial, 2-year PFS was 70% in 39 stage III/IVA-B patients who received cisplatin/docetaxel/cetuximab as induction therapy followed by cisplatin/cetuximab/radiotherapy and who then continued cetuximab for a maximum of 6 months.[35] Further trials are needed.

The role of anti-epidermal growth factor receptor monoclonal antibodies in recurrent and/or metastatic disease
First-line treatment in combination with platinum-based chemotherapy Burtness and colleagues[36] conducted a randomized trial (ECOG E5397) comparing cisplatin and placebo with cisplatin and cetuximab in chemotherapy-naïve SCCHN patients with incurable SCCHN. There was a statistically significant higher response rate in the cetuximab arm, 26% versus 10% ($P = .03$), but no difference in PFS (the primary endpoint) or OS.

The phase III EXTREME trial[37] randomized 442 patients with recurrent or metastatic SCCHN to receive 5-fluorouracil and platinum-based therapy alone or in combination with cetuximab as a first-line palliative regimen. In the experimental arm, patients who had at least stable disease after a maximum of 6 cycles of chemotherapy received cetuximab monotherapy until the disease progressed or occurrence of unacceptable toxic effects. This study demonstrated a benefit of cetuximab with an improvement in median OS from 7.4 to 10.1 months ($P = .04$). An unplanned retrospective analysis assessed the outcome by tumor p16 status (as a surrogate marker for HPV) and concluded that the survival benefit of adding cetuximab to chemotherapy was independent of tumor p16 status, and that patients with p16-positive tumors had a more favorable outcome than those with p16-negative tumors. However, this last analysis is limited by the low number of patients with p16-positive disease.[38]

The SPECTRUM trial[39] randomized 657 patients with recurrent and/or metastatic SCCHN to cisplatin and 5-fluorouracil alone or with panitumumab, every 3 weeks. Panitumumab did not significantly improve the primary endpoint of OS (median, 11.1 vs 9.0 months; $P = .14$), but did yield significantly higher objective response rate (ORR; 36% vs 25%; $P = .007$) and PFS (5.8 vs 4.6 months; $P = .004$). An analysis of the results stratified by tumor p16 status suggested that panitumumab improved OS and PFS in patients with p16-negative tumors but not in those with p16-positive disease. These results should be interpreted with caution because of the low number of patients with p16-positive tumors as well as the definition of p16 positivity (>10% of the tumor cells expressing p16 in contrast with the more commonly accepted criterion of >70%). In addition, as mentioned, a similar analysis in the EXTREME study, using the 70% cutoff point, did not show the same results. Therefore, further evaluation is needed to better understand the impact of HPV and/or p16 status on the activity of anti-EGFR mAbs.

A randomized (1:1) phase II study investigated docetaxel and cisplatin with or without panitumumab in the first-line palliative treatment.[40] Median PFS, median OS, and overall response rate were 6.9 months, 12.9 months, and 44% in the panitumumab arm versus 5.5 months, 13.8 months, and 37% in the arm without panitumumab, respectively. Crossover to panitumumab monotherapy was allowed in the docetaxel/cisplatin arm and occurred in 57% of the patients, which may have impaired the OS analysis.

Second-line treatment after platinum-based chemotherapy The results of 2 phase II trials investigating the addition of cetuximab to carboplatin or cisplatin in patients with platinum-refractory SCCHN showed an ORR of 10% and a median survival of 5.2 to 6.1 months.[41,42] Another phase II study with similar inclusion criteria evaluated cetuximab as monotherapy and reported an ORR of 13% with a median OS of 5.9 months.[43] This last study suggests that single agent cetuximab, in this platinum-refractory population, can offer similar results to those obtained when the drug is used in combination with a platinum compound. A pooled analysis of these three phase II trials (n = 278)[44] was performed and the results were compared with those from Leon's retrospective study in which patients (n = 151)[45] were treated with best supportive care or various second-line treatments. This indirect comparison suggests that cetuximab has the potential to increase median OS by approximately 2 months. Although a randomized trial is missing in the recurrent, metastatic or palliative setting, cetuximab was approved by the US Food and Drug Administration as monotherapy in recurrent and/or metastatic disease after platinum-based treatment (www.fda.gov).

The ZALUTE trial[46] randomized 286 patients with recurrent and/or metastatic SCCHN that progressed within 6 months of platinum-based therapy to receive either zalutumumab plus best supportive care with optional methotrexate in a 2:1 ratio. This study did not meet its primary endpoint of improving OS (median of 6.7 months in the zalutumumab group vs 5.2 months in the control group; $P = .06$). However, PFS was significantly higher in the zalutumumab group ($P = .001$), suggesting clinical activity of this agent.

Cetuximab therapy in the recurrent and/or metastatic setting is considered standard of care by many clinicians. In Europe, cetuximab is mainly used in first-line in combination with platinum-based chemotherapy and in United States it is frequently used in monotherapy, as second-line treatment after platinum failure. However, the cost of anti-EGFR mAbs should be balanced with the limited benefit of this compound. Therefore, some countries do not provide health insurance coverage for cetuximab in noncurable SCCHN.

Other anti-epidermal growth factor receptor monoclonal antibodies with preliminary results

Nimotuzumab (h-R3mAb) is another mAb that bivalently binds to the extracellular domain of the EGFR that overlaps with the binding site of cetuximab and EGF. Different phase II studies also investigated this agent in combination either with radiation or chemoradiation in advanced SCCHN. A randomized, phase II trial[47] compared radiotherapy and nimotuzumab with radiotherapy and placebo in a group of 106 patients with unresectable SCCHN who were unfit for concurrent chemoradiation. Toxicities were limited to almost only grade I/II. The complete response rate was significantly higher in the nimotuzumab group (59.5%) versus the placebo group (34.2%; $P = .038$), as was survival ($P = .0491$). However, the radiation dose used in this study was low and could be questioned. Another phase II study[48] randomized 92 patients with (LA) SCCHN to receive radiotherapy alone or radiotherapy plus nimotuzumab (arm A) or chemoradiation without or with nimotuzumab (arm B). Locoregional response was better in the nimotuzumab arms: 76% versus 37% in arm A, and 100% versus 70% in arm B. The corresponding OS rates at 48 months were 34% versus 13% (nonsignificant) in group A, and 47% versus 21% in group B ($P = .01$). The addition of nimotuzumab to chemoradiation resulted in a significant reduction in the risk of death by 65% (hazard ratio, 0.35; $P = .01$). These results should, however, be interpreted with caution owing to the low number of patients included.

Epidermal Growth Factor Receptor Tyrosine Kinase Inhibitors

Reversible "selective" EGFR tyrosine kinase inhibitors, such as gefitinib and erlotinib, have been investigated in SCCHN (**Table 2**).

The role of anti-epidermal growth factor receptor tyrosine kinase inhibitors in multimodal curative treatment

Some investigators have attempted to add EGFR tyrosine kinase inhibitors to chemoradiation in LA SCCHN. Martins and colleagues[49] randomized 204 patients in a phase II study with LA SCCHN to receive radiotherapy and cisplatin without (arm A) or with erlotinib (arm B) starting 1 week before and during chemoradiation. Arm A had a complete response rate of 40% and arm B had a complete response rate of 52% ($P = .08$). With a median follow-up of 26 months and 54 progression events, there was no difference in PFS.

In a randomized phase II trial, Gregoire and colleagues[50] enrolled 226 patients to receive either gefitinib 250 mg/d, 500 mg/d, or placebo in 2 phases: a concomitant phase (gefitinib or placebo with chemoradiotherapy) followed by a maintenance phase (gefitinib or placebo alone). The investigators concluded that gefitinib did not improve the 2-year LCR compared with placebo, when given either concomitantly with chemoradiation (32.7% vs 33.6%, respectively; $P = .607$) or as maintenance therapy (28.8% vs 37.4%; $P = .894$). Another phase II study showed that feasibility of administrating gefitinib as maintenance therapy during 2 years after chemoradiation.[51]

The role of anti-epidermal growth factor receptor tyrosine kinase inhibitors in recurrent and/or metastatic disease

A phase III trial (IMEX) compared methotrexate alone with gefitinib alone as palliative therapy for incurable, recurrent SCCHN.[52] Four hundred eighty-six patients were

Table 2
Selected trials with anti-EGFR or HER tyrosine kinase inhibitors

Trial	Regimens	N	Disease Stage	Complete (CRR) or Objective Response Rate (ORR)	Disease-free Survival	Overall Survival
Anti-EGFR or HER TKIs in the multimodal curative treatment						
Martins (phase III)[49]	Chemoradiation (high-dose cisplatin) versus	99	Stage III or IV squamous cell carcinoma of the head and neck	CRR: 40%	Hazard ratio: 0.9	Hazard ratio: 1.05
	Chemoradiation (high-dose cisplatin) plus erlotinib	105		CRR: 52%		
Harrington (phase III)[59]	Postoperative chemoradiation (high-dose cisplatin) versus	342	Resected stage II or IVA squamous cell carcinoma of the head and neck with surgical margin ≤5 mm and/or extracapsular extension	NA	Not reached (median)	Hazard ratio: 0.96
	Postoperative chemoradiation plus lapatinib (lapatinib during chemoradiation and as maintenance during 1 y)	346			53.6 mo (median)	
Anti-EGFR or HER TKIs in recurrent and/or metastatic (R/M) disease						
IMEX (phase III)[52]	Methotrexate versus	161	R/M squamous cell carcinoma after radical radiotherapy	ORR: 3.9%	NA	5.6 mo (median)
	Gefitinib 250 mg/d versus	158		ORR: 2.7%		6 mo (median)
	Gefitinib 500 mg/d	167		ORR: 7.6%		6.7 mo (median)
Argiris (phase III)[53]	Docetaxel + placebo versus	136	R/M squamous cell carcinoma	ORR: 6.2%	NA	6 mo (median)
	Docetaxel + gefitinib	134		ORR: 12.5%		7.3 mo (median)
LUX-H&N 1 (phase III)[62]	Methotrexate versus	161	R/M squamous cell carcinoma: second-line after platinum therapy	ORR: 5.6%	1.7 mo[a] (median)	6 mo (median)
	Afatinib	322		ORR: 10.2%	2.6 mo[a] (median)	6.8 mo (median)

Abbreviations: EGFR, epidermal growth factor receptor; HER, human epidermal receptor; NA, nonavailable or not applicable; R/M, recurrent and/or metastatic; TKI, tyrosine kinase inhibitor.

[a] $P < .05$.

Data from Refs. [49,52,53,59,62]

assigned randomly to oral gefitinib at 250 mg/d, oral gefitinib at 500 mg/d, or weekly intravenous methotrexate at 40 mg/m^2. No differences between the gefitinib regimen and methotrexate were found. The median OS were 5.6, 6.0, and 6.7 months and the ORR were 2.7%, 7.6%, and 3.9%, respectively. No unexpected adverse events were observed, except for more tumor hemorrhage events in the gefitinib arms (8.9% in gefitinib 250 mg/d, 11.4% in gefitinib 500 mg/d, and 1.9% in methotrexate).

In another phase III trial,[53] 270 patients were assigned randomly to receive docetaxel plus placebo (arm A) or plus daily gefitinib 250 mg given orally (arm B) until disease progression. The study was stopped at the interim analysis in November 2008 because of the low likelihood of meeting the primary endpoint. Median OS was 6 months in arm A versus 7.3 months in arm B ($P = .60$). Median time to progression was 2.1 and 3.5 months ($P = .19$), respectively.

STRATEGIES TO OVERCOME RESISTANCE TO ANTI-EPIDERMAL GROWTH FACTOR RECEPTOR THERAPY
Blockage of Multiple Human Epidermal Receptors

Background
C-erbB-2/HER-2-neu, c-erbB-3/HER-3, and c-erbB4/HER-4 are other members of the HER tyrosine kinase receptor family. Targeting these receptors, in addition to the EGFR, has been an area of recent clinical studies (see **Fig. 1**).

The *HER-2/neu* gene encodes a transmembrane protein of 185 kDa. HER-2 has no ligand, but the intracellular part of this receptor has tyrosine kinase activity. It can dimerize spontaneously or form heterodimers with other members of the EGFR family to activate some of the downstream signal transduction pathways implicated in carcinogenesis. HER-3 does not have intrinsic tyrosine kinase activity but can be transphosphorylated by EGFR and HER-2/neu. HER-4, the fourth member of the family, encodes a 180-kDa transmembrane tyrosine kinase that can also form heterodimers with the other HER receptors.

The overexpression rates of HER-2, HER-3, and HER-4 in SCCHN have been reported by different groups. However, conflicting results exist and their value as a prognostic tool remains unclear.[54–56]

Heterodimerization of EGFR with HER-2, HER-3 or HER-4 induced by ligand binding may be responsible for the limited activity of EGFR targeted mAbs or tyrosine kinase inhibitors. The ability to block more than just one HER receptors could therefore be of interest.

Lapatinib is an oral reversible dual tyrosine kinase inhibitor of epidermal growth factor receptor and HER2. More recently, a new generation of HER inhibitors, the irreversible small molecule pan-HER inhibitors including afatinib and dacomitinib, have been developed. By covalently binding and irreversibly blocking all kinase receptors from the ErbB family, a prolonged inhibition is obtained with the aim of improving clinical activity.

The role of human epidermal receptor inhibitors in the multimodal curative treatment
Adding lapatinib to TPF induction chemotherapy followed by chemoradiation was found to be too toxic. Of the 7 patients with LA larynx or hypopharynx SCC enrolled, 4 experienced DLTs at the first dose level of lapatinib. Therefore, the trial was terminated.[57]

Harrington and colleagues[58] treated 67 patients with LA SCCHN with either daily lapatinib or placebo plus 3 cycles of high-dose cisplatin, and radiotherapy followed by maintenance lapatinib/placebo. This study showed that lapatinib was well-tolerated when combined with chemoradiation. The complete response rates at

6 months were 53% with lapatinib and 36% with placebo. The PFS and OS rates at 18 months were 55% versus 41% and 68% versus 57%, respectively.

The same investigators presented recently the results of a phase III study (NCT00424255) combining lapatinib with chemoradiation in resected high-risk patients. They did not observe differences in disease-free survival for any of the prespecified subgroups (nodal status, primary tumor location, geographic region, and ErbB1 expression), including HPV.[59]

The role of human epidermal receptor inhibitors in recurrent and/or metastatic disease

Lapatinib used in the setting of recurrent and/or metastatic SCCHN yielded no objective response[60] in either EGFR inhibitor naive or refractory patients. Seiwert and colleagues[61] randomized 124 patients with metastatic or recurrent SCCHN who progressed after platinum-containing therapy to receive afatinib (50 mg/d) or cetuximab. ORRs were 8.1% for afanitib and 9.7% for cetuximab. Median PFS times were 13 and 15 weeks in the afatinib and cetuximab arms, respectively. For the 32 patients crossing from afatinib to cetuximab, the disease control rate was 19% and the median PFS of 5.7, weeks whereas for the 36 patients switching from cetuximab to afatinib, the disease control rate was 33% and the median PFS was 9.3 weeks.

The phase III trial LUX-Head & Neck 1 randomized 483 patients with recurrent and/or metastatic SCCHN progressing after first-line platinum regimens to oral afatinib (40 mg/d) or intravenous methotrexate (40 mg/m^2/wk). Afatinib statistically improved PFS versus methotrexate by only 0.9 months (median 2.6 vs 1.7 months; $P = .030$) without improvement in OS.[62]

Dacomitinib (PF00299804) is also an irreversible, small molecule inhibitor of EGFR, HER-2, and HER-4 tyrosine kinases. A phase II study of 69 patients with recurrent or metastatic SCCHN showed a PR rate of 12.7% and stable disease of 57.1%, which lasted for 24 weeks or longer in 14.3% of patients. The median PFS was 12.1 weeks and the median OS was 34.6 weeks.[63]

Dual Targeting Monoclonal Antibodies or Mixture of Monoclonal Antibodies

A large variety of bispecific antibodies are under development. The goal of such antibodies is to simultaneously block 2 receptors or mediators to overcome resistance or to stimulate immune effector cells.

The IgG1 antibody *MEHD7945A* inhibits both EGFR- and HER3-mediated signaling and mediates antibody-dependent cellular cytotoxicity in vitro and in vivo.[64] A phase I study of 36 patients showed an encouraging safety profile and evidence of antitumor activity when given at a dose of 14 mg/kg every 2 weeks.[65] Best response by RECIST criteria included 2 PRs (both SCCHN) and 6 stable disease ≥8 weeks (2 non–small cell lung cancer and 4 colorectal cancer). Seven out of 8 patients were treated previously with EGFR inhibitors. A randomized, phase II trial compared MEHD7945A with cetuximab in patients with recurrent/metastatic SCCHN that progressed during or shortly after platinum-based chemotherapy. No difference between the 2 arms could be detected in this trial.[66]

Finally, *Sym004* is a drug mixture of 2 IgG1 mAbs targeting nonoverlapping epitopes on the EGFR. In preclinical models, Sym004 exhibited more pronounced EGFR internalization, degradation, and tumor growth inhibition than cetuximab.[67] Sym004 was recently investigated as palliative monotherapy in patients with SCCHN.[68] Twenty-six patients, of whom 23 (88%) had progressed while on anti-EGFR mAb treatment, were included. Median PFS and OS were 82 days and 156 days, respectively. No

Table 3
Selected ongoing clinical trials

Trial	N	Main Inclusion Criteria	Treatment	Primary Endpoint/Objective
Chemoradiation vs (chemo)radiation plus anti-EGFR therapy				
GORTEC 2007-01 NCT00609284 (phase III)	406	Stage III or IV (T0-4, N0-N2b) squamous cell carcinoma of the head and neck	Radiation therapy (70 Gy) + carboplatin/ 5-fluorouracil versus Radiotherapy (70 Gy) + weekly cetuximab	Progression-free survival
NCT01216020 (phase II)	140	Stage III or IV squamous cell carcinoma of the head and neck	Radiation therapy (70 Gy) + cisplatin 40 mg/m²/wk versus Radiotherapy (70 Gy) + weekly cetuximab	Evaluation and comparison of the compliance
RTOG 1016	706	Stage III or IV squamous cell carcinoma of the oropharynx (p16-positive, T1-2 N2a-N3 or T3-4 any N).	Accelerated radiotherapy (70 Gy) + cisplatin 100 mg/m² days 1 and 22 versus Accelerated radiotherapy + cetuximab	To determine whether substitution of cisplatin with cetuximab will result in comparable 5-y overall survival
NCT01711658 (phase II)	176	Non-HPV stage III or IV squamous cell carcinoma of the head and neck	Radiation therapy (70 Gy) + cisplatin 100 mg/m² days 1, 22, 43 versus Radiation therapy (70 Gy) + cisplatin 100 mg/m² days 1, 22, 43 + lapatinib for 3 mo	Progression-free survival
RTOG 0920 NCT00956007 (phase III)	700	Resected squamous cell carcinoma of the head and neck with intermediate risk of recurrence	Postoperative radiotherapy (IMRT) versus Postoperative radiotherapy (IMRT) plus weekly cetuximab	Overall survival
Anti-EGFR therapy in p16-positive disease				
RTOG 1016 NCT01302834 (phase III)	706	p16-positive oropharyngeal cancer (T1-2 N2a-N3 or T3-4 any N)	Accelerated radiotherapy (6 wk) + cisplatin 100 mg/m² (days 1 and 22) versus Accelerated radiotherapy (6 wk) + Weekly cetuximab	Overall survival
De-ESCALaTE NCT01874171 (phase III)	304	p16-positive and HPV positive by PCR oropharyngeal cancer (T3-3 N0, T1-4 N1-2) Exclusion: N2b, N2c or N3 and ≥10 pack-years	Radiation therapy (70 Gy) + cisplatin 100 mg/m² days 1, 22, and 43 versus Radiotherapy (70 Gy) + weekly cetuximab	Severe toxicity

(continued on next page)

Table 3
(continued)

Trial	N	Main Inclusion Criteria	Treatment	Primary Endpoint/Objective
TROG12.01 NCT01855451 (phase III)	200	p16-positive oropharyngeal cancer: Stage III (excluding T1-2 N1) or stage IV if smoking history of ≤10 pack-years Exclusion: T4N3 and N2b, N2c or N3 and > 10 pack-years	Radiation therapy (70 Gy) + cisplatin 40 mg/m²/wk versus Radiotherapy (70 Gy) + weekly cetuximab	Symptom severity
Anti-EGFR therapy in the context of induction chemotherapy				
NCT00999700 (phase III)	278	Stage III and IV squamous cell carcinoma of the head and neck	TPF followed by radiotherapy (70 Gy) + weekly cetuximab versus Radiotherapy (70 Gy) + cisplatin 100 mg/m² (days 1, 22, and 43)	Overall survival
NCT00716391 (phase III)	458	Stage III and IV squamous cell carcinoma of the head and neck	TPF followed by radiotherapy (70 Gy) + weekly cetuximab versus TPF followed by radiotherapy (70 Gy)+ cisplatin 100 mg/m² (days 1, 22, and 43)	Overall survival
GORTEC 2007-02 NCT01233843 (phase III)	370	Locally advanced squamous cell carcinoma of the head and neck	TPF followed by radiotherapy (70 Gy) + weekly cetuximab versus Radiotherapy (70 Gy)+ carboplatin/ 5-fluorouracil	Complete response rate
Anti-EGFR therapy in recurrent and metastatic disease				
CetuGEX NCT02052960 (phase III)	240	Recurrent and/or metastatic squamous cell carcinoma of the head and neck: first-line	Cisplatin/5-fluorouracil + cetuximab versus Cisplatin/5-fluorouracil + cetuGEX	Progression-free survival
NCT01884623 (phase III)	164	Recurrent and/or metastatic squamous cell carcinoma of the head and neck: first-line and unfit for platinum-based therapy and >70 y old	Methotrexate versus Methotrexate plus cetuximab	Failure-free survival
GORTEC 2014-01 NCT02268695 (phase III)	416	Recurrent and/or metastatic squamous cell carcinoma of the head and neck: first-line	Cisplatin/5-fluorouracil + cetuximab versus Cisplatin/docetaxel + cetuximab	Overall survival

HER inhibitors as maintenance therapy

NCT01427478 (phase III)	315	Resected squamous cell carcinoma of the head and neck with high risk of recurrence	Postoperative chemoradiation plus maintenance placebo for 1 y versus Postoperative chemoradiation plus maintenance afatinib for 1 y	Disease-free survival at 2 y
LUX-H&N2 NCT013456669 (phase III)	669	Stage III or IVb squamous cell carcinoma of the head and neck.	Chemoradiation plus maintenance placebo for 18 mo versus Chemoradiation plus maintenance afatinib for 18 mo	Disease-free survival

Abbreviations: EGFR, epidermal growth factor receptor; Gy, Gray; HER, human epidermal receptor; HPV, human papillomavirus; IMRT, intensity-modulated radiation therapy; PCR, polymerase chain reaction; TPF, induction with cisplatin, docetaxel, and 5-fluorouracil.

objective responses were recorded and 13 (50%) patients had stable disease as best response. Minor tumor shrinkages were observed in 8 (31%) patients.

SUMMARY

The anti-EGFR mAb cetuximab has been shown to improve OS either as curative treatment in combination with radiation therapy or as palliative treatment in combination with chemotherapy. Although some patients benefit from anti-EGFR mAbs, some tumors have primary resistance already, and ultimately all develop acquired resistance. A better understanding of the molecular mechanisms involved in treatment resistance is therefore crucial in SCCHN, as is the identification of predictive parameters. The use of combination or sequential targeted therapies may ultimately be necessary to abrogate treatment resistance.

Today, important clinical questions are addressed in clinical trials to optimize the utilization of anti-EGFR therapy (**Table 3**). Among these unresolved questions are the impact of HPV positivity on anti-EGFR therapy efficacy, the role of irreversible pan-HER inhibitors, the activity of concurrent anti-EGFR therapy and radiotherapy compared with chemoradiation as well as in the context of induction chemotherapy.

REFERENCES

1. Normanno N, De Luca A, Bianco C, et al. Epidermal growth factor receptor (EGFR) signaling in cancer. Gene 2006;366:2–16.
2. Kalyankrishna S, Grandis JR. Epidermal growth factor receptor biology in head and neck cancer. J Clin Oncol 2006;24:2666–72.
3. Ang KK, Berkey BA, Tu X, et al. Impact of epidermal growth factor receptor expression on survival and pattern of relapse in patients with advanced head and neck carcinoma. Cancer Res 2002;62:7350–6.
4. Wheeler S, Siwak DR, Chai R, et al. Tumor epidermal growth factor receptor and EGFR PY1068 are independent prognostic indicators for head and neck squamous cell carcinoma. Clin Cancer Res 2012;18:2278–89.
5. Rubin Grandis J, Melhem MF, Gooding WE, et al. Levels of TGF-alpha and EGFR protein in head and neck squamous cell carcinoma and patient survival. J Natl Cancer Inst 1998;90:824–32.
6. Jedlinski A, Ansell A, Johansson AC, et al. EGFR status and EGFR ligand expression influence the treatment response of head and neck cancer cell lines. J Oral Pathol Med 2013;42:26–36.
7. Bentzen SM, Atasoy BM, Daley FM, et al. Epidermal growth factor receptor expression in pretreatment biopsies from head and neck squamous cell carcinoma as a predictive factor for a benefit from accelerated radiation therapy in a randomized controlled trial. J Clin Oncol 2005;23:5560–7.
8. Temam S, Kawaguchi H, El-Naggar AK, et al. Epidermal growth factor receptor copy number alterations correlate with poor clinical outcome in patients with head and neck squamous cancer. J Clin Oncol 2007;25:2164–70.
9. Mrhalova M, Plzak J, Betka J, et al. Epidermal growth factor receptor–its expression and copy numbers of EGFR gene in patients with head and neck squamous cell carcinomas. Neoplasma 2005;52:338–43.
10. Chung CH, Ely K, McGavran L, et al. Increased epidermal growth factor receptor gene copy number is associated with poor prognosis in head and neck squamous cell carcinomas. J Clin Oncol 2006;24:4170–6.

11. Chiang WF, Liu SY, Yen CY, et al. Association of epidermal growth factor receptor (EGFR) gene copy number amplification with neck lymph node metastasis in areca-associated oral carcinomas. Oral Oncol 2008;44:270–6.
12. Lynch TJ, Bell DW, Sordella R, et al. Activating mutations in the epidermal growth factor receptor underlying responsiveness of non-small-cell lung cancer to gefitinib. N Engl J Med 2004;350:2129–39.
13. Bigner SH, Humphrey PA, Wong AJ, et al. Characterization of the epidermal growth factor receptor in human glioma cell lines and xenografts. Cancer Res 1990;50:8017–22.
14. Sok JC, Coppelli FM, Thomas SM, et al. Mutant epidermal growth factor receptor (EGFRvIII) contributes to head and neck cancer growth and resistance to EGFR targeting. Clin Cancer Res 2006;12:5064–73.
15. Chau NG, Perez-Ordonez B, Zhang K, et al. The association between EGFR variant III, HPV, p16, c-MET, EGFR gene copy number and response to EGFR inhibitors in patients with recurrent or metastatic squamous cell carcinoma of the head and neck. Head Neck Oncol 2011;3:11.
16. Cancer Genome Atlas Network. Comprehensive genomic characterization of head and neck squamous cell carcinomas. Nature 2015;517:576–82.
17. Torres S, Bartolome RA, Mendes M, et al. Proteome profiling of cancer-associated fibroblasts identifies novel proinflammatory signatures and prognostic markers for colorectal cancer. Clin Cancer Res 2013;19:6006–19.
18. Ferris RL, Jaffee EM, Ferrone S. Tumor antigen-targeted, monoclonal antibody-based immunotherapy: clinical response, cellular immunity, and immunoescape. J Clin Oncol 2010;28:4390–9.
19. Chen DJ, Nirodi CS. The epidermal growth factor receptor: a role in repair of radiation-induced DNA damage. Clin Cancer Res 2007;13:6555–60.
20. Bonner JA, Harari PM, Giralt J, et al. Radiotherapy plus cetuximab for squamous-cell carcinoma of the head and neck. N Engl J Med 2006;354:567–78.
21. Bonner JA, Harari PM, Giralt J, et al. Radiotherapy plus cetuximab for locoregionally advanced head and neck cancer: 5-year survival data from a phase 3 randomised trial, and relation between cetuximab-induced rash and survival. Lancet Oncol 2010;11:21–8.
22. Rosenthal DI, Harari PM, Giralt J, et al. Impact of p16 status on the results of the phase III cetuximab (cet)/radiotherapy (RT). J Clin Oncol 2014;32 [abstract: 6001].
23. Ghi MG, Paccagnella A, Ferrari D, et al. A phase II-III study comparing concomitant chemoradiotherapy (CRT) versus cetuximab/RT (CET/RT) with or without induction docetaxel/cisplatin/5-fluorouracil (TPF) in locally advanced head and neck squamous cell carcinoma (LASCCHN): efficacy results (NCT01086826). J Clin Oncol 2013;31 [abstract: 6003].
24. Giralt J, Trigo J, Nuyts S, et al. Panitumumab plus radiotherapy versus chemoradiotherapy in patients with unresected, locally advanced squamous-cell carcinoma of the head and neck (CONCERT-2): a randomised, controlled, open-label phase 2 trial. Lancet Oncol 2015;16:221–32.
25. Siu L, Waldron J, Chen B, et al. Phase III randomized trial of standard fractionation radiotherapy (SFX) with concurrent cisplatin (CIS) versus accelerated fractionation radiotherapy (AFX) with panitumumab (PMab) in patients (pts) with locoregionally advanced squamous cell carcinoma of the head and neck (LA-SCCHN): NCIC Clinical Trials Group HN.6 trial. J Clin Oncol 2015; 33(Suppl) [abstract: 6000].
26. Pignon JP, Bourhis J, Domenge C, et al. Chemotherapy added to locoregional treatment for head and neck squamous-cell carcinoma: three meta-analyses of

updated individual data. MACH-NC Collaborative Group. Meta-Analysis of Chemotherapy on Head and Neck Cancer. Lancet 2000;355:949–55.

27. Lefebvre JL, Pointreau Y, Rolland F, et al. Induction chemotherapy followed by either chemoradiotherapy or bioradiotherapy for larynx preservation: the TREMPLIN randomized phase II study. J Clin Oncol 2013;31:853–9.

28. Ghi MG, Paccagnella A, Ferrari D, et al. Concomitant chemoradiation (CRT) or cetuximab/RT (CET/RT) versus induction Docetaxel/Cisplatin/5-Fluorouracil (TPF) followed by CRT or CET/RT in patients with Locally Advanced Squamous Cell Carcinoma of Head and Neck (LASCCHN). A randomized phase III factorial study (NCT01086826). J Clin Oncol 2014;32 [abstract: 6004].

29. Ang KK, Zhang Q, Rosenthal DI, et al. Randomized phase III trial of concurrent accelerated radiation plus cisplatin with or without cetuximab for stage III to IV head and neck carcinoma: RTOG 0522. J Clin Oncol 2014;32:2940–50.

30. Giralt J, Fortin A, Mesia R, et al. A phase II, randomized trial (CONCERT-1) of chemoradiotherapy (CRT) with or without panitumumab (pmab) in patients (pts) with unresected, locally advanced squamous cell carcinoma of the head and neck (LASCCHN). J Clin Oncol 2012;30 [abstract: 5502].

31. Mesia R, Henke M, Fortin A, et al. Chemoradiotherapy with or without panitumumab in patients with unresected, locally advanced squamous-cell carcinoma of the head and neck (CONCERT-1): a randomised, controlled, open-label phase 2 trial. Lancet Oncol 2015;16:208–20.

32. Eriksen JG, Maare C, Johansen J, et al. Update of the randomized phase III trial DAHANCA 19: primary C-RT or RT and zalutumumab for squamous cell carcinomas of the head and neck. Radiotherapy and Oncology 2015;114(S1):10 (abstract OC-009).

33. Harari PM, Harris J, Kies MS, et al. Postoperative chemoradiotherapy and cetuximab for high-risk squamous cell carcinoma of the head and neck: Radiation Therapy Oncology Group RTOG-0234. J Clin Oncol 2014;32:2486–95.

34. Mesia R, Rueda A, Vera R, et al. Adjuvant therapy with cetuximab for locally advanced squamous cell carcinoma of the oropharynx: results from a randomized, phase II prospective trial. Ann Oncol 2013;24:448–53.

35. Argiris A, Heron DE, Smith RP, et al. Induction docetaxel, cisplatin, and cetuximab followed by concurrent radiotherapy, cisplatin, and cetuximab and maintenance cetuximab in patients with locally advanced head and neck cancer. J Clin Oncol 2010;28:5294–300.

36. Burtness B, Goldwasser MA, Flood W, et al. Phase III randomized trial of cisplatin plus placebo compared with cisplatin plus cetuximab in metastatic/recurrent head and neck cancer: an Eastern Cooperative Oncology Group study. J Clin Oncol 2005;23:8646–54.

37. Vermorken JB, Mesia R, Rivera F, et al. Platinum-based chemotherapy plus cetuximab in head and neck cancer. N Engl J Med 2008;359:1116–27.

38. Vermorken JB, Psyrri A, Mesia R, et al. Impact of tumor HPV status on outcome in patients with recurrent and/or metastatic squamous cell carcinoma of the head and neck receiving chemotherapy with or without cetuximab: retrospective analysis of the phase III EXTREME trial. Ann Oncol 2014;25:801–7.

39. Vermorken JB, Stohlmacher-Williams J, Davidenko I, et al. Cisplatin and fluorouracil with or without panitumumab in patients with recurrent or metastatic squamous-cell carcinoma of the head and neck (SPECTRUM): an open-label phase 3 randomised trial. Lancet Oncol 2013;14:697–710.

40. Wirth LJ, Dakhil SR, Kornek G, et al. A randomized phase II study of docetaxel/cisplatin (doc/cis) chemotherapy with or without panitumumab (pmab) as

first-line treatment (tx) for recurrent or metastatic squamous cell carcinoma of the head and neck (R/M SCCHN). J Clin Oncol 2013;31 [abstract: 6029].

41. Baselga J, Trigo JM, Bourhis J, et al. Phase II multicenter study of the antiepidermal growth factor receptor monoclonal antibody cetuximab in combination with platinum-based chemotherapy in patients with platinum-refractory metastatic and/or recurrent squamous cell carcinoma of the head and neck. J Clin Oncol 2005;23:5568–77.

42. Herbst RS, Arquette M, Shin DM, et al. Phase II multicenter study of the epidermal growth factor receptor antibody cetuximab and cisplatin for recurrent and refractory squamous cell carcinoma of the head and neck. J Clin Oncol 2005;23:5578–87.

43. Vermorken JB, Trigo J, Hitt R, et al. Open-label, uncontrolled, multicenter phase II study to evaluate the efficacy and toxicity of cetuximab as a single agent in patients with recurrent and/or metastatic squamous cell carcinoma of the head and neck who failed to respond to platinum-based therapy. J Clin Oncol 2007;25: 2171–7.

44. Vermorken JB, Herbst RS, Leon X, et al. Overview of the efficacy of cetuximab in recurrent and/or metastatic squamous cell carcinoma of the head and neck in patients who previously failed platinum-based therapies. Cancer 2008;112:2710–9.

45. Leon X, Hitt R, Constenla M, et al. A retrospective analysis of the outcome of patients with recurrent and/or metastatic squamous cell carcinoma of the head and neck refractory to a platinum-based chemotherapy. Clin Oncol (R Coll Radiol) 2005;17:418–24.

46. Machiels JP, Subramanian S, Ruzsa A, et al. Zalutumumab plus best supportive care versus best supportive care alone in patients with recurrent or metastatic squamous-cell carcinoma of the head and neck after failure of platinum-based chemotherapy: an open-label, randomised phase 3 trial. Lancet Oncol 2011; 12:333–43.

47. Rodriguez MO, Rivero TC, Del Castillo Bahi R, et al. Nimotuzumab plus radiotherapy for unresectable squamous-cell carcinoma of the head and neck. Cancer Biol Ther 2010;9:343–9.

48. Babu KG, Viswanath L, Reddy BK, et al. An open-label, randomized, study of h-R3mAb (nimotuzumab) in patients with advanced (stage III or IVa) squamous cell carcinoma of head and neck (SCCHN): four-year survival results from a phase IIb study. J Clin Oncol 2010;28 [abstract: 5530].

49. Martins RG, Parvathaneni U, Bauman JE, et al. Cisplatin and radiotherapy with or without erlotinib in locally advanced squamous cell carcinoma of the head and neck: a randomized phase II trial. J Clin Oncol 2013;31:1415–21.

50. Gregoire V, Hamoir M, Chen C, et al. Gefitinib plus cisplatin and radiotherapy in previously untreated head and neck squamous cell carcinoma: a phase II, randomized, double-blind, placebo-controlled study. Radiother Oncol 2011;100: 62–9.

51. Cohen EE, Haraf DJ, Kunnavakkam R, et al. Epidermal growth factor receptor inhibitor gefitinib added to chemoradiotherapy in locally advanced head and neck cancer. J Clin Oncol 2010;28:3336–43.

52. Stewart JS, Cohen EE, Licitra L, et al. Phase III study of gefitinib compared with intravenous methotrexate for recurrent squamous cell carcinoma of the head and neck [corrected]. J Clin Oncol 2009;27:1864–71.

53. Argiris A, Ghebremichael M, Gilbert J, et al. Phase III randomized, placebo-controlled trial of docetaxel with or without gefitinib in recurrent or metastatic head and neck cancer: an eastern cooperative oncology group trial. J Clin Oncol 2013;31:1405–14.

54. Del Sordo R, Angiero F, Bellezza G, et al. HER family receptors expression in squamous cell carcinoma of the tongue: study of the possible prognostic and biological significance. J Oral Pathol Med 2010;39:79–86.

55. Cavalot A, Martone T, Roggero N, et al. Prognostic impact of HER-2/neu expression on squamous head and neck carcinomas. Head Neck 2007;29:655–64.

56. Ekberg T, Nestor M, Engstrom M, et al. Expression of EGFR, HER2, HER3, and HER4 in metastatic squamous cell carcinomas of the oral cavity and base of tongue. Int J Oncol 2005;26:1177–85.

57. Lalami Y, Specenier PM, Awada A, et al. EORTC 24051: unexpected side effects in a phase I study of TPF induction chemotherapy followed by chemoradiation with lapatinib, a dual EGFR/ErbB2 inhibitor, in patients with locally advanced resectable larynx and hypopharynx squamous cell carcinoma. Radiother Oncol 2012;105:238–40.

58. Harrington K, Berrier A, Robinson M, et al. Randomised Phase II study of oral lapatinib combined with chemoradiotherapy in patients with advanced squamous cell carcinoma of the head and neck: rationale for future randomised trials in human papilloma virus-negative disease. Eur J Cancer 2013;49:1609–18.

59. Harrington KJ, Temam S, D'Cruz AK, et al. Final analysis: a randomized, blinded, placebo (P)-controlled phase III study of adjuvant postoperative lapatinib (L) with concurrent chemotherapy and radiation therapy (CH-RT) in high-risk patients with squamous cell carcinoma of the head and neck (SCCHN). J Clin Oncol 2014;32 [abstract: 6005].

60. De Souza JA, Davis DW, Zhang Y, et al. A phase II study of lapatinib in recurrent/metastatic squamous cell carcinoma of the head and neck. Clin Cancer Res 2012;18:2336–43.

61. Seiwert TY, Fayette J, Cupissol D, et al. A randomized, phase 2 study of afatinib versus cetuximab in metastatic or recurrent squamous cell carcinoma of the head and neck. Ann Oncol 2014;25(9):1813–20.

62. Machiels JP, Haddad RI, Fayette J, et al. Afatinib versus methotrexate (MTX) as second-line treatment for patients with recurrent and/or metastatic (R/M) head and neck squamous cell carcinoma. Lancet Oncol 2015;16:583–94.

63. Abdul Razak AR, Soulieres D, Laurie SA, et al. A phase II trial of dacomitinib, an oral pan-human EGF receptor (HER) inhibitor, as first-line treatment in recurrent and/or metastatic squamous-cell carcinoma of the head and neck. Ann Oncol 2013;24:761–9.

64. Schaefer G, Haber L, Crocker LM, et al. A two-in-one antibody against HER3 and EGFR has superior inhibitory activity compared with monospecific antibodies. Cancer Cell 2011;20:472–86.

65. Cervantes-Ruiperez A, Juric D, Hidalgo M, et al. A phase I study of MEHD7945A (MEHD), a first-in-class HER3/EGFR dual-action antibody, in patients (pts) with refractory/recurrent epithelial tumors: expansion cohorts. J Clin Oncol 2009;27 [abstract: 2565].

66. Fayette J, Wirth LJ, Oprean C, et al. Randomized phase II study of MEHD7945A (MEHD) vs cetuximab (Cet) in >= 2nd-line recurrent/metastatic squamous cell Carcinoma of the head & neck. Ann Oncol 2014;25:iv340–56.

67. Pedersen MW, Jacobsen HJ, Koefoed K, et al. Sym004: a novel synergistic anti-epidermal growth factor receptor antibody mixture with superior anticancer efficacy. Cancer Res 2010;70:588–97.

68. Machiels JP, Specenier PM, Krauss J, et al. A proof of concept trial of the anti-EGFR antibody mixture Sym004 in patients with squamous cell carcinoma of the head and neck. Cancer Chemother Pharmacol 2015;76(1):13–20.

Immunotherapy for Head and Neck Squamous Cell Carcinoma

 CrossMark

David W. Schoppy, MD, PhD, John B. Sunwoo, MD*

KEYWORDS

- HNSCC • Immunotherapy • CTLA-4 • PD-1 • Cetuximab • Vaccine
- Chimeric antigen receptor

KEY POINTS

- Checkpoint blockade of the PD-1:PD-L1 axis has significant activity against head and neck squamous cell carcinoma (HNSCC).
- The mechanism of cetuximab is, at least in part, due antibody-induced cell-mediated cytotoxicity by immune effector cells, such as natural killer (NK) cells. This response by NK cells can be enhanced by additional immune-stimulatory mechanisms, such as activation of CD137.
- Vaccines can further augment recognition of tumor cells by the adaptive immune system, and a variety of approaches are being investigated for use against HNSCC. This strategy may ultimately be useful in combination with checkpoint blockade strategies.
- T cells engineered with chimeric antigen receptors (CARs) are being developed for use in HNSCC.

INTRODUCTION

Advanced head and neck squamous cell carcinoma (HNSCC) can involve multiple sites of the upper aerodigestive tract, often precluding surgical intervention with curative intent. Additionally, a substantial proportion of patients with HNSCC will progress despite traditional cytotoxic chemotherapy and radiation therapy, and locoregional recurrence following any initial treatment of advanced tumors is relatively common.[1–3] In concert with efforts to develop new chemotherapy regimens, radiation protocols, and surgical approaches, much work has been focused on understanding the immunobiology of HNSCC and on developing strategies to promote an antitumor immune response.[4]

Disclosures: The authors have no financial or commercial conflicts of interest.
Division of Head and Neck Surgery, Department of Otolaryngology, Stanford University School of Medicine, Stanford, CA 94305, USA
* Corresponding author. 801 Welch Road, 2nd Floor, Stanford, CA 94305.
E-mail address: sunwoo@stanford.edu

Hematol Oncol Clin N Am 29 (2015) 1033–1043
http://dx.doi.org/10.1016/j.hoc.2015.07.009
0889-8588/15/$ – see front matter © 2015 Elsevier Inc. All rights reserved.

The idea that the immune system may be able to recognize and control cells undergoing malignant transformation has been around for more than a century.[5,6] Recent robust and durable clinical responses with immune checkpoint blocking antibodies have led to a resurgence in enthusiasm for this therapeutic strategy for solid malignancies.

IMMUNE CHECKPOINT BLOCKADE

Immune checkpoints are inhibitory pathways critical for self-tolerance under normal circumstances. It is now clear that tumors often co-opt these pathways by expressing cognate ligands for inhibitory checkpoint receptors and are thus able to induce immune tolerance and suppress responses by tumor-infiltrating lymphocytes (TIL), which would otherwise be activated in the tumor microenvironment. Antibodies that block the interaction between these immune checkpoint receptors and their ligands have demonstrated significant clinical efficacy in recent trials. The first of this class of drugs to be approved by the Food and Drug Administration (FDA) in 2011 was ipilimumab, an antibody to the cytotoxic T-lymphocyte–associated antigen 4 (CTLA-4), designed for use in unresectable or metastatic melanoma. This came following the landmark phase III clinical trial, demonstrating a survival benefit with ipilimumab in this disease.[7] As a single agent, however, a role for anti–CTLA-4 antibodies has not yet been reported in HNSCC.

More recently, another checkpoint inhibitory receptor, the programmed cell death protein 1 (PD-1), has garnered significant interest as a therapeutic target. Expression of PD-1 is induced on activated T cells and, on binding its ligands, PD-L1 (also known as B7-H1 and CD274) or PD-L2 (also known as B7-DC and CD273), inhibits T-cell receptor–induced signaling. Although PD-L2 is primarily expressed on activated macrophages and dendritic cells, PD-L1 expression is induced on both hematopoietic and nonhematopoietic cells, including epithelial cells, both benign and malignant, of head and neck mucosa.[8] Inflammatory cytokines, particularly interferon-γ (IFNγ), upregulate PD-L1 expression on these cells, further promoting an immunosuppressive environment.

Phase I studies of blocking antibodies to either PD-1 or PD-L1 showed surprising responses in solid tumor malignancies, including melanoma, renal cell carcinoma, and traditionally nonimmunogenic cancers, such as non–small cell lung cancer (NSCLC).[9,10] In 2014, accelerated approval of pembrolizumab, an antibody that blocks PD-1, was granted by the FDA for advanced melanoma. This followed significant responses seen in an open-label, multicenter expansion cohort of a phase I trial (KEYNOTE-001), in which 173 patients with advanced melanoma, who were refractory to ipilimumab, were randomized to either 2 mg/kg or 10 mg/kg every 3 weeks.[11] At both dosing regimens, there was an objective response rate of 26%, and the toxicity profile was similar between the 2 arms, with the most common adverse reactions being fatigue, pruritus, and rash. More recently, a phase III study of patients with previously untreated BRAF wild-type advanced melanoma compared nivolumab (another antibody to PD-1) with dacarbazine. The patients receiving nivolumab had significantly greater overall (72.9%) and median progression-free (5.1 months) survival compared with those receiving dacarbazine (42.1% and 2.2 months).[12]

As part of the phase I KEYNOTE-001 trial previously mentioned, an expansion cohort of patients with NSCLC receiving pembrolizumab also was analyzed.[13] An objective response rate of 19.4% and a median duration of response of 12.5 months were observed. Of note, in this study, the proportion of tumor cells expressing PD-L1 correlated with improved efficacy of pembrolizumab. In a randomized phase III trial of advanced NSCLC, in which 272 patients were randomized to nivolumab or docetaxel, the response rate, overall survival, and progression-free survival were significantly greater in the nivolumab cohort.[14] The patients included in this study had recurrent disease after 1 previous platinum-containing regimen. Unlike the phase I trial, PD-L1 expression did not correlate with response.

The histologic similarities between NSCLC and HNSCC and the recent success observed in NSCLC and other solid malignancies have generated much hope for similar success of PD-1:PD-L1 blockade in the treatment of the HNSCC. Of an interesting historical note, the initial preclinical studies demonstrating the blockade of this immune checkpoint axis in the treatment of cancer was actually shown in preclinical models of HNSCC.[15]

Clinical studies of HNSCC have reported that PD-L1 is expressed in 68% to 77% of HNSCC tumors, although different thresholds and antibodies have been used.[15–17] At the American Society of Clinical Oncology (ASCO) annual meeting in 2015, Seiwert and colleagues[17] presented on an HNSCC expansion cohort of KEYNOTE-012 (NCT01848834), in which pembrolizumab was given to patients with recurrent/metastatic HNSCC. In the study, 132 patients were enrolled; 99 were available for preliminary analysis. The objective response rate per RECIST 1.1 criteria was 18.2% with 18 partial responses and 31.3% with stable disease. Drug-related adverse events of any grade occurred in 47% of patients; the most common were fatigue, decreased appetite, pyrexia, and rash. Adverse events of grade ≥ 3 occurred in only 7.6%. Another study reported by Segal and colleagues[18] at the ASCO annual meeting in 2015 was of an ongoing phase I/II, multicenter, open-label study that is evaluating the safety and efficacy of MEDI4736, a human immunoglobulin (Ig)G1 monoclonal antibody against PD-L1 (NCT01693562). In this study, 62 patients were enrolled, and 51 with 24 months or more of follow-up were analyzed. The overall objective response rate was 12% and was 25% for patients with tumors that stained positive for PD-L1. The overall disease control rate was 16% at 24 months and 25% for PD-L1+ tumors. The median duration of response had not been reached at the time of the report, indicating meaningful durability of the responses. These promising results have led to an ongoing international open-label phase III trial (KEYNOTE-040, NCT02252042) in which 466 patients with recurrent/metastatic HNSCC, whose tumors had progressed following a platinum-based regimen, will be randomized to receive either pembrolizumab or the investigator's choice of standard-of-care single systemic agent (methotrexate, docetaxel, or cetuximab), and a similar trial of nivolumab versus standard chemotherapy is under way as well (NCT02105636).[19]

While the effect of PD-1:PD-L1 blockade and the durability of response in the approximately 20% of patients who benefit from this treatment is remarkable, a clearer understanding of the precise mechanism is needed to better select patients to treat and improve response rates. There is a growing sense that greater PD-1 and PD-L1 expression by the tumor-infiltrating immune cells correlates with a greater response to PD-1:PD-L1 blockade.[20–22] This may reflect a state of activation of the tumor-infiltrating immune effector cells that can be released from inhibition by blocking the PD-1 checkpoint. A novel window-of-opportunity study (NCT02296684), in which neoadjuvant pembrolizumab is given approximately 2 to 3 weeks before standard-of-care surgery for locally advanced, surgically resectable HNSCC, is currently being conducted. Preinfusion and postinfusion biopsies of the tumors will hopefully provide important insight into biologic parameters that can predict responses to PD-1 blockade.

Enhancement of response to PD-1:PD-L1 blockade may potentially occur with tumor antigen vaccines (discussed later), in combination with radiation therapy, and/or in combination with other checkpoint inhibitors. The idea that combination of immune checkpoint inhibitors with radiation may be synergistic comes from observations of an abscopal effect against lesions outside of the radiation field when a patient with melanoma was treated with ipilimumab.[23] By modeling of this abscopal response in mice, it was observed that the upregulation of PD-L1 following treatment is a dominant component of immune evasion and that dual blockade of PD-L1 and CTLA-4 significantly augments the therapeutic effect of radiation.[24] This effect was related to an increase in the CD8[+]/regulatory T-cell (Treg) ratio promoted by CTLA-4 blockade and a reinvigoration of exhausted CD8[+] T cells by PD-L1 blockade. Thus, combination checkpoint blockade, possibly with radiation (which presumably promotes release of tumor antigens) or vaccine strategies, may prove to be promising therapeutic strategies in the future.

Finally, activation of the innate immune system may also enhance the response to the PD-1:PD-L1 blockade. As an example, activation of the stimulator of interferon genes (STING) pathway appears to augment the response to anti-PD-1 antibodies. STING is a cytosolic receptor that senses exogenous and endogenous cyclic dinucleotides (CDN). In preclinical models of poorly immunogenic solid tumor malignancies, an engineered CDN designed to have greater in vivo stability and formulated with a GM-CSF secreting whole-cell vaccine (STINGVAX) is able to induce regression of solid tumors alone and synergize with anti-PD-1 antibodies in tumors resistant to PD-1 blockade.[25] It will be interesting to see if these observations are translated to the clinic and if other combinations, which include activation of the innate immune system (such as antibody-induced natural killer [NK] cell activation), can synergize with checkpoint blockade.

AUGMENTING CETUXIMAB-BASED IMMUNOTHERAPY

Cetuximab is a human-mouse chimeric IgG1 antibody directed against an epidermal growth factor receptor (EGFR); it has been shown to be a useful adjunct to standard therapeutic regimens in patients with recurrent or metastatic HNSCC.[26–31] Although direct inhibition of EGFR signaling may contribute to the antitumor effect of cetuximab, appreciable evidence indicates that a prominent component of any therapeutic effect can be attributed to the extracellular consequences of antibody binding to EGFR.[27,32] For instance, the constant region (Fc) of cetuximab can bind to Fc receptors on a variety of immune cells, including the low-affinity, activating Fc receptor expressed on NK cells (CD16/FcγRIII). This interaction induces antibody-dependent cell-mediated cytotoxicity (ADCC), and the degree to which ADCC occurs has been correlated with clinical responses.[33] Thus, cetuximab is actually the first "immunotherapeutic" agent approved for use in HNSCC.

Augmentation of ADCC induced by cetuximab is possible and is a focus of recent clinical investigation. One way in which cetuximab-induced ADCC can be augmented is by the activation of CD137 (also known as 4-1BB), which is an inducible, costimulatory molecule that is upregulated on activated NK cells and T cells following exposure to certain cytokines and Fc fragments.[34,35] CD137 expression is induced on NK cells following exposure to cetuximab and EGFR-expressing targets.[36] The addition of an agonist CD137 antibody can augment NK cell–mediated, cetuximab-dependent cytotoxicity, resulting in apoptosis of cultured cells, inhibition of tumor growth in vivo, and prolonged survival of tumor-bearing mice.[36] This effect was largely dependent on NK cells, although depletion of CD8[+] T cells partially abrogated the observed response.[36] Several additional findings further indicated that treatment with cetuximab followed by CD137 stimulation was capable of concurrently stimulating an adaptive immune response. Specifically, mice previously cured with cetuximab/anti-CD137 agonist therapy rejected further tumor engraftment and additionally rejected tumors with coincident epitopes, indicating both immunologic memory and epitope spreading.[36] Previous work had demonstrated that CD8[+] T cells significantly contribute to the antitumor effect of cetuximab,[37] and this reaction can be elicited through NK cell–mediated dendritic cell maturation and their subsequent interface with CD8[+] T cells.[38] As a result of these findings, a phase Ib open-label, multicenter trial (NCT02110082) of combination cetuximab and anti-CD137 antibody (urelumab) in patients with advanced/metastatic colorectal cancer or advanced/metastatic head and neck cancer is currently under way.

Similarly, Toll-like receptor (TLR)-8 stimulation of peripheral blood mononuclear cells has been shown to enhance cetuximab-induced NK cell–mediated ADCC of HNSCC cells and lead to dendritic cell maturation and priming of EGFR-specific CD8[+] T cells.[39] These findings have led to a phase I dose-escalation study (NCT01334177) of a TLR8 agonist (VTX-2337) given in conjunction with cetuximab in patients with locally advanced, recurrent, or metastatic HNSCC.

Tregs (CD4[+]FOXP3[+]) can constitute a significant proportion of the TIL population following cetuximab therapy. The presence of Tregs correlates with a functional impairment of NK cells.[40] Depletion of these Tregs with anti-CTLA-4 antibody can partially correct this immunosuppressive environment and restore NK-mediated cytotoxicity.[40] This provides rationale for the combination of cetuximab and ipilimumab in the clinic. A phase I trial of cetuximab, ipilimumab, and intensity-modulated radiation therapy is currently under way.

VACCINES

There is abundant evidence that the adaptive immune system actively participates in the elimination of susceptible cells (a process termed "editing") during tumor formation, and that the more resistant cells may achieve a state of equilibrium with the host immune system. One principal goal of immunotherapy is to bias an immune response toward elimination of these more resistant cells. This can be achieved, in part, through augmenting the recognition of cancer cells through therapeutic vaccination, with the intent to induce an antigen-specific, cytotoxic CD8[+] T-cell response.[41] Practically, this involves promoting the uptake and presentation of antigen by antigen-presenting cells, the most efficient of which are dendritic cells.[41] Following antigen capture and processing, maturation, and recruitment of CD4[+] T cells, dendritic cells prime a CD8[+] T-cell response, which is then integrally involved in the antitumor immune response. There are several different approaches to using dendritic cells in tumor vaccination, ranging from direct delivery of antigen to loading of autologous dendritic cells with tumor antigen ex vivo, followed by maturation and reintroduction. These strategies have been used in various ways to target HNSCC[42] and, in most studies, are predicated on the availability of a specific tumor-associated antigen.[4]

A potential source of antigens in a substantial proportion of HNSCC is the human papilloma virus (HPV) virus. HPV is a double-stranded DNA virus that can infect the epithelium of the upper aerodigestive tract and significantly contribute to malignant transformation.[43] Typical infection can elicit a T-cell–mediated immune response and subsequent clearance, and much work has centered on understanding and adapting this response to the treatment of HPV[+] HNSCC. Previous studies have confirmed that patients with HPV[+] HNSCC have a significantly higher number of E7-specific cytotoxic CD8[+] T cells than patients with HPV[+] HNSCC or healthy controls, demonstrating a preexisting level of endogenous immunity.[44] Interestingly, this study also demonstrated that components of the antigen-processing machinery were relatively lower in HPV$^+$ HNSCC compared with surrounding squamous epithelium, suggesting a degree of immune escape in the development of these malignancies and underscoring the complexity of the immune response to developing tumors.[44,45] There have subsequently been varied efforts to augment the immune response to HPV-associated HNSCC.[45] One study of peptide/protein vaccines used a "Trojan peptide" approach, in which HPV-16 and MAGE-A3 tumor-associated antigens were engineered to contain sequences intended to promote modified processing and subsequent generation of HLA-I and HLA-II responses.[46] Patients with advanced recurrent or metastatic HNSCC were injected with either the HPV-16 or MAGE-A3 Trojan peptide vaccine at 4-week intervals for up to 4 total doses. Although no complete or partial responses were documented, apart from 1 serious adverse event associated toxicities were generally well tolerated. Interestingly, although there was an appreciable response to the HLA-II restricted epitopes in most patients, there was no detectable response to the HLA-I restricted epitopes. In 1 of the 2 patients treated with the HPV-16 vaccine who underwent a neck dissection 3 months after vaccination, there was marked a CD4$^+$ and CD8$^+$ infiltrate that was notably enriched for HPV-specific T cells.[46] This study illustrates that peptide/protein vaccines targeting HPV-16 can induce an immune reaction to HNSCCs, although the response can be relatively complex and may bias toward HLA-II–restricted epitopes and is not yet of clinical utility in its present form.[46]

In addition to peptide-based vaccines, there have been several preclinical studies focused on the development of DNA-based vaccine strategies to induce tumor-specific immunity in HPV$^+$ HNSCC.[47] For instance, treatment of tumor-bearing mice with a construct containing the HPV-16 E7 gene modified to disrupt Rb-binding and transforming capability was shown to result in a significant inhibition of tumor growth and an induction of antigen-specific CD8$^+$ T cells.[48] This effect was further augmented by cyclophosphamide administration, which correlated with a reduction in regulatory T cells.[48] This finding suggests an inherent constraint on vaccine effect and again highlights the relatively complex nature of the immune response to cancer vaccines.[48]

Another potential source of antigen in HNSCC is p53, a central component of the cellular response to a diverse array of stressors and an essential tumor suppressor. Mutations in p53 can be detected in just more than half of patients with HNSCC undergoing definitive surgical resection, and the presence of disruptive p53 mutations is associated with significantly decreased overall survival.[49] Subsequent studies have confirmed the frequent occurrence of p53 mutations in HNSCC, as well as an inverse relationship between p53 mutations and HPV infection.[50,51] There has thus been much interest in developing strategies to elicit an immune reaction toward p53. The frequency of p53 antigen-specific CD8$^+$ T cells is higher in the peripheral blood of patients with HNSCC than healthy controls, though this relative enrichment interestingly does not correlate with overexpression of p53 in the tumor itself.[52,53] Subsequent studies have demonstrated that p53-specific T cells are not only found in the circulation, but are appreciably enriched in primary tumors or tumor-involved lymph nodes.[44] Again, this accumulation of TILs was not necessarily related to p53 overexpression, as it was seen in several tumors with no notable p53 staining.[44] This population of TILs is, however, functionally deficient, as demonstrated by a relative inability to secrete interferon-gamma after stimulation.[44]

Building on this previous work, a dendritic cell–based vaccine strategy was developed and used in a recent phase 1 trial.[54] The study accrued 16 patients with advanced HNSCC treated with either surgery alone (10 patients) or surgery and adjuvant chemotherapy (6 patients). These patients were then randomized to receive 1 of 3 different vaccines by ultrasound-guided inguinal lymph node injection: autologous dendritic cells loaded with 2 optimized p53 peptides, dendritic cells loaded with optimized p53 peptides and tetanus helper peptide, or dendritic cells loaded with optimized p53 peptides and HLA class II p53 helper peptide. Apart from a local injection site reaction in 2 patients, the vaccines were well tolerated and disease-free survival compared favorably with a historical cohort. After vaccination, 69% of patients showed some peptide-specific response, with 38% developing cytotoxic T lymphocytes (CTLs) reactive to either optimized peptide and another 31% developing CTLs reactive to either peptide.[54] One additional, notable finding was the effect of vaccination on Treg populations. The average frequency and absolute number of Tregs was significantly reduced after vaccination, and this outcome was postulated to be a component of any potential benefit.

In addition to vaccination centered on a clearly defined, specific antigen, there has been interest in a broader approach using dendritic cells loaded with antigens derived from autologous apoptotic tumor cells.[55] One study enrolled patients with operable stage III or IV HNSCC.[55] Tumor cells harvested during surgical resection were purified and stored. Approximately 2 months following conventional therapy, monocytes were harvested from these patients and coincubated with the previously harvested autologous tumor cells induced to undergo apoptosis by UV treatment. Dendritic cells exposed to apoptotic tumor cells were then induced to undergo maturation and administered to disease-free patients by ultrasound-guided intranodal injection in 2 separate doses 6 weeks apart. Because of strict inclusion criteria and appreciable issues with the number and sterility of autologous tumor cells, 4 patients could be given the planned 2 doses of the dendritic cell–based vaccine. Apoptotic tumor cell–reactive T cells were detected after vaccination in 3 patients, and no adverse events occurred, illustrating that, in principle, this strategy was immunogenic.[55]

ENGINEERED T CELLS

Vaccination relies on the natural induction of an antigen-specific adaptive immune response, which can be constrained by a number of factors inherent to the immune system. There are several strategies being developed to circumvent these limitations, one of which incorporates synthetic T cells engineered to express either enhanced T-cell receptors or chimeric antigen receptors (CARs).[56,57] CARs are composed of an antibody-based cell surface receptor linked to intracellular signaling domains on T cells.[58,59] Adoptive therapy with CAR-modified T cells was effective at achieving remission in chronic lymphocytic leukemia and relapsed acute lymphoblastic leukemia, and preclinical data suggest this therapy may additionally be useful in solid malignancies, such as glioblastoma.[60,61] These watershed trials have led to an interest in adapting CAR therapy to HNSCC, and several preclinical studies suggest this may be a viable therapeutic option.[42] For instance, T cells have been engineered to express a CAR targeting ErbB receptors, often overexpressed in HNSCC.[62,63] These T cells have shown antitumor activity in a murine model, and there are current plans for a clinical trial using this CAR therapy in patients with HNSCC.[64] In addition, on the heels of a successful clinical demonstration that TILs isolated from patients with HPV+ cervical cancer and selected for reactivity against HPV-16 and HPV-18 E6 and E7 can induce durable, complete regression following a single infusion of these cells,[65] a new clinical trial, using CARs engineered with a T-cell receptor specifically targeting HPV-16 E6, has been initiated (NCT02280811). This is a phase I/II trial to determine the safe number of cells to infuse and to assess response in a variety of HPV-16–associated malignancies, including oropharyngeal squamous cell carcinoma. The results of this trial will be extremely interesting, as it may open avenues of targeting other cancer-associated antigens in this disease.

SUMMARY

Although HNSCC has traditionally been considered to be a very immunosuppressive, or at least nonimmunogenic, tumor type, recent results from clinical studies of immune checkpoint blockade strategies have led to resurgence in the enthusiasm for immuno-therapeutic approaches. Additional strategies for immunotherapy that are under active investigation include enhancement of cetuximab-mediated ADCC, tumor vaccines, and engineered T cells for adoptive therapy. All of these studies have early-phase clinical trials under way, and the next several years will be exciting as the results of these studies are reported.

REFERENCES

1. Ho AS, Kraus DH, Ganly I, et al. Decision making in the management of recurrent head and neck cancer. Head Neck 2014;36:144–51.
2. Vermorken JB, Specenier P. Optimal treatment for recurrent/metastatic head and neck cancer. Ann Oncol 2010;21(Suppl 7):vii252–61.
3. Argiris A, Karamouzis MV, Raben D, et al. Head and neck cancer. Lancet 2008; 371:1695–709.
4. Galluzzi L, Vacchelli E, Bravo-San Pedro JM, et al. Classification of current anti-cancer immunotherapies. Oncotarget 2014;5:12472–508.
5. Ehrlich P. Uber den jetzigen Stand der Karzinomforschung. Ned Tijdschr Gen-eeskd 1909;5:273–90.
6. Manjili MH. Revisiting cancer immunoediting by understanding cancer immune complexity. J Pathol 2011;224:5–9.
7. Hodi FS, O'Day SJ, McDermott DF, et al. Improved survival with ipilimumab in patients with metastatic melanoma. N Engl J Med 2010;363:711–23.
8. Ritprajak P, Azuma M. Intrinsic and extrinsic control of expression of the immuno-regulatory molecule PD-L1 in epithelial cells and squamous cell carcinoma. Oral Oncol 2015;51:221–8.
9. Topalian SL, Hodi FS, Brahmer JR, et al. Safety, activity, and immune correlates of anti-PD-1 antibody in cancer. N Engl J Med 2012;366:2443–54.
10. Brahmer JR, Tykodi SS, Chow LQ, et al. Safety and activity of anti-PD-L1 antibody in patients with advanced cancer. N Engl J Med 2012;366:2455–65.
11. Robert C, Ribas A, Wolchok JD, et al. Anti-programmed-death-receptor-1 treat-ment with pembrolizumab in ipilimumab-refractory advanced melanoma: a rand-omised dose-comparison cohort of a phase 1 trial. Lancet 2014;384:1109–17.
12. Robert C, Long GV, Brady B, et al. Nivolumab in previously untreated melanoma without BRAF mutation. N Engl J Med 2015;372:320–30.
13. Garon EB, Rizvi NA, Hui R, et al. Pembrolizumab for the treatment of non-small-cell lung cancer. N Engl J Med 2015;372:2018–28.
14. Brahmer J, Reckamp KL, Baas P, et al. Nivolumab versus docetaxel in advanced squamous-cell non-small-cell lung cancer. N Engl J Med 2015;373(2):123–35.
15. Strome SE, Dong H, Tamura H, et al. B7-H1 blockade augments adoptive T-cell immunotherapy for squamous cell carcinoma. Cancer Res 2003;63:6501–5.
16. Kim HS, et al. The prevalence and prognostic relevance of PD-L1 expression in patients with HPV-negative and HPV-positive oropharyngeal cancer. ASCO Meeting Abstracts 2015;33:e14003.

17. Seiwert TY, et al. Antitumor activity and safety of pembrolizumab in patients (pts) with advanced squamous cell carcinoma of the head and neck (SCCHN): preliminary results from KEYNOTE-012 expansion cohort. ASCO Meeting Abstracts 2015;33:LBA6008.
18. Segal NH, et al. Safety and efficacy of MEDI4736, an anti-PD-L1 antibody, in patients from a squamous cell carcinoma of the head and neck (SCCHN) expansion cohort. ASCO Meeting Abstracts 2015;33:3011.
19. Cohen EEW, et al. KEYNOTE-040: a phase III randomized trial of pembrolizumab (MK-3475) versus standard treatment in patients with recurrent or metastatic head and neck cancer. ASCO Meeting Abstracts 2015;33:TPS6084.
20. Tumeh PC, Harview CL, Yearley JH, et al. PD-1 blockade induces responses by inhibiting adaptive immune resistance. Nature 2014;515:568–71.
21. Powles T, Eder JP, Fine GD, et al. MPDL3280A (anti-PD-L1) treatment leads to clinical activity in metastatic bladder cancer. Nature 2014;515:558–62.
22. Herbst RS, Soria JC, Kowanetz M, et al. Predictive correlates of response to the anti-PD-L1 antibody MPDL3280A in cancer patients. Nature 2014;515:563–7.
23. Postow MA, Callahan MK, Barker CA, et al. Immunologic correlates of the abscopal effect in a patient with melanoma. N Engl J Med 2012;366:925–31.
24. Twyman-Saint Victor C, Rech AJ, Maity A, et al. Radiation and dual checkpoint blockade activate non-redundant immune mechanisms in cancer. Nature 2015; 520(7547):373–7.
25. Fu J, Kanne DB, Leong M, et al. STING agonist formulated cancer vaccines can cure established tumors resistant to PD-1 blockade. Sci Transl Med 2015;7:283ra52.
26. Arteaga CL, Engelman JA. ERBB receptors: from oncogene discovery to basic science to mechanism-based cancer therapeutics. Cancer Cell 2014;25: 282–303.
27. Bauman JE, Ferris RL. Integrating novel therapeutic monoclonal antibodies into the management of head and neck cancer. Cancer 2014;120:624–32.
28. Bernier J. Incorporation of molecularly targeted agents in the primary treatment of squamous cell carcinomas of the head and neck. Hematol Oncol Clin North Am 2008;22:1193–208, ix.
29. Reeves TD, Hill EG, Armeson KE, et al. Cetuximab therapy for head and neck squamous cell carcinoma: a systematic review of the data. Otolaryngol Head Neck Surg 2011;144:676–84.
30. Bonner JA, Harari PM, Giralt J, et al. Radiotherapy plus cetuximab for squamous-cell carcinoma of the head and neck. N Engl J Med 2006;354:567–78.
31. Vermorken JB, Mesia R, Rivera F, et al. Platinum-based chemotherapy plus cetuximab in head and neck cancer. N Engl J Med 2008;359:1116–27.
32. Ferris RL, Jaffee EM, Ferrone S. Tumor antigen-targeted, monoclonal antibody-based immunotherapy: clinical response, cellular immunity, and immunoescape. J Clin Oncol 2010;28:4390–9.
33. Taylor RJ, Saloura V, Jain A, et al. Ex vivo antibody-dependent cellular cytotoxicity inducibility predicts efficacy of cetuximab. Cancer Immunol Res 2015;3:567–74.
34. Wilcox RA, Tamada K, Strome SE, et al. Signaling through NK cell-associated CD137 promotes both helper function for CD8[+] cytolytic T cells and responsiveness to IL-2 but not cytolytic activity. J Immunol 2002;169:4230–6.
35. Lin W, Voskens CJ, Zhang X, et al. Fc-dependent expression of CD137 on human NK cells: insights into "agonistic" effects of anti-CD137 monoclonal antibodies. Blood 2008;112:699–707.
36. Kohrt HE, Colevas AD, Houot R, et al. Targeting CD137 enhances the efficacy of cetuximab. J Clin Invest 2014;124:2668–82.

37. Yang X, Zhang X, Mortenson ED, et al. Cetuximab-mediated tumor regression depends on innate and adaptive immune responses. Mol Ther 2013;21:91–100.
38. Srivastava RM, Lee SC, Andrade Filho PA, et al. Cetuximab-activated natural killer and dendritic cells collaborate to trigger tumor antigen-specific T-cell immunity in head and neck cancer patients. Clin Cancer Res 2013;19:1858–72.
39. Stephenson RM, Lim CM, Matthews M, et al. TLR8 stimulation enhances cetuximab-mediated natural killer cell lysis of head and neck cancer cells and dendritic cell cross-priming of EGFR-specific CD8[+] T cells. Cancer Immunol Immunother 2013;62:1347–57.
40. Jie HB, Schuler PJ, Lee SC, et al. CTLA-4+ regulatory T cells are increased in cetuximab treated head and neck cancer patients, suppress NK cell cytotoxicity and correlate with poor prognosis. Cancer Res 2015;75(11):2200–10.
41. Palucka K, Banchereau J. Dendritic-cell-based therapeutic cancer vaccines. Immunity 2013;39:38–48.
42. Li Q, Prince ME, Moyer JS. Immunotherapy for head and neck squamous cell carcinoma. Oral Oncol 2015;51:299–304.
43. Leemans CR, Braakhuis BJ, Brakenhoff RH. The molecular biology of head and neck cancer. Nat Rev Cancer 2011;11:9–22.
44. Albers A, Abe K, Hunt J, et al. Antitumor activity of human papillomavirus type 16 E7-specific T cells against virally infected squamous cell carcinoma of the head and neck. Cancer Res 2005;65:11146–55.
45. Gildener-Leapman N, Lee J, Ferris RL. Tailored immunotherapy for HPV positive head and neck squamous cell cancer. Oral Oncol 2014;50:780–4.
46. Voskens CJ, Sewell D, Hertzano R, et al. Induction of MAGE-A3 and HPV-16 immunity by Trojan vaccines in patients with head and neck carcinoma. Head Neck 2012;34:1734–46.
47. Lin K, Roosinovich E, Ma B, et al. Therapeutic HPV DNA vaccines. Immunol Res 2010;47:86–112.
48. Peng S, Lyford-Pike S, Akpeng B, et al. Low-dose cyclophosphamide administered as daily or single dose enhances the antitumor effects of a therapeutic HPV vaccine. Cancer Immunol Immunother 2013;62:171–82.
49. Poeta ML, Manola J, Goldwasser MA, et al. TP53 mutations and survival in squamous-cell carcinoma of the head and neck. N Engl J Med 2007;357:2552–61.
50. Agrawal N, Frederick MJ, Pickering CR, et al. Exome sequencing of head and neck squamous cell carcinoma reveals inactivating mutations in NOTCH1. Science 2011;333:1154–7.
51. Stransky N, Egloff AM, Tward AD, et al. The mutational landscape of head and neck squamous cell carcinoma. Science 2011;333:1157–60.
52. Hoffmann TK, Donnenberg AD, Finkelstein SD, et al. Frequencies of tetramer+ T cells specific for the wild-type sequence p53(264-272) peptide in the circulation of patients with head and neck cancer. Cancer Res 2002;62:3521–9.
53. Hoffmann TK, Nakano K, Elder EM, et al. Generation of T cells specific for the wild-type sequence p53(264-272) peptide in cancer patients: implications for immunoselection of epitope loss variants. J Immunol 2000;165:5938–44.
54. Schuler PJ, Harasymczuk M, Visus C, et al. Phase I dendritic cell p53 peptide vaccine for head and neck cancer. Clin Cancer Res 2014;20:2433–44.
55. Whiteside TL, Ferris RL, Szczepanski M, et al. Dendritic cell-based autologous tumor vaccines for head and neck squamous cell carcinoma: promise vs reality. Head Neck 2015. [Epub ahead of print].
56. Vonderheide RH, June CH. Engineering T cells for cancer: our synthetic future. Immunol Rev 2014;257:7–13.

57. June CH, Maus MV, Plesa G, et al. Engineered T cells for cancer therapy. Cancer Immunol Immunother 2014;63:969–75.
58. Maus MV, June CH. CARTs on the road for myeloma. Clin Cancer Res 2014;20: 3899–901.
59. Barrett DM, Singh N, Porter DL, et al. Chimeric antigen receptor therapy for cancer. Annu Rev Med 2014;65:333–47.
60. Maude SL, Frey N, Shaw PA, et al. Chimeric antigen receptor T cells for sustained remissions in leukemia. N Engl J Med 2014;371:1507–17.
61. Johnson LA, Scholler J, Ohkuri T, et al. Rational development and characterization of humanized anti-EGFR variant III chimeric antigen receptor T cells for glioblastoma. Sci Transl Med 2015;7:275ra22.
62. Davies DM, Foster J, Van Der Stegen SJ, et al. Flexible targeting of ErbB dimers that drive tumorigenesis by using genetically engineered T cells. Mol Med 2012; 18:565–76.
63. van der Stegen SJ, Davies DM, Wilkie S, et al. Preclinical in vivo modeling of cytokine release syndrome induced by ErbB-retargeted human T cells: identifying a window of therapeutic opportunity? J Immunol 2013;191:4589–98.
64. van Schalkwyk MC, Papa SE, Jeannon JP, et al. Design of a phase I clinical trial to evaluate intratumoral delivery of ErbB-targeted chimeric antigen receptor T-cells in locally advanced or recurrent head and neck cancer. Hum Gene Ther Clin Dev 2013;24:134–42.
65. Stevanovic S, Draper LM, Langhan MM, et al. Complete regression of metastatic cervical cancer after treatment with human papillomavirus-targeted tumor-infiltrating T cells. J Clin Oncol 2015;33:1543–50.

Anticipation of the Impact of Human Papillomavirus on Clinical Decision Making for the Head and Neck Cancer Patient

Maura L. Gillison, MD, PhD[a],*, Carlo Restighini, MD[b]

KEYWORDS

- Human papillomavirus • Clinical decision making • Head and neck cancer • Patient
- Survival • Prognosis

KEY POINTS

- Human papillomavirus (HPV) is a common sexually transmitted infection that is the cause of a distinct subset of oropharyngeal cancer (OPC) rising in incidence in the United States and other developed countries.
- This increased incidence, combined with the strong effect of tumor HPV status on survival, has had a profound effect on the head and neck cancer (HNC) discipline.
- The multidisciplinary field of HNC clinicians is in the midst of re-evaluating evidence-based algorithms for clinical decision making, developed from clinical trials conducted in an era when HPV-negative cancer predominated.
- This article reviews relationships between tumor HPV status and gender, cancer incidence trends, overall survival, treatment response, racial disparities, tumor staging, risk stratification, survival post disease progression, and clinical trial design.
- Elucidation of the causal role for HPV in HNC has already altered the understanding of risk factors for HNC, and we anticipate a time in the near future when it will have a tremendous impact on clinical decision making.

INTRODUCTION

Human papillomavirus (HPV) is a common sexually transmitted infection that is the cause of a distinct subset of oropharyngeal cancer (OPC) rising in incidence in the United States and other developed countries. This increased incidence, combined

[a] Cancer Control and Prevention Program, The Ohio State University Comprehensive Cancer Center, The Ohio State University, 420 West 12th Avenue, Room 620, Columbus, OH 43210, USA; [b] Medical Oncology, Istituto Nazionale dei Tumori, Via G. Venezian, 1, Milano 20133, Italy
* Corresponding author.
E-mail address: Maura.gillison@osumc.edu

Hematol Oncol Clin N Am 29 (2015) 1045–1060
http://dx.doi.org/10.1016/j.hoc.2015.08.003   hemonc.theclinics.com
0889-8588/15/$ – see front matter © 2015 Elsevier Inc. All rights reserved.

with the strong effect of tumor HPV status on survival, has had a profound effect on the head and neck cancer (HNC) discipline. The multidisciplinary field of HNC is in the midst of re-evaluating evidence-based algorithms for clinical decision making, developed from clinical trials conducted in an era when HPV-negative cancer predominated. This article reviews relationships between tumor HPV status and gender, cancer incidence trends, overall survival, treatment response, racial disparities, tumor staging, risk stratification, survival post disease progression, and clinical trial design. Elucidation of the causal role for HPV in HNC has already altered the understanding of risk factors for HNC, and we anticipate a time in the near future when it will have a tremendous impact on clinical decision making.

HUMAN PAPILLOMAVIRUS BIOLOGY

HPVs are small, nonenveloped, double-stranded DNA viruses of approximately 8000 base-pairs in size that have a distinct tropism for human epidermal and mucosal epithelium.[1] More than 150 HPV types, distinguished by viral sequence variation, have been isolated from humans to date. Most infections spread by direct human-to-human contact are asymptomatic. Viruses with low oncogenic potential, called low-risk types, may cause benign hyperproliferation of the epithelium that manifests as skin warts, genital warts, or oral papillomas. The viral genome encodes early proteins that promote viral maintenance in the infected cell nuclei and viral replication (E1, E2, E4, E5, E6, and E7). Late proteins L1 and L2 encode the viral capsid proteins.

HPV types are classified as oncogenic or "high-risk" based on case-control studies demonstrating significant associations with cervical cancer.[2,3] High-risk types include 16, 18, 31, 33, 35, 39, 45, 51, 52, 56, 58, 59, and 66. However, HPV types 16 and 18 are accountable for approximately 70% of cervical and greater than 90% of noncervical cancers (eg, vaginal, vulvar, penile, anal) caused by HPV, including HNCs. The transforming ability of high-risk HPV types has been attributed to myriad functions of the classic viral oncoproteins E6 and E7,[4] which disrupt regulation of cellular replication and differentiation to facilitate viral replication. HPV E7 oncoprotein disrupts control of the G1 to S phase of the cell cycle through interactions with pRb family members (p105, p107, p130),[5] and HPV E6 prevents apoptosis by inducing degradation of p53.[6,7] HPV16 E6 and E7 expression is sufficient to immortalize human keratinocytes, but insufficient for malignant progression. HPV E6 and E7 promote genomic instability,[8] leading to secondary genetic events necessary for malignant progression. However, these secondary events remain poorly defined.

Early in infection, HPV genomes replicate as extrachromosomal elements in the nucleus. The frequency of viral integration increases with severity of precancerous lesions,[9] and most cervical cancers harbor HPV integrants.[10] The literature suggests approximately 20% to 48% of HPV-positive OPC have HPV integrants,[11-13] but the sensitivity of assays used to detect HPV integrants in these studies has been called into question. HPV integration imparts genomic instability and a selective growth advantage on infected cells.[14-18] Enhanced expression and stabilization of viral oncogene transcripts[17] and disruption of the viral repressor HPV E2 contribute to such clonal selection.[19]

Until recently, insertional mutagenesis has not been widely accepted as a functionally important consequence of HPV infection.[10] However, Akagi and colleagues[20] recently reported a striking association between HPV integrants and focal host alterations in genomic structures, frequently disrupting the expression and function of cancer-associated genes. Subsequently, HPV integration was associated with copy number variation in cervical cancer.[21] Moreover, expression of genes neighboring HPV integration sites was significantly higher than that found in tumors without HPV integration. Recently, HPV integration analysis in cervical dysplasias, cancers, and cell lines identified recurrent genomic HPV integration hotspots.[9] Analysis of 35 HPV-positive OPC in the TCGA dataset revealed an association between HPV integration and genomic structural variation and alterations in host cell gene transcription.[22] The potential role of HPV integration and associated alterations of the host cell genome in cancer progression and the malignant phenotype is an active area of investigation.

EPIDEMIOLOGY OF HUMAN PAPILLOMAVIRUS–POSITIVE OROPHARYNGEAL CANCER

In 2007, the International Agency for Research on Cancer stated that there was sufficient evidence to conclude that HPV16 is a cause of OPC and oral cavity cancers in humans.[3] A review of the molecular and epidemiologic evidence in support of this causal association was updated by Gillison and colleagues in 2012[23] and 2015.[24] In brief, strong and consistent associations between high-risk HPV infection and OPC have been observed in numerous case-control studies.[23] In nested case-control studies, serologic evidence of HPV16 infection has been estimated to elevate risk of OPC by 14[25] to 270 times.[26] The original observations reported by Gillison and colleagues[27] of a causal association between predominantly HPV16 and a distinct molecular, clinical, and pathologic subset of OPC with an improved prognosis have now been reproduced on a global scale.[23,28] Castellsague and colleagues[28] collected 3741 HNCs diagnosed after 1990 from 32 countries and have reported preliminary analysis of tumor HPV status by HPV DNA, E6/E7 mRNA, and p16 immunohistochemistry. Most (~88%) HPV-positive samples had type HPV16 DNA. HPV presence was associated with nonkeratinizing histopathology and location in the lingual and palatine tonsils of the oropharynx. This study estimated that approximately 18% of all OPCs worldwide were attributable to HPV infection (as defined by combined HPV DNA, E6/E7 mRNA, and p16 IHC positivity).[28]

Case-control studies have estimated individuals with an oral HPV16 infection to have a 50- to 200-fold increased risk of OPC.[23] The behavior most strongly associated with odds of OPC[29] and prevalent oral HPV infection[30] is oral-genital sex. The odds of cancer[29] and infection[30] increase with increased number of lifetime partners for oral-genital sex. Prospective studies of the natural history of oral HPV infection have now temporally linked oral-genital sex with risk of acquiring an oral HPV infection.[31–34]

Recent studies of the epidemiology of oral HPV infection in the US population have observed the distribution of high-risk HPV infection to mirror incidence and risk for OPC in the United States.[30,35,36] In 2009 to 2012, the prevalence of oral high-risk and HPV16 infections in the United States was three- to five-fold higher among men than women,[29,34] consistent with a three- to five-fold relative risk for OPC among men versus women.[35] Prevalence also increased with age,[34] as does risk of OPC.[35] Male gender, increasing age, intensity of current cigarette smoking, and number of lifetime oral-genital sexual partners were independently associated with prevalent high-risk oral HPV infection.[29,34] Prevalence was therefore highest among men, aged 60 to 69 years, who were current smokers of greater than 20 cigarettes per day with a history of greater than 20 lifetime sexual partners. However, the number of individuals who fit this risk-profile in the US population was low. When the absolute number of individuals in the US population with an oral high-risk infection was considered, the burden of infections was greatest among men aged 40 to 59 years who were never or former smokers with a moderate number of sexual partners (2–19). This explains the frequent presentation of HPV-positive OPC in this subgroup of the US population.

Importantly, the study of oral high-risk HPV infection in the US population also provided a possible explanation for the escalating risk of OPC since 1984 in the United States[36] (and other developed countries[37]) among men, but not women. Although men reported a higher median lifetime number of sexual partners than women, oral HPV prevalence differences by gender were largely attributable to stronger associations between sexual behavior and infection among men.[35] For example, the increase in HPV prevalence per oral-genital sexual partner was three-times stronger in men versus women, and prevalence plateaued after 15 partners among men in comparison with only five partners among women. That is, women seemed to be protected from increased HPV exposure after five sexual partners, whereas men were not.[35] Lower rates of seroconversion and development of protective neutralizing antibodies in response to genital HPV infection in men versus women are hypothesized to explain this observation.[38] Thus, recent birth cohorts of men may have experienced a disproportionately greater impact than women of sexual behavioral changes associated with oral HPV exposure, resulting in disproportionate increased OPC incidence largely among men.

Tumor Human Papillomavirus Status and Disease: Survival and Overall Survival

Tumor HPV status is now established as an important prognostic factor for HNC based on consistently higher survival rates for HPV-positive versus HPV-negative HNC in retrospective analyses of randomized controlled clinical trials of primary (chemo) radiotherapy.[39–43] Despite significant heterogeneity in treatment platforms (eg, radiotherapy alone, platinum-based chemoradiotherapy, or induction chemotherapy followed by platinum-based chemoradiotherapy), patients with HPV-positive tumors have at least a 50% reduction in risk of disease progression and death when compared with HPV-negative patients. In a meta-analysis summarizing data from 1130 OPC patients within these five trials, HPV-positive patients had a 51% (hazard ratio [HR], 0.49; 95% confidence interval [CI], 0.35–0.69) reduction in risk of death and a 35% (HR, 0.65; 95% CI, 0.4–1.06) reduction in risk of death from cancer when compared with patients with HPV-negative HNC.[44] The improved outcomes for HPV-positive patients are attributable to higher rates of local-regional control, reduced rates of second primary tumors, and reduced frequency of poor prognostic factors (eg, performance status, advanced T stage, younger age, reduced smoking trials) relative to the HPV-negative patient.[39–43]

Although not performed within the context of prospective clinical trials, single-institutional case series also observed survival to be superior for HPV-positive versus HPV-negative OPC treated with primary surgical resection, largely in univariate analyses.[45–47]

Molecular Mechanisms, Human Papillomavirus Status, and Prognosis

The underlying molecular basis for the increased survival for patients with HPV-positive versus HPV-negative HNC remains unclear, despite considerable data that gene expression profiles in HPV-positive and HPV-negative HNC significantly differ.[48,49] Increased apoptosis of p53 wild-type tumors in response to radiotherapy and increased immune surveillance to HPV-specific tumor antigens have been proposed as possible explanations.[27] There are now data to support both hypotheses (reviewed in[50]). Several investigators have reported relatively increased radiation sensitivity in HPV-positive versus negative HNC cell lines,[51–54] and support different molecular mechanisms for this increase radiation sensitivity. Kimple and colleagues[54] observed upregulation of p53 expression and related genes in HPV-positive cell lines in response to radiation therapy, despite expression of HPV E6, leading to cell death. An alternative explanation of a relative impairment of double strand break repair and G2-cell cycle arrest, and not induction of apoptosis, was observed in response to radiotherapy in five HPV-positive versus five HPV-negative HNC cell lines.[51] Sorensen and colleagues[53] observed similar increased sensitivity to radiotherapy among HPV-positive versus HPV-negative HNC cell lines in vitro, but found no difference in upregulation of hypoxia-associated genes in the two groups. However, an in vivo model found decreased proliferation and hypoxia in HPV-positive tumors in comparison with HPV-negative tumor xenografts in response to radiation. The improved response to radiotherapy thus seems to be multifactorial.

Evidence to support enhanced immune-mediated clearance of HPV-positive tumors was observed in an in vivo mouse model.[55] Enhanced clearance among transformed HPV-positive versus HPV-negative mouse tonsillar epithelial cells in response to radiation and/or cisplatin therapy was dependent on immune-competence or adoptive transfer of splenocytes to immune-incompetent mice.[55] $CD4^+$ and $CD8^+$ T cells were necessary to mount this antitumor response.[56] This effect was mediated in part by down-regulation of CD47 expression in response to radiation.[57] Expression of CD47 by cancer cells has been shown to be a mechanism of immune evasion by suppressing phagocytosis.[58] In agreement with this animal model are consistent findings that high levels of tumor-infiltrating lymphocytes are associated with improved survival relative to low levels for HPV-positive[59,60] and HPV-negative patients.[61]

HUMAN PAPILLOMAVIRUS TUMOR STATUS, RACE, AND SURVIVAL

In the 1970s, incidence rates for OPC were significantly higher among black persons than white persons in the United States.[62] Over the four subsequent decades, rates significantly declined for black men but increased for white men, resulting in significantly higher rates among white men by 2013.[63] An analysis of tumors collected through US Surveillance, Epidemiology, and End Results (SEER) registries from 1984 to 1999 revealed nonsignificant increases in HPV-prevalence of OPC among black persons in the United States, in contrast to strong increases among white persons.[36] These data indicate that increased HPV prevalence in OPC over time among black persons reported by some institutions[64] was likely attributable in large part to reduced incidence rates for HPV-negative cancers. By contrast, increased HPV prevalence in OPC among white persons was attributable to increased incidence for HPV-positive OPC.[36] In agreement with these data, several single-institutional case series[64–67] (but not all[68,69]) have observed higher HPV prevalence among OPC diagnosed among white than black persons. Indeed, an analysis of 557 OPC collected by US SEER cancer registries from 1995 to 2005 observed lower prevalence of high-risk HPV DNA among non-Hispanic blacks (~50%) than all other races (>73%).[70]

Historically, survival rates from HNC have been lower among black persons in comparison with white persons in the United States.[71–76] These differences have been attributed to higher stage at presentation, comorbidities, and socioeconomic factors that affect access and delivery of care.[71–76] Recently, several single-institutional analyses have investigated the impact of tumor HPV status on survival outcomes from HNC by race (black vs white). Generally, HPV-positive tumors were more frequent in white than black persons and were associated with a strong survival benefit.[64–67] Most of these studies conclude that race was not an independent predictor of poor survival for OPC after accounting for tumor HPV status.[65,66,68,69] For example, a shorter median survival among black than white persons with HNC enrolled in the TAX 324 was not observed after stratification by tumor HPV status.[77] Similarly, among OPC patients treated in the Veterans Affairs system, race was not associated with survival after accounting for HPV status.[69] It should be noted, however, that many of these studies either did not investigate (or were underpowered to do so) the independent effect of race after adjustment for known prognostic factors (including HPV) in multivariate models.

Several studies suggest that differences in tumor HPV status by race do not entirely explain survival differences, even in patients with OPC. In a prospective analysis of a uniformly treated patient population enrolled in Radiation Therapy Oncology Group (RTOG) 0129, black race remained associated with significantly lower survival after chemoradiotherapy for OPC patients and HNC patients overall, after adjustment for tumor HPV status, tumor and nodal stage, age, and treatment assignment.[39] A simulated analysis of US SEER data observed that differences in survival by race observed for OPC patients may be attributable to differences in tumor HPV status by race, but that survival differences by race persisted for most non-OPC sites.[71] Indeed, differences in tumor HPV status and smoking by race accounted for the differences in survival for OPC patients, but not for non-OPC cancers in another analysis.[67] An analysis of a case series conducted at the University of Maryland also observed that HPV-negative tumor status and black race remained independently associated with less favorable survival, largely because of poorer survival among black persons with HPV-negative tumors.[64] There is thus a growing consensus across studies that race remains a negative prognostic factor for survival for patients with HPV-negative cancers.[64,67,78] Although differences in survival by race for patients with OPC are in large part attributable to differences in tumor HPV status by race (with HPV-positive status more common among white persons), racial disparities in outcome are still present for patients with OPC, but seem significantly larger in absolute magnitude for non-OPC.

The underlying reasons for the difference in HPV prevalence in OPC by race are in large part explained by higher incidence for HPV-negative cancer among black persons and HPV-positive OPC among white persons. In 1993, Day and colleagues[79] reported that higher incidence rates for oral cancers among black than white persons was caused by a higher frequency of heavy drinking and current smoking among black persons and found no differences in estimates for relative risks for these exposures by race. Although current tobacco smoking declined from 1965 to 2007 in the United States for black and white persons, smoking rates remain higher for black persons.[62] These declines are consistent with declining incidence rates for HPV-negative OPC in the United States.[36] At this time, the relative increase of HPV-positive OPC among white versus black persons remains unexplained. Interestingly, increasing incidence trends from 1978 to 2007 in the United States for HPV-related preinvasive and invasive anogenital (eg, cervical, anal, vulvar, penile) cancers were similar among white and black persons.[80] These data suggest changes in genital HPV infection trends were similar over time among black and white persons. Although ever performance of oral-genital sex and number of lifetime oral sex partners were higher for white than black persons in the United States, the prevalence of HPV16 or high-risk oral HPV infections in 2009 to 2010 was nonsignificantly higher in white persons.[30] Frequent, concomitant age at first experience of oral and genital sexual behaviors among white persons, in contrast to sole genital or sequential behaviors in black persons,[81] could in theory result in higher protective seroconversion rates after genital infection in black persons, resulting in relative protection from subsequent oral HPV infection.

HUMAN PAPILLOMAVIRUS STATUS, TUMOR STAGING, AND PROGNOSIS

An analysis by Ang and colleagues[39] conducted within RTOG 0129 demonstrated that tumor HPV status and tobacco smoking history had a more significant impact on patient prognosis than American Joint Committee on Cancer (AJCC) TNM stage. These data raise the question as to whether or not the current staging system should be modified to reflect differences in survival for HPV-positive versus HPV-negative OPC by stage. Single institutional retrospective analyses at MD Anderson Cancer Center[82] and Princess Margaret Hospital[83] revealed the current AJCC TNM stage to inaccurately reflect survival rates for all patients with OPC. Survival rates declined in a stepwise manner as a function of advancing AJCC TNM stage for HPV-negative OPC patients, but not for HPV-positive OPC patients (using p16 IHC as a surrogate for HPV tumor status).[83] Recursive partitioning analysis demonstrated that survival was superior for patients diagnosed with HPV-positive, low-volume (eg, T1-T3, N0-N2c) as compared with high-volume local-regional disease (eg, T4 or N3[83]). Tobacco smoking and age further stratified survival: tobacco smoking history greater than 20 pack-years reduced survival for low-volume disease, whereas age greater than 70 years similarly affected high-volume disease.[83]

Although there is growing consensus that the AJCC staging system will require modification to reflect the differences in prognosis by stage for HPV-positive and HPV-negative OPC, additional research is needed to determine specifics of these modifications. Notably, the different prognostic groups defined within retrospective analysis of clinical trials and single-institutional case series are being used to determine clinical trial eligibility for treatment deintensification protocols. For example, only patients with low-volume (eg, T1-T3, N0-N2b) HPV-positive OPC with low tobacco smoking exposure (<10 pack-years) are eligible for treatment deintensification protocols currently being conducted by NRG Oncology and Eastern Cooperative Oncology Group (ECOG)/American College of Radiology Imaging Network. Therefore, we can anticipate that additional data relevant to AJCC staging categories together with results from these clinical trials will eventually result in stratification by tumor HPV status of the AJCC staging system and National Comprehensive Cancer Center practice guidelines.

HUMAN PAPILLOMAVIRUS STATUS, SURGICAL RESECTION, EXTRACAPSULAR EXTENSION, AND RISK OF CANCER PROGRESSION

The presence of extracapsular extension (ECE) in surgically resected cervical lymph nodes is a well-established biomarker for risk of local-regional recurrence, distant metastases, and reduced survival.[84–86] Randomized controlled trials (RTOG 9501 and European Organization for Research and Treatment of Cancer [EORTC] 22931) demonstrated significantly improved local-regional control and disease-free survival for adjuvant cisplatin-based chemoradiotherapy in comparison with radiotherapy alone for patients treated with primary surgical resection found to have high-risk pathologic features, including positive margins, ECE, two or more nodal metastases, level 4 or 5 nodal involvement (EORTC only), or perineural or vascular invasion (EORTC only).[87–89] Combined analysis of the two trials demonstrated improved survival only among patients with positive margins or ECE when treated with adjuvant chemoradiotherapy versus radiotherapy alone.[90] Notably, 10-year data from RTOG 9501 confirmed benefit for OPC and non-OPC patients.[89]

Recently, several retrospective analyses of single-institutional case series have called into question whether or not ECE is a biomarker for high-risk of disease recurrence for HPV-positive OPC. In a University of Pittsburgh series of 214 oral cavity and 137 OPC patients, the frequency of ECE in nodal metastases was similar in the two groups. However, ECE was associated with disease-specific survival in oral cavity, but not OPC.[91] Similarly, a case-series at Washington University did not observe the presence of ECE (present in 80% of patients with nodal metastases) to be associated with recurrence among 220 p16-positive OPC patients treated with primary surgical resection.[92] At a median follow-up of 59 months, 5-year disease-specific survival for all patients in this series was 93%. Disease recurrence was observed in 22 patients (10%), with only four patients experiencing regional recurrence. Factors found to be associated with recurrence in univariate analysis included age, T3-4 versus T1-T2 stage, five or more metastatic nodes, and the presence of lymphovascular invasion. However, because of the small number of events, the independent predictors of disease recurrence could not be determined. Notably, in an earlier analysis, ECE was positively associated with several other adverse pathologic features, including number and level of involved lymph nodes, perineural invasion, angioinvasion, and lymphatic invasion.[93] Thus, the independent effects of ECE on local-regional recurrence would be difficult to evaluate in a study with few events. Because of the high disease control rates among patients with HPV-positive OPC, these studies had very low power to detect prognostic differences among groups.

These retrospective analyses appropriately call into question the definition and use of "high-risk" features for selection of HPV-positive OPC patients for benefit from adjuvant chemoradiotherapy. The effect of ECE on disease progression clearly differs by HPV status, at least in terms of absolute magnitude. It must be noted, however, that all of the studies had very low power, and therefore estimated HRs are more important for inferences from the data than tests of significance (eg, P values). These suggest that the relative benefit from chemotherapy may be similar among HPV-positive and HPV-negative patients with ECE. In the first report of the Washington University series, ECE seemed associated with diminished disease-free survival (HR, 2.54; 95% CI, 0.88–7.34) and diminished overall survival (HR, 4.22; 95% CI, 1.17–12.1) in univariate analysis.[93] Gross soft tissue extension also seemed associated with worse disease-free survival (HR, 2.1; 95% CI, 0.63–7.4) and benefit from chemoradiotherapy (HR, 2.78; 95% CI, 0.14–54.68).[93] A case-series from Memorial Sloan Kettering Cancer Center observed a significantly worse survival among HPV-negative OPC patients with than without ECE (41.2 vs 76.1%; $P = .002$) together with nonsignificant differences for HPV-positive patients (74 vs 91.2%; $P = .12$).[45] Additionally, these retrospective analyses are subject to bias by indication, and therefore it is difficult to evaluate the effect of chemoradiotherapy versus radiotherapy on disease control. A multicenter, randomized clinical trial comparing adjuvant chemoradiotherapy with radiotherapy for p16-positive OPC patients with ECE led by Washington University is ongoing. Until the results from that clinical trial become available, National Comprehensive Cancer Center guidelines recommend the use of adjuvant chemoradiotherapy for patients with ECE, regardless of tumor HPV status.[87–89]

TUMOR HUMAN PAPILLOMAVIRUS STATUS AND OVERALL SURVIVAL POSTPROGRESSION

It is now clear that HPV-positive OPC is a distinct entity when compared with HPV-negative HNC with regard to risk factors,[94] treatment response,[95] and prognosis.[39,40] Distinctions between these two diseases may also extend to natural history post primary chemoradiotherapy. Observational studies suggest that time to resolution of cervical adenopathy is more prolonged among patients with HPV-positive OPC and that measurable nodal disease 8 to 12 weeks post chemoradiotherapy may not have detrimental effects on survival rates.[96] Cautious interpretation of these data is warranted because of selection bias for decisions regarding continued observation versus immediate salvage neck dissection. Preliminary observational data indicate that overall survival may also be significantly longer among patients with HPV-positive versus HPV-negative HNC found to have residual disease on salvage neck dissections performed within 20 weeks of completion of primary (chemo) radiotherapy.[97]

According to recent analysis of RTOG 0129 and 0522, median time to first local-regional or distant progression after primary chemoradiotherapy is similar for HPV-positive and HPV-negative OPC patients.[98] Prospective clinical trials have observed nonsignificantly lower rates for distant metastases among HPV-positive patients.[39,40,43] Lung, liver, and bone are the most frequent sites of first distant metastases in both HPV-positive and HPV-negative OPC patients.[98] Nevertheless, clinicians frequently perceive distant metastases to be more frequent for HPV-positive cancers. Two factors likely contribute to this misperception. First, local-regional disease control is significantly greater for HPV-positive versus HPV-negative HNC,[39,40,43] and therefore distant failures comprise a higher proportion of progression events among HPV-positive patients. Second, the RTOG analysis demonstrated median survival after disease progression to be almost 2 years longer for HPV-positive versus HPV-negative OPC patients (2.6 vs 0.8 years; log-rank $P<.001$).[98] Retrospective, single-institutional observational studies have also observed median survival after development of distant metastases to be longer for HPV-positive versus HPV-negative patients.[99] This 1- to 2-year prolongation in survival postprogression likely provides the opportunity for unusual patterns of continued disease progression, such as soft tissue and brain metastases.[99–101] This is analogous to increased rates of brain metastases among long-term survivors of breast cancer.[102]

The underlying reasons for improved prognosis postprogression for HPV-positive OPC are unclear. However, preliminary data indicate that improved response rates to palliative chemotherapy may contribute.[103,104] Combined analysis of two ECOG clinical trials of palliative chemotherapy (cisplatin/5-fluorouracil or docetaxel/irinotecan) for recurrent metastatic disease revealed response rates (55% vs 19%; $P = .02$) and median survival (12.9 vs 6.7 months; $P = .014$) were higher for HPV-positive versus HPV-negative patients.[103] Combined analysis of these data with results from the EXTREME and SPECTRUM trials also demonstrated an approximately 40% reduction in the hazard of death for HPV-positive versus HPV-negative patients when treated with cisplatin/5-fluorouracil.[105] These data are consistent with results from a prospective phase II trial conducted by ECOG, in which patients with newly diagnosed HPV-positive HNC had significantly improved response rates to induction chemotherapy when compared with HPV-negative patients.[95] The molecular reasons underlying increased sensitivity to radiotherapy noted previously may be relevant to chemotherapeutics that induce double-strand breaks.

HUMAN PAPILLOMAVIRUS STATUS AND CLINICAL TRIAL DESIGN

The improved survival for HPV-positive versus HPV-negative HNC patients has had a profound effect on clinical trial design over the last 5 years. Tumor HPV status is now used as a stratification factor for all HNC trials for which patients with newly diagnosed locoregionally advanced cancer are eligible. Recent findings on improved prognosis for HPV-positive patients after cancer progression will likely result in stratification by tumor HPV status in trials for patients with recurrent or metastatic HNC.

However, most cooperative groups have elected to design clinical trials specifically for the HPV-positive or HPV-negative patient, because of contrasting goals in the two populations. Ang and colleagues[39] first reported that tumor HPV status (positive vs negative), smoking history (<10 vs ≥10 pack-years), and tumor (T2-3 vs T4) and nodal stage (N0-N2A vs N2B-N3) could be used to classify OPC patients as low-, intermediate-, or high-risk of death when treated by cisplatin-based chemoradiotherapy. Because of high survival rates for nonsmoking HPV-positive patients, this subgroup is being targeted for protocols investigating whether reductions in total radiotherapy dose or elimination of chemotherapy can be performed without compromising survival. Ongoing clinical trials have recently been summarized by Masterson and coworkers[44] and Mirghani and coworkers.[106] To date, preliminary results of only one of these trials have been reported. The study design was based on results from a phase II trial conducted by ECOG investigating induction paclitaxel and carboplatin followed by concomitant weekly paclitaxel and radiotherapy.[95] In that trial, patients with HPV-positive tumors were found to have improved response rates after induction chemotherapy and chemoradiotherapy.[95] Therefore, the ECOG 1308 protocol investigated whether improved response to induction chemotherapy (paclitaxel, cisplatin, cetuximab) could be used to select HPV-positive patients for dose-reduced radiotherapy (from 69 to 54 Gy) without compromising 2-year progression-free survival.[107] The trial included smokers and all stage III-IV patients with resectable disease. A subset of patients (T1-T3, N0-N2b, < 10 pack-years) for whom excellent disease control (23-month progression-free survival, 0.96; 95% CI, 0.82–0.99) was maintained with reduced radiotherapy was identified.[107] This patient population is therefore the target of an ongoing trial conducted by NRG oncology comparing disease control in patients treated with reduced-dose radiotherapy with or without weekly cisplatin (NRG HN002).

In conclusion, the HNC field is in the midst of a fascinating transition, conducting active investigations that will soon result in tumor HPV status altering numerous decision points for HNC patients.

REFERENCES

1. zur Hausen H. Papillomaviruses and cancer: from basic studies to clinical application. Nat Rev Cancer 2002;2(5):342–50.
2. Munoz N, Bosch FX, de Sanjose S, et al. Epidemiologic classification of human papillomavirus types associated with cervical cancer. N Engl J Med 2003; 348(6):518–27.
3. International Agency for Research on Cancer, editor. IARC monographs on the evaluation of carcinogenic risks to humans, vol. 90. Lyon (France): World Health Organization; 2007. p. 670.
4. Yugawa T, Kiyono T. Molecular mechanisms of cervical carcinogenesis by high-risk human papillomaviruses: novel functions of E6 and E7 oncoproteins. Rev Med Virol 2009;19(2):97–113.
5. Moody CA, Laimins LA. Human papillomavirus oncoproteins: pathways to transformation. Nat Rev Cancer 2010;10(8):550–60.
6. Werness BA, Levine AJ, Howley PM. Association of human papillomavirus types 16 and 18 E6 proteins with p53. Science 1990;248(4951):76–9.
7. Veldman T, Horikawa I, Barrett JC, et al. Transcriptional activation of the telomerase hTERT gene by human papillomavirus type 16 E6 oncoprotein. J Virol 2001; 75(9):4467–72.

8. Duensing S, Munger K. The human papillomavirus type 16 E6 and E7 oncoproteins independently induce numerical and structural chromosome instability. Cancer Res 2002;62(23):7075–82.

9. Hu Z, Zhu D, Wang W, et al. Genome-wide profiling of HPV integration in cervical cancer identifies clustered genomic hot spots and a potential microhomology-mediated integration mechanism. Nat Genet 2015;47(2):158–63.

10. Wentzensen N, Vinokurova S, von Knebel Doeberitz M. Systematic review of genomic integration sites of human papillomavirus genomes in epithelial dysplasia and invasive cancer of the female lower genital tract. Cancer Res 2004;64(11):3878–84.

11. Olthof NC, Speel EJ, Kolligs J, et al. Comprehensive analysis of HPV16 integration in OSCC reveals no significant impact of physical status on viral oncogene and virally disrupted human gene expression. PLoS One 2014;9(2): e88718.

12. Deng Z, Hasegawa M, Kiyuna A, et al. Viral load, physical status, and E6/E7 mRNA expression of human papillomavirus in head and neck squamous cell carcinoma. Head Neck 2013;35(6):800–8.

13. Gao G, Johnson SH, Kasperbauer JL, et al. Mate pair sequencing of oropharyngeal squamous cell carcinomas reveals that HPV integration occurs much less frequently than in cervical cancer. J Clin Virol 2014;59(3):195–200.

14. Pett MR, Alazawi WO, Roberts I, et al. Acquisition of high-level chromosomal instability is associated with integration of human papillomavirus type 16 in cervical keratinocytes. Cancer Res 2004;64(4):1359–68.

15. Winder DM, Pett MR, Foster N, et al. An increase in DNA double-strand breaks, induced by Ku70 depletion, is associated with human papillomavirus 16 episome loss and de novo viral integration events. J Pathol 2007;213(1): 27–34.

16. Dall KL, Scarpini CG, Roberts I, et al. Characterization of naturally occurring HPV16 integration sites isolated from cervical keratinocytes under noncompetitive conditions. Cancer Res 2008;68(20):8249–59.

17. Jeon S, Lambert PF. Integration of human papillomavirus type 16 DNA into the human genome leads to increased stability of E6 and E7 mRNAs: implications for cervical carcinogenesis. Proc Natl Acad Sci U S A 1995;92(5):1654–8.

18. Pett MR, Herdman MT, Palmer RD, et al. Selection of cervical keratinocytes containing integrated HPV16 associates with episome loss and an endogenous antiviral response. Proc Natl Acad Sci U S A 2006;103(10):3822–7.

19. Thierry F, Yaniv M. The BPV1-E2 trans-acting protein can be either an activator or a repressor of the HPV18 regulatory region. EMBO J 1987;6(11):3391–7.

20. Akagi K, Li J, Broutian TR, et al. Genome-wide analysis of HPV integration in human cancers reveals recurrent, focal genomic instability. Genome Res 2014; 24(2):185–99.

21. Ojesina AI, Lichtenstein L, Freeman SS, et al. Landscape of genomic alterations in cervical carcinomas. Nature 2014;506(7488):371–5.

22. Parfenov M, Pedamallu CS, Gehlenborg N, et al. Characterization of HPV and host genome interactions in primary head and neck cancers. Proc Natl Acad Sci U S A 2014;111(43):15544–9.

23. Gillison ML, Alemany L, Snijders PJ, et al. Human papillomavirus and diseases of the upper airway: head and neck cancer and respiratory papillomatosis. Vaccine 2012;30(Suppl 5):F34–54.

24. Gillison M, Chaturvedi A, Anderson W, et al. The epidemiology of HPV-positive head and neck squamous cell carcinoma. J Clin Oncol, in press.

25. Mork J, Lie AK, Glattre E, et al. Human papillomavirus infection as a risk factor for squamous-cell carcinoma of the head and neck. N Engl J Med 2001;344(15): 1125–31.
26. Kreimer AR, Johansson M, Waterboer T, et al. Evaluation of human papillomavirus antibodies and risk of subsequent head and neck cancer. J Clin Oncol 2013;31(21):2708–15.
27. Gillison ML, Koch WM, Capone RB, et al. Evidence for a causal association between human papillomavirus and a subset of head and neck cancers. J Natl Cancer Inst 2000;92(9):709–20.
28. Castellsague X, Alemany L, Holzinger D, et al. Estimation of the HPV etiological fraction in over 4,000 head and neck cancers worldwide. International Human Papillomavirus Conference. Seattle (WA), 2014. p. 224.
29. D'Souza G, Kreimer AR, Viscidi R, et al. Case-control study of human papillomavirus and oropharyngeal cancer. N Engl J Med 2007;356(19):1944–56.
30. Gillison ML, Broutian T, Pickard RK, et al. Prevalence of oral HPV infection in the United States, 2009-2010. JAMA 2012;307(7):693–703.
31. Beachler DC, Sugar EA, Margolick JB, et al. Risk factors for acquisition and clearance of oral human papillomavirus infection among HIV-infected and HIV-uninfected adults. Am J Epidemiol 2015;181(1):40–53.
32. Edelstein ZR, Schwartz SM, Hawes S, et al. Rates and determinants of oral human papillomavirus infection in young men. Sex Transm Dis 2012;39(11):860–7.
33. Pickard R, Xiao W, Broutian T, et al. The prevalence and incidence of oral human papillomavirus infection among young men and women, age 18-30 years. Sex Transm Dis 2012;39(7):559–66.
34. Kreimer AR, Pierce Campbell CM, Lin HY, et al. Incidence and clearance of oral human papillomavirus infection in men: the HIM cohort study. Lancet 2013; 382(9895):877–87.
35. Chaturvedi A, Graubard B, Broutian T, et al. NHANES 2009-2012 Findings: Sexual behaviors and higher prevalence of oral oncogenic human papillomavirus infection among men in the U.S. population. Cancer Res 2015;75(12):2468–77.
36. Chaturvedi AK, Engels EA, Pfeiffer RM, et al. Human papillomavirus and rising oropharyngeal cancer incidence in the United States. J Clin Oncol 2011;29(32): 4294–301.
37. Chaturvedi AK, Anderson WF, Lortet-Tieulent J, et al. Worldwide trends in incidence rates for oral cavity and oropharyngeal cancers. J Clin Oncol 2013; 31(36):4550–9.
38. Giuliano AR, Nyitray AG, Kreimer AR, et al. EUROGIN 2014 roadmap: differences in human papillomavirus infection natural history, transmission and human papillomavirus-related cancer incidence by gender and anatomic site of infection. Int J Cancer 2015;136(12):2752–60.
39. Ang KK, Harris J, Wheeler R, et al. Human papillomavirus and survival of patients with oropharyngeal cancer. N Engl J Med 2010;363(1):24–35.
40. Rischin D, Young R, Fisher R, et al. Prognostic significance of HPV and p16 status in patients with oropharyngeal cancer treated on a large international phase III trial. J Clin Oncol 2009;27(15S):302.
41. Ang KK, Zhang Q, Rosenthal DI, et al. Randomized phase III trial of concurrent accelerated radiation plus cisplatin with or without cetuximab for stage III to IV head and neck carcinoma: RTOG 0522. J Clin Oncol 2014;32(27):2940–50.
42. Gillison ML, Zhang Q, Jordan R, et al. Tobacco smoking and increased risk of death and progression for patients with p16-positive and p16-negative oropharyngeal cancer. J Clin Oncol 2012;30(17):2102–11.

43. Posner M, Lorch J, Goloubeva O, et al. Survival and human papillomavirus in oropharynx cancer in TAX 324: a subset analysis from an international phase III trial. Ann Oncol 2011;22(5):1071-7.
44. Masterson L, Moualed D, Liu ZW, et al. De-escalation treatment protocols for human papillomavirus-associated oropharyngeal squamous cell carcinoma: a systematic review and meta-analysis of current clinical trials. Eur J Cancer 2014;50(15):2636-48.
45. Iyer NG, Dogan S, Palmer F, et al. Detailed analysis of clinicopathologic factors demonstrate distinct difference in outcome and prognostic factors between surgically treated hpv-positive and negative oropharyngeal cancer. Ann Surg Oncol 2015. [Epub ahead of print].
46. Ljokjel B, Lybak S, Haave H, et al. The impact of HPV infection on survival in a geographically defined cohort of oropharynx squamous cell carcinoma (OPSCC) patients in whom surgical treatment has been one main treatment. Acta Otolaryngol 2014;134(6):636-45.
47. Geiger JL, Lazim AF, Walsh FJ, et al. Adjuvant chemoradiation therapy with high-dose versus weekly cisplatin for resected, locally-advanced HPV/p16-positive and negative head and neck squamous cell carcinoma. Oral Oncol 2014; 50(4):311-8.
48. Pyeon D, Newton MA, Lambert PF, et al. Fundamental differences in cell cycle deregulation in human papillomavirus-positive and human papillomavirus-negative head/neck and cervical cancers. Cancer Res 2007;67(10):4605-19.
49. Schlect N, Burk R, Adrien L, et al. Gene expression profiles in HPV-infected head and neck cancer. J Pathol 2007;213(3):283-93.
50. Bol V, Gregoire V. Biological basis for increased sensitivity to radiation therapy in HPV-positive head and neck cancers. Biomed Res Int 2014;2014:696028.
51. Rieckmann T, Tribius S, Grob TJ, et al. HNSCC cell lines positive for HPV and p16 possess higher cellular radiosensitivity due to an impaired DSB repair capacity. Radiother Oncol 2013;107(2):242-6.
52. Arenz A, Ziemann F, Mayer C, et al. Increased radiosensitivity of HPV-positive head and neck cancer cell lines due to cell cycle dysregulation and induction of apoptosis. Strahlenther Onkol 2014;190(9):839-46.
53. Sorensen BS, Busk M, Olthof N, et al. Radiosensitivity and effect of hypoxia in HPV positive head and neck cancer cells. Radiother Oncol 2013;108(3):500-5.
54. Kimple RJ, Smith MA, Blitzer GC, et al. Enhanced radiation sensitivity in HPV-positive head and neck cancer. Cancer Res 2013;73(15):4791-800.
55. Spanos WC, Nowicki P, Lee DW, et al. Immune response during therapy with cisplatin or radiation for human papillomavirus-related head and neck cancer. Arch Otolaryngol Head Neck Surg 2009;135(11):1137-46.
56. Williams R, Lee DW, Elzey BD, et al. Preclinical models of HPV+ and HPV-HNSCC in mice: an immune clearance of HPV+ HNSCC. Head Neck 2009; 31(7):911-8.
57. Vermeer DW, Spanos WC, Vermeer PD, et al. Radiation-induced loss of cell surface CD47 enhances immune-mediated clearance of human papillomavirus-positive cancer. Int J Cancer 2013;133(1):120-9.
58. Soto-Pantoja DR, Stein EV, Rogers NM, et al. Therapeutic opportunities for targeting the ubiquitous cell surface receptor CD47. Expert Opin Ther Targets 2013;17(1):89-103.
59. Ward MJ, Thirdborough SM, Mellows T, et al. Tumour-infiltrating lymphocytes predict for outcome in HPV-positive oropharyngeal cancer. Br J Cancer 2014; 110(2):489-500.

60. Nordfors C, Grun N, Tertipis N, et al. CD8+ and CD4+ tumour infiltrating lymphocytes in relation to human papillomavirus status and clinical outcome in tonsillar and base of tongue squamous cell carcinoma. Eur J Cancer 2013; 49(11):2522–30.

61. Wansom D, Light E, Thomas D, et al. Infiltrating lymphocytes and human papillomavirus-16–associated oropharyngeal cancer. Laryngoscope 2012;122(1): 121–7.

62. Brown LM, Check DP, Devesa SS. Oropharyngeal cancer incidence trends: diminishing racial disparities. Cancer Causes Control 2011;22(5):753–63.

63. Jemal A, Simard EP, Dorell C, et al. Annual Report to the Nation on the Status of Cancer, 1975-2009, featuring the burden and trends in human papillomavirus(HPV)-associated cancers and HPV vaccination coverage levels. J Natl Cancer Inst 2013;105(3):175–201.

64. Zandberg DP, Liu S, Goloubeva OG, et al. Emergence of HPV16-positive oropharyngeal cancer in Black patients over time: University of Maryland 1992-2007. Cancer Prev Res (Phila) 2015;8(1):12–9.

65. Chernock RD, Zhang Q, El-Mofty SK, et al. Human papillomavirus-related squamous cell carcinoma of the oropharynx: a comparative study in whites and African Americans. Arch Otolaryngol Head Neck Surg 2011;137(2):163–9.

66. Weinberger PM, Merkley MA, Khichi SS, et al. Human papillomavirus-active head and neck cancer and ethnic health disparities. Laryngoscope 2010; 120(8):1531–7.

67. Jiron J, Sethi S, Ali-Fehmi R, et al. Racial disparities in human papillomavirus (HPV) associated head and neck cancer. Am J Otolaryngol 2014;35(2): 147–53.

68. Isayeva T, Xu J, Dai Q, et al. African Americans with oropharyngeal carcinoma have significantly poorer outcomes despite similar rates of human papillomavirus-mediated carcinogenesis. Hum Pathol 2014;45(2):310–9.

69. Zevallos JP, Sandulache VC, Hamblin J, et al. Impact of race on oropharyngeal squamous cell carcinoma presentation and outcomes among veterans. Head Neck 2014. [Epub ahead of print].

70. Steinau M, Saraiya M, Goodman MT, et al. Human papillomavirus prevalence in oropharyngeal cancer before vaccine introduction, United States. Emerg Infect Dis 2014;20(5):822–8.

71. Schrank TP, Han Y, Weiss H, et al. Case-matching analysis of head and neck squamous cell carcinoma in racial and ethnic minorities in the United States: possible role for human papillomavirus in survival disparities. Head Neck 2011;33(1):45–53.

72. Shavers VL, Harlan LC, Winn D, et al. Racial/ethnic patterns of care for cancers of the oral cavity, pharynx, larynx, sinuses, and salivary glands. Cancer Metastasis Rev 2003;22(1):25–38.

73. Mahal BA, Inverso G, Aizer AA, et al. Impact of African-American race on presentation, treatment, and survival of head and neck cancer. Oral Oncol 2014; 50(12):1177–81.

74. Molina MA, Cheung MC, Perez EA, et al. African American and poor patients have a dramatically worse prognosis for head and neck cancer: an examination of 20,915 patients. Cancer 2008;113(10):2797–806.

75. Zakeri K, MacEwan I, Vazirnia A, et al. Race and competing mortality in advanced head and neck cancer. Oral Oncol 2014;50(1):40–4.

76. Ragin CC, Langevin SM, Marzouk M, et al. Determinants of head and neck cancer survival by race. Head Neck 2011;33(8):1092–8.

77. Settle K, Posner MR, Schumaker L, et al. Racial survival disparity in head and neck cancer results from low prevalence of human papillomavirus infection in black oropharyngeal cancer patients. Cancer Prev Res 2009;2:769–72.
78. Worsham MJ, Stephen JK, Chen KM, et al. Improved survival with HPV among African Americans with oropharyngeal cancer. Clin Cancer Res 2013;19(9):2486–92.
79. Day GL, Blot WJ, Austin DF, et al. Racial differences in risk of oral and pharyngeal cancer: alcohol, tobacco, and other determinants. J Natl Cancer Inst 1993; 85(6):465–73.
80. Kurdgelashvili G, Dores GM, Srour SA, et al. Incidence of potentially human papillomavirus-related neoplasms in the United States, 1978 to 2007. Cancer 2013;119(12):2291–9.
81. D'Souza G, Cullen K, Bowie J, et al. Differences in oral sexual behaviors by gender, age, and race explain observed differences in prevalence of oral human papillomavirus infection. PLoS One 2014;9(1):e86023.
82. Dahlstrom KR, Calzada G, Hanby JD, et al. An evolution in demographics, treatment, and outcomes of oropharyngeal cancer at a major cancer center: a staging system in need of repair. Cancer 2013;119(1):81–9.
83. Huang SH, Xu W, Waldron J, et al. Refining American Joint Committee on Cancer/Union for International Cancer Control TNM Stage and Prognostic Groups for Human Papillomavirus-Related Oropharyngeal Carcinomas. J Clin Oncol 2015;33(8):836–45.
84. Cooper JS, Pajak TF, Forastiere A, et al. Precisely defining high-risk operable head and neck tumors based on RTOG #85-03 and #88-24: targets for postoperative radiochemotherapy? Head Neck 1998;20(7):588–94.
85. Langendijk JA, Slotman BJ, van der Waal I, et al. Risk-group definition by recursive partitioning analysis of patients with squamous cell head and neck carcinoma treated with surgery and postoperative radiotherapy. Cancer 2005; 104(7):1408–17.
86. Myers JN, Greenberg JS, Mo V, et al. Extracapsular spread. A significant predictor of treatment failure in patients with squamous cell carcinoma of the tongue. Cancer 2001;92(12):3030–6.
87. Bernier J, Domenge C, Ozsahin M, et al. Postoperative irradiation with or without concomitant chemotherapy for locally advanced head and neck cancer. N Engl J Med 2004;350(19):1945–52.
88. Cooper JS, Pajak TF, Forastiere AA, et al. Postoperative concurrent radiotherapy and chemotherapy for high-risk squamous-cell carcinoma of the head and neck. N Engl J Med 2004;350(19):1937–44.
89. Cooper JS, Zhang Q, Pajak TF, et al. Long-term follow-up of the RTOG 9501/intergroup phase III trial: postoperative concurrent radiation therapy and chemotherapy in high-risk squamous cell carcinoma of the head and neck. Int J Radiat Oncol Biol Phys 2012;84(5):1198–205.
90. Bernier J, Cooper JS, Pajak TF, et al. Defining risk levels in locally advanced head and neck cancers: a comparative analysis of concurrent postoperative radiation plus chemotherapy trials of the EORTC (#22931) and RTOG (# 9501). Head Neck 2005;27(10):843–50.
91. Maxwell JH, Ferris RL, Gooding W, et al. Extracapsular spread in head and neck carcinoma: impact of site and human papillomavirus status. Cancer 2013; 119(18):3302–8.
92. Sinha P, Kallogjeri D, Gay H, et al. High metastatic node number, not extracapsular spread or N-classification is a node-related prognosticator in transorally-resected, neck-dissected p16-positive oropharynx cancer. Oral Oncol 2015;51(5):514–20.

93. Sinha P, Lewis JS Jr, Piccirillo JF, et al. Extracapsular spread and adjuvant therapy in human papillomavirus-related, p16-positive oropharyngeal carcinoma. Cancer 2012;118(14):3519–30.

94. Gillison M, D'souza G, Westra W, et al. Distinct risk factor profiles for human papillomavirus type 16-positive and human papillomavirus 16-negative head and neck cancers. J Natl Cancer Inst 2008;100(6):407–20.

95. Fakhry C, Westra WH, Li S, et al. Improved survival of patients with human papillomavirus-positive head and neck squamous cell carcinoma in a prospective clinical trial. J Natl Cancer Inst 2008;100(4):261–9.

96. Huang SH, O'Sullivan B, Xu W, et al. Temporal nodal regression and regional control after primary radiation therapy for N2-N3 head-and-neck cancer stratified by HPV status. Int J Radiat Oncol Biol Phys 2013;87(5):1078–85.

97. Huang SH, Patel S, O'Sullivan B, et al. Longer survival in patients with human papillomavirus-related head and neck cancer after positive postradiation planned neck dissection. Head Neck 2015;37(7):946–52.

98. Fakhry C, Zhang Q, Nguyen-Tan PF, et al. Human papillomavirus and overall survival after progression of oropharyngeal squamous cell carcinoma. J Clin Oncol 2014;32(30):3365–73.

99. Trosman SJ, Koyfman SA, Ward MC, et al. Effect of human papillomavirus on patterns of distant metastatic failure in oropharyngeal squamous cell carcinoma treated with chemoradiotherapy. JAMA Otolaryngol Head Neck Surg 2015; 141(5):457–62.

100. Huang SH, Perez-Ordonez B, Weinreb I, et al. Natural course of distant metastases following radiotherapy or chemoradiotherapy in HPV-related oropharyngeal cancer. Oral Oncol 2013;49(1):79–85.

101. Huang SH, Perez-Ordonez B, Liu FF, et al. Atypical clinical behavior of p16-confirmed HPV-related oropharyngeal squamous cell carcinoma treated with radical radiotherapy. Int J Radiat Oncol Biol Phys 2012;82(1):276–83.

102. Tabouret E, Chinot O, Metellus P, et al. Recent trends in epidemiology of brain metastases: an overview. Anticancer Res 2012;32(11):4655–62.

103. Argiris A, Li S, Ghebremichael M, et al. Prognostic significance of human papillomavirus in recurrent or metastatic head and neck cancer: an analysis of Eastern Cooperative Oncology Group trials. Ann Oncol 2014;25(7):1410–6.

104. Misiukiewicz K, Camille N, Gupta V, et al. The role of HPV status in recurrent/metastatic squamous cell carcinoma of the head and neck. Clin Adv Hematol Oncol 2014;12(12):812–9.

105. Spreafico A, Amir E, Siu LL. Demystifying the role of tumor HPV status in recurrent and/or metastatic squamous cell carcinoma of the head and neck. Ann Oncol 2014;25(4):760–2.

106. Mirghani H, Amen F, Blanchard P, et al. Treatment de-escalation in HPV-positive oropharyngeal carcinoma: ongoing trials, critical issues and perspectives. Int J Cancer 2015;136(7):1494–503.

107. Cmelak A, Li S, Marur S, et al. E1308: reduced-dose IMRT in human papillomavirus (HPV)-associated resectable oropharyngeal squamous cell carcinomas (OPSCC) after clinical complete response (cCR) to induction chemotherapy (IC). J Clin Oncol 2014;32(5 Suppl).

Sequential and Concurrent Chemoradiation

State of the Art

Nicole G. Chau, MD[a,b,c], Robert I. Haddad, MD[a,b,c],*

KEYWORDS

- Head and neck cancer • Chemoradiation • Induction chemotherapy
- Sequential therapy • Treatment

KEY POINTS

- Sequential chemoradiotherapy (ST) and concurrent chemoradiotherapy (CRT) are accepted nonsurgical, curative-intent treatment strategies for locally advanced head and neck cancer (LAHNC).
- Head-to-head comparison of ST and CRT in randomized phase III trials has not definitively shown which approach is superior, and patient selection remains controversial.
- Definitive management of LAHNC is evolving with increasing efforts to tailor therapy according to patient risk.
- Patients with low-risk LAHNC may benefit from deintensification of therapy. Strategies currently being tested include chemosparing CRT with the use of biologic agents instead of cisplatin, and the use of ST to select patients for subsequent reduced-dose radiation.
- In contrast, patients with high-risk LAHNC require novel strategies to improve therapeutic efficacy. Approaches under investigation include adding novel agents to the backbone of CRT, and intensification with ST incorporating novel induction regimens.

INTRODUCTION

Head and neck cancer is the seventh most common cancer worldwide, with an estimated 686,328 new cases diagnosed in 2012.[1] Most patients present with locally advanced disease (stage III or IVA-B). Nonsurgical management using radiation-based therapy is a definitive curative-intent treatment strategy in patients with unresectable disease and is often favored as an organ-sparing strategy. The benefit of

[a] Center for Head and Neck Oncology, Dana-Farber Cancer Institute, Harvard Medical School, 450 Brookline Avenue, Boston, MA 02115, USA; [b] Department of Medical Oncology, Dana-Farber Cancer Institute, 450 Brookline Avenue, Boston, MA 02115, USA; [c] Department of Medicine, Brigham and Women's Hospital, 75 Francis Street, Boston, MA 02115, USA
* Corresponding author. Dana-Farber Cancer Institute, 450 Brookline Avenue, Boston, MA 02215.
E-mail address: Robert_haddad@dfci.harvard.edu

Hematol Oncol Clin N Am 29 (2015) 1061–1074
http://dx.doi.org/10.1016/j.hoc.2015.07.005
0889-8588/15/$ – see front matter © 2015 Elsevier Inc. All rights reserved.

chemotherapy delivered concurrently with radiation is well established in locally advanced head and neck cancer (LAHNC). The addition of chemotherapy concomitant with radiation improves survival and locoregional control compared with radiation alone.[2,3] Multiple meta-analyses have shown the superiority of chemoradiation compared with radiation alone in LAHNC, with an absolute survival benefit at 5 years of 5% to 9% depending on anatomic location.[2–4] Concurrent chemoradiotherapy (CRT) consisting of bolus cisplatin 100 mg/m^2 is an established regimen in LAHNC.

Sequential chemoradiotherapy (ST) integrates induction chemotherapy followed by CRT with the goal of reducing distant metastases and maximizing local regional control and organ preservation. The optimal induction chemotherapy regimen was defined by 2 landmark randomized phase III trials, TAX 323 and TAX 324, which showed superiority of docetaxel, cisplatin, and 5-fluorouracil (TPF) compared with cisplatin/5-fluorouracil (PF) with respect to improved survival, progression-free survival (PFS), and locoregional and distant failure.[5,6] Subsequently the GORTEC study in larynx cancer also confirmed the superiority of TPF compared with PF.[7] Based on these results, TPF is the induction chemotherapy regimen for comparison in randomized trials evaluating ST versus CRT.

Several randomized clinical trials comparing head-to-head ST and CRT have had methodological limitations, including poor accrual, leading to equivocal results.[8–10] Most recently, one randomized trial showed a survival advantage with ST compared with CRT, fueling further controversy and debate.[11] This article discusses the latest evidence and state-of-the-art approaches to ST and CRT, highlighting ongoing controversies and future directions.

SUMMARY OF RECENT RANDOMIZED CLINICAL TRIALS COMPARING SEQUENTIAL CHEMORADIOTHERAPY VERSUS CONCURRENT CHEMORADIOTHERAPY

The head-to-head comparison of ST and CRT in LAHNC has recently been reported in 4 randomized phase III clinical trials (**Table 1**).[9–12] Notably, of the 4 studies, 3 were methodologically underpowered to detect a survival benefit. Two studies, PARADIGM and DeCIDE, lacked statistical power for their primary end point, overall survival (OS), because of early closure and a higher than expected survival in the control arm (3-year OS ~78% compared with 55% at the time of study design) likely secondary to a large proportion of human papillomavirus (HPV)–related oropharynx cases.[8,9] Only 1 trial was methodologically powered to detect a survival difference and this study showed a survival benefit favoring the ST arm compared with CRT.[11]

PARADIGM is a randomized phase III trial of ST versus CRT in patients with LAHNC.[8] In the ST arm, patients who achieved complete clinical response at the primary site following induction chemotherapy received weekly carboplatin (area under the curve, 1.5) and daily radiation fractionation, whereas the remaining patients received weekly docetaxel (20 mg/m^2) with accelerated radiation therapy (RT). Patients in the CRT-alone arm received 2 cycles of bolus cisplatin with accelerated concomitant boost over 6 weeks (as in RTOG 0129). No differences in PFS (hazard ratio [HR], 1.07; confidence interval [CI], 0.59–1.92; $P = .82$) or OS (HR, 1.09; CI, 0.59–2.03; $P = .77$) were detected, although statistical power was limited because only 145 of the 300 planned patients enrolled. In an unplanned subset analysis, there were non–statistically significant trends noted favoring ST in nonoropharynx sites and CRT for the oropharynx sites. ST did not significantly reduce distant recurrence rates; however, distant recurrences were rare. Patients who did not achieve complete clinical response to induction chemotherapy seemed to have much poorer survival, suggesting that TPF may be used to identify biologically bad cancers and subsequent novel salvage regimens in this patient population are needed. No significant differences in toxicity were noted between the arms and no treatment-related deaths occurred in the study.

DeCIDE is a multicenter phase III study comparing CRT consisting of docetaxel, 5-fluorouracil (5-FU), hydroxyurea, and hyperfractionated radiotherapy (DFHX-RT) versus 2 cycles of TPF induction followed by DFHX-RT.[9] Eligibility required N2 and N3 disease, and prior organ-sparing surgery was allowed. This study enrolled 280 patients (initially planned for 400 patients). No significant difference was identified between the 2 arms for the primary end point, OS (HR, 0.91; CI, 0.59–1.41; $P = .68$), or for recurrence-free survival or distant failure-free survival. There was no difference in survival between the 2 treatment arms in oropharynx patients or nonoropharynx patients, or among patients with N2a or N2b disease. The cumulative incidence of distant recurrence without prior locoregional recurrence favored the ST arm ($P = .043$). Toxicities were higher in the ST arm, with increased severe neutropenia during CRT (14% vs 4%, $P = .023$) and more deaths during treatment (13 deaths [13.5%] in the ST arm versus 4 deaths [3.8%] in the CRT arm).

The Spanish Head and Neck Cancer Cooperative Group conducted a 3-arm phase III trial of 439 patients with previously untreated unresectable LAHNC comparing TPF followed by CRT versus PF followed by CRT versus CRT alone.[10] This study was designed before the establishment of TPF as superior to PF. The primary end point was PFS and time to treatment failure (TTF). This study was not powered to detect survival differences. The initial abstract presentation reported a significant reduction in TTF favoring ST compared with CRT; however, subsequent published intent-to-treat analysis found no difference in PFS, TTF, or OS. Notably, CRT consisted of conventional bolus cisplatin every 3 weeks for all treatment arms. Deaths caused by study treatment toxicity were reported as 7 in the TPF ST arm, 4 in the PF ST arm, and 2 in the CRT arm, raising concerns for excessive toxicity with concurrent bolus cisplatin-radiation following induction chemotherapy. Forty-five patients (29%) in the TPF ST arm and 33 patients (21%) in the PF ST arm did not received CRT for reasons other than disease progression.

The GSTTC Italian Study Group is the only randomized phase III trial showing an improvement in OS with ST compared with CRT.[11] This multicenter study of 421 patients with LAHNC was designed to evaluate (1) OS benefit of ST versus CRT, and (2) grade 3 to 4 in-field mucosal toxicity of CRT versus cetuximab-radiation. The 2×2 factorial design consisted of 4 arms as follows: (1) A1, CRT (PF $\times$ 2 concomitant to standard radiation fractionation); (2) A2, cetuximab concomitant to radiation; (3) B1, 3 cycles of TPF followed by CRT; (4) B2, 3 cycles of TPF followed by cetuximab-radiation. ST significantly improved PFS (HR, 0.73; 95% CI, 0.57–0.94; $P = .015$), and OS (HR, 0.72; 95% CI, 0.55–0.96; $P = .025$) compared with CRT. Superiority of ST compared with CRT was independent of type of CRT; however, in an unplanned subgroup analysis, greater OS benefit was observed with ST using concurrent cetuximab-radiation (HR, 0.57; 95% CI, 0.34–0.93), rather than cisplatin/5-FU–radiation (HR, 0.8; 95% CI, 0.56–1.15). There was no difference in grade 3 to 4 nonhematologic toxicities, including stomatitis, between the ST and CRT arms. Compliance with CRT was not affected by induction TPF. These results, presented in abstract form, are noteworthy and further the argument that ST may be superior to CRT. Controversy still remains because definitive conventional bolus cisplatin-radiation was not a comparator arm in this trial. These results also raise the question of what is the optimal CRT following TPF induction. Further evaluation is required to determine whether TPF followed by cetuximab-radiation (bioradiation) is a preferred ST regimen for therapeutic efficacy and tolerance. Subset analysis to identify which patients are most likely to benefit from ST is of great interest.

Table 1
Completed randomized phase III trials comparing ST and CRT in LAHNC

Study	n	Eligibility	Treatment Arms	Primary End Point	Summary of Results
PARADIGM[12]	145	Stage III/IV LAHNC unresectable or advanced resectable	A: TPF × 3 → CRT B: CRT TPF = docetaxel 75 mg/m² + cisplatin 100 mg/m² + 5-FU 1000 mg/m² days 1–5 A1: if no CR → accelerated concomitant boost × 6 w (72 Gy in 1.8/1.5 Gy#) + docetaxel 20 mg/m² × 4 w A2: if CR → RT once daily × 7 w (70 Gy in 2 Gy#) + carboplatin AUC 1.5 weekly B: accelerated boost RT × 6 w + cisplatin 100 mg/m² on days 1 and 28	OS	No difference in 3-y OS (73% vs 78%) No difference in 3-y PFS (67% vs 69%) No difference in 3-y LR failure (16% vs 15%) Underpowered because of failure to meet accrual target of 200 pts
DeCIDE[8]	285	N2 or N3 LAHNC Prior organ-sparing surgery allowed	A: TPF × 2 → DFHX-RT B: DFHX-RT TPF = docetaxel 75 mg/m² + cisplatin 75 mg/m² + 5-FU 750 mg/m² days 1–5 DFHX-RT: 0.15 Gy twice per day every other week	OS	No difference in OS No difference in recurrence-free survival No difference in distant failure-free survival Underpowered because of failure to meet accrual target of 400 pts

Trial	N	Population	Treatment	Endpoint	Results
Spanish Trial[11]	439	Unresectable LAHNC No prior treatment	A: TPF × 3 → CRT (bolus cis-RT); B: PF × 3-CRT; C: CRT; TPF = docetaxel 75 mg/m² + cisplatin 75 mg/m² + 5-FU 750 mg/m² days 1-5; PF = cisplatin 100 mg/m² + 5-FU 1000 mg/m² days 1-5; CRT = cisplatin 100 mg/m² days 1, 22, 43	PFS and TTP	No difference in PFS (median, mo): 14.6 vs 14.3 vs 13.8; No difference in TTF (median, mo): 7.9 vs 7.9 vs 8.2; No difference in OS (median, mo): 27 vs 27.2 vs 26.2
GSTTC H&N07[9]	421	Stage III–IV LAHNC (larynx excluded)	A1: CRT; A2: cetuximab-RT; B1: TPF × 3 → CRT; B2: TPF × 3 → cetuximab-RT; TPF = docetaxel 75 mg/m² + cisplatin 80 mg/m² + 5-FU 800 mg/m² days 1-5; CRT = cisplatin 20 mg/m² + 5-FU 800 mg/m² days 1-5 wk 1 and 6 of RT 70 Gy (2 Gy/d, 5 d/wk); Cetuximab-RT = cetuximab 400 mg/m² d 7, 250 mg/m² × 7 w RT = 70 Gy (2 Gy/d, 5 d/wk)	3-y OS of A1 + A2 vs B1 + B2 G3–G4 in-field toxicity A1 + B1 vs A2 + B2	OS favors ST more than CRT; ST vs CRT: median OS 53.7 mo vs 30.3 mo; 3-y OS 58% vs 46%; HR 0.72, 95% CI 0.55–0.96, $P = .025$; PFS favors ST more than CRT; ST vs CRT: median PFS 29.7 mo vs 18.5 mo; 3-y PFS 47% vs 37%; HR 0.73, 95% CI 0.57–0.94, $P = .0155$; No difference in G3–G4 nonhematologic toxicity including stomatitis (35% vs 42%, $P = .15$) dermatitis (14% vs 18% $P = .17$) during CRT

Abbreviations: AUC, area under the curve; CI, confidence interval; cis-RT, cisplatin-radiation; CR, complete response; DFHX-RT, docetaxel, 5-FU, hydroxyurea, and hyperfractionated radiotherapy; HR, hazard ratio; LR, locoregional; OS, overall survival; PF, cisplatin/5-fluorouracil; PFS, progression-free survival; pts, patients; RT, radiation therapy; TTP, time to progression.

Data from Refs.[9–12]

LARYNX PRESERVATION RANDOMIZED TRIALS: SEQUENTIAL CHEMORADIOTHERAPY VERSUS CONCURRENT CHEMORADIOTHERAPY

ST and CRT are both validated as organ preservation strategies in locally advanced larynx cancer. Induction chemotherapy was first established as part of an organ preservation strategy following the landmark Department of Veterans' Affairs Laryngeal Cancer Study Group larynx trial in 1991, which randomized patients to either 3 cycles of PF induction chemotherapy followed by definitive RT or primary surgery followed by postoperative RT.[13] Patients without at least a partial response to induction chemotherapy, and those with evidence of disease progression during or after induction, were managed with surgery and postoperative RT. The larynx preservation rate was 64% in the induction chemotherapy group. The 2-year survival rate was equivalent in both treatment arms (68%).

Concurrent chemoradiotherapy was subsequently evaluated as an alternative to induction chemotherapy followed by RT alone in the RTOG 91-11 study.[14] RTOG 91-11 randomized 547 patients with T2, T3, or low-volume T4 supraglottic or glottic larynx cancer to CRT with bolus cisplatin, PF induction chemotherapy followed by RT alone in responders, or RT alone. In all 3 groups, definitive RT consisted of 70 Gy in 35 fractions. The initial report in 2003 after a median follow-up of 3.8 years concluded that CRT was superior to PF followed by RT, or RT alone for larynx preservation rate (88% vs75% vs70% respectively) at 2 years.[14] CRT and induction chemotherapy were equivalent for the primary end point of laryngectomy-free survival (LFS). OS rates were similar among all 3 groups. Following RTOG 91-11, CRT was adopted in North America, whereas induction chemotherapy continued to be favored in Europe.

Notably, the updated long-term results of RTOG 91-11, with a median of 10.8 years' follow-up, support a more favorable role of induction compared with CRT.[15] The 10-year LFS and OS rates for CRT and induction chemotherapy were similar, and both were superior to RT alone. However, after about 4.5 years, the Kaplan-Meier curves for LFS and OS show clear separation favoring induction chemotherapy compared with CRT (10-year OS 39% vs 28%). This trial was not designed to assess whether this difference was statistically significant but it represents a potentially clinically meaningful difference. Although CRT was associated with a superior larynx preservation rate compared with induction, this was coupled with a statistically significant increase in non-larynx cancer–related deaths in the CRT arm compared with the induction chemotherapy arm (69.8% vs 52.8% at 10 years; $P = .03$). This finding highlights that larynx preservation is an imperfect end point and ultimately success cannot be claimed if many patients succumb to late treatment toxicity that compromises the function of a preserved larynx or ultimately survival.

For larynx cancer, it remains unclear whether an ST approach using modern induction chemotherapy regimens of TPF would result in greater survival benefit or reduction in distant metastases compared with CRT alone. The superiority of TPF compared with PF induction in larynx preservation has been shown,[7] but the optimal CRT regimen following TPF induction chemotherapy is less defined. TREMPLIN is a phase II trial in locally advanced larynx/hypopharynx squamous cell carcinoma that randomized 153 patients to TPF (docetaxel and cisplatin 75 mg/m^2 each on day 1 and fluorouracil 750 mg/m^2 on days 1–5) followed by conventional bolus cisplatin concurrent with radiation or TPF followed by cetuximab-radiation.[16] The primary end point of larynx preservation at 3 months was similar, as were larynx function preservation and OS. Compliance was higher with cetuximab-RT, but there were fewer local failures in the cisplatin-RT arm. Despite this, after salvage surgery (which only occurred in the cetuximab-RT arm) the ultimate local failure rates were comparable between both arms.

CLOSING THE CONTROVERSY: ONGOING RANDOMIZED PHASE III TRIALS OF SEQUENTIAL CHEMORADIOTHERAPY VERSUS CONCURRENT CHEMORADIOTHERAPY

Two ongoing randomized phase III trials may help to settle the debate regarding the superiority of ST versus CRT in LAHNC (**Table 2**). ST consisting of TPF followed by cetuximab-RT is being tested in 2 large phase III trials against either definitive CRT using standard 70-Gy RT concurrent with conventional bolus cisplatin (INTERCEPTOR, NCT00999700) or carboplatin and 5-FU (GORTEC 2007-02, NCT01233843). The ongoing Italian multicenter INTERCEPTOR study has a primary end point of OS. The French multicenter GORTEC study has completed accrual with a primary end point of complete response rate and secondary end point of OS. If results of these studies show the superiority of ST compared with CRT, which would be in keeping with the results of GTTSC,[11] it will be imperative to identify which patient population within LAHNC is most likely to benefit from ST, in order to make progress.

Table 2
Ongoing randomized phase III trials comparing ST and CRT

Study	n (Target)	Eligibility	Treatment Arms	Primary End Point	Secondary End Point
GORTEC 2007-02 (NCT01233843)	370	Unresectable, no prior treatment	A: CRT B: TPF × 3 → cetuximab-RT CRT = carboplatin 70 mg/m² days 1–4, 5-FU 600 mg/m² days 1–4 every 3 wk concurrent with 70 Gy in 2 Gy/d, 5 d/wk × 7 w TPF = docetaxel 100 mg/m² + cisplatin 100 mg/m² + 5-FU 1000 mg/m² days 1–5 Cetuximab-RT = cetuximab 400 mg/m² day 7, 250 mg/m² × 7 wk (RT 70 Gy in 2 Gy/d, 5 d/wk)	Complete response rate	OS
INTERCEPTOR trial (NCT00999700)	278	Unresectable or unsuitable for surgery Stage III/IV LAHNC	A: TPF × 3 → cetuximab + RT B: CRT TPF = docetaxel 75 mg/m² + cisplatin 75 mg/m² + 5-FU 750 mg/m² days 1–5 Cetuximab-RT = cetuximab 400 mg/m² day 7, 250 mg/m² × 7 wk (RT 70 Gy in 2 Gy/d, 5 d/wk) CRT = cisplatin 100 mg/m² every 3 wk concurrent with 70 Gy RT	OS	Toxicity PFS Locoregional control Response rate

PATIENT SELECTION AND RISK STRATIFICATION IN LOCALLY ADVANCED HEAD AND NECK CANCER: ONE SIZE DOES NOT FIT ALL

Routine administration of ST for all patients with LAHNC is not warranted. However, it is likely that a subset of patients is more likely to benefit from ST compared with CRT. LAHNC is heterogeneous and personalized definitive treatment approaches are presently lacking. Patient selection and further tailoring of ST or CRT approaches according to patient risk are desperately needed to improve efficacy and avoid toxicity. Presently, risk stratification and treatment selection are primarily based on anatomic location and traditional tumor, node, metastasis staging. In clinical practice, patients who may be considered for ST are those deemed at high risk for failure because of factors such as extensive primary tumors (T4) and/or advanced nodal involvement (N2, N3), those with significant local symptoms, and those with anticipated delay in initiation of RT. Robust performance status and careful consideration of comorbidities are prerequisites for ST.

Unlike other tumors, validated biomarkers to select patients for therapy are lacking in LAHNC. The presence of HPV is the only validated biomarker and predictor of response to both ST[17] and CRT[18]; however, its prognostic value is limited to oropharynx squamous cell carcinoma and is tempered by tobacco use.[18,19] Distinct genomic differences exist between HPV-positive and HPV-negative LAHNC, and targetable candidate biomarkers exist within both groups.[20] Outcomes compared with the last 2 decades have significantly improved for oropharynx LAHNC, but have improved less for nonoropharynx LAHNC.[21] Most patients with low-risk HPV-related LAHNC are cured, and strategies to reduce long-term treatment toxicities are warranted.[18,22] In contrast, most patients with high-risk LAHNC relapse, suggesting that current approaches are inadequate.[18,22] Taken together, this highlights the rationale to investigate deintensification treatment strategies for HPV-positive low-risk LAHNC, and to test novel approaches for therapeutic intensification for high-risk LAHNC.

STATE OF THE ART: FUTURE DIRECTIONS
Deintensification Strategies for Low-risk Locally Advanced Head and Neck Cancer

Deintensification is intended to reduce toxicity without compromising therapeutic efficacy. Definitive CRT-based strategies include chemosparing by substituting cisplatin with a radiosensitizing epidermal growth factor receptor (EGFR) inhibitor for bioradiation instead. RTOG-1016 is an ongoing randomized phase III trial testing cetuximab with accelerated, intensity-modulated therapy (IMRT) versus 2 cycles of bolus cisplatin with accelerated IMRT in HPV-positive patients with locally advanced oropharyngeal cancer stratified by stage and smoking history (**Table 3**). The primary outcome is survival at 5 years. Similarly, other phase III trials comparing cetuximab-radiation with weekly cisplatin (TROG12.01) or bolus cisplatin (De-ESCALATE) are ongoing in HPV-positive oropharynx cancer (see **Table 3**). Another EGFR monoclonal antibody, panitumumab, combined with accelerated fractionation RT is being tested against conventional high-dose cisplatin concurrent with standard radiation in an ongoing phase III trial, HN.6 (NCT00820248) in LAHNC and may determine whether bioradiation maintains efficacy (PFS primary end point) with reduced toxicity (quality of life is a secondary end point). Notably, a phase II trial (CONCERT-2) of 152 patients comparing panitumumab concurrent with RT versus CRT consisting of 2 cycles of bolus cisplatin showed inferior locoregional control at 2 years in the panitumumab arm.[23]

Deintensification has also been attempted using induction chemotherapy to select patients for reduced-dose radiation as part of ST (see **Table 3**). Dose reduction in radiation from 69.3 Gy to 54 Gy substantially decreases the dose delivered to the pharyngeal constrictor muscles, which may translate into reduction of late swallowing complications. ECOG-1308 is a phase II trial in patients with stage III/IVA HPV-positive oropharynx disease using induction chemotherapy consisting of paclitaxel, cisplatin, and cetuximab to select patients for response-adapted RT with standard or low-dose IMRT concurrent with cetuximab.[24] The complete clinical response rate to induction was 71%, and low-dose radiation (54 Gy IMRT) resulted in 2-year PFS of 80% and 2-year survival of 93%.[24] PFS in patients who had less than a complete clinical response to induction therapy was 65% and the 2-year OS was 87%. Patients with the best outcomes with 54 Gy were those with smoking history of less than 10 pack years, non-T4 and non-N2c disease (2-year PFS and OS of 96%), suggesting that this patient population may be most suitable for deintensification. Induction chemotherapy consisting of TPF is being used to assign patients for subsequent deintensification of RT in an ongoing phase III trial (Quarterback Trial) (see **Table 3**). Nonresponders to induction will receive standard chemoradiation, whereas patients with a complete or partial response will be randomized 2:1 to weekly carboplatin concurrent with low-dose radiation (56 Gy) versus weekly carboplatin with standard-dose radiation (70 Gy).

Intensification Strategies for High-risk Locally Advanced Head and Neck Cancer

In high-risk LAHNC, therapeutic intensification is being explored with the addition of novel agents to the definitive CRT backbone. Progress in this arena has been disappointing, and this may in part be because of early combined toxicities,[25] limited preclinical data, and evaluation of targeted therapies in unselected patient populations. RTOG 0522, a large randomized phase III trial in LAHNC, found that the addition of cetuximab accelerated radiation compared with concurrent bolus cisplatin-radiation, which resulted in no difference in PFS and OS, but increased serious adverse events.[26] The addition of panitumumab to standard fractionation RT and bolus cisplatin in a randomized phase II trial (CONCERT-1) was also negative.[27] The oral EGFR and ErbB2 tyrosine kinase inhibitor, lapatinib, is being tested in similar fashion in a randomized phase II trial (TRYHARD, NCT01711658). Dacomitinib, an oral second-generation EGFR tyrosine kinase inhibitor, is being evaluated concurrently with radiation, with or without cisplatin, in a phase I trial in LAHNC, with the plan for dose expansion of dacomitinib plus chemoradiation in HPV-negative LAHNC (NCT01737008). Beyond EGFR, alterations in the phosphatidylinositol 3 kinase (PI3K) pathway are frequently observed in LAHNC. A phase Ib study of the addition of the PI3K inhibitor, BKM120, to concurrent cisplatin-radiation in high-risk LAHNC is underway (NCT02113878). Other novel strategies in phase I testing include the addition of the poly(ADP-ribose) polymerase-1 inhibitor, olaparib, to cisplatin-radiation in high-risk LAHNC (NCT01758731), and also olaparib added to cetuximab-radiation in heavy smokers (NCT01758731). In addition, immune checkpoint inhibition combining ipilimumab, cetuximab, and radiation is also in phase Ib testing in the intermediate to high-risk LAHNC population (NCT01860430, NCT01935921).

Novel ST regimens testing new induction regimens are also under investigation as a strategy to intensify therapy in high-risk LAHNC. The addition of cetuximab to TPF induction in the context of ST, with subsequent platinum-radiation[12] or cetuximab-radiation is feasible.[28] Cetuximab-TPF followed by carboplatin-radiation is being compared with another ST approach consisting of cetuximab-paclitaxel-carboplatin[29] followed by weekly cisplatin-radiation in a large randomized phase II trial in stage IV LAHNC (NCT01154920) (see **Table 3**). Study accrual is complete and data are maturing for the primary end point of PFS at 2 years. Alternatively, other modifications

Table 3
Examples of clinical trials using CRT or ST as potential strategies to deintensify therapy for low-risk patients with LAHNC or intensify therapeutic efficacy for high-risk LAHNC

	Chemoradiation				Sequential Therapy			
	Trial	n	Phase	Treatment	Trial	n	Phase	Treatment
Deintensification for low-risk LAHNC	RTOG-1016 (NCT01302834)	706	3	Cetuximab vs bolus cisplatin concurrent with accelerated IMRT (70 Gy in 6 wk)	ECOG-1308[a] (NCT01084083)	83	2	Induction chemotherapy followed by response-adapted RT (54 or 66–70 Gy) with cetuximab
	TROG12.01 (NCT01855451)	200	3	Cetuximab vs weekly cisplatin concurrent with RT (70 Gy)	The Quarterback Trial (NCT01706939)	365	3	Induction chemotherapy with TPF: pts with CR or PR will be randomized 2:1 to weekly carboplatin concurrent with RT (56 Gy) vs weekly carboplatin concurrent with RT (70 Gy). Nonresponders will receive standard chemoradiation
	De-ESCALATE (NCT01874171)	304	3	Cetuximab vs bolus cisplatin concurrent with RT (70 Gy)	—	—	—	—
	CONCERT-2[23,a]	152	2	Panitumumab vs bolus cisplatin concurrent with RT	—	—	—	—

Category	Trial	No.	Phase	Regimen
Intensification for high-risk LAHNC	RTOG 0522[26,a]	940	3	Bolus cisplatin concurrent with accelerated IMRT with or without cetuximab
	CONCERT-1[27,a]	153	2	Bolus cisplatin concurrent with RT (70 Gy) with or without panitumumab
	TRYHARD (NCT01711658)	176	2	Bolus cisplatin concurrent with IMRT with or without lapatinib (1500 mg daily 1 wk before radiation, followed by 1500 mg daily concurrent with radiation, followed by 1500 mg daily for 3 mo)
	NCT01737008	34	1	Dacomitinib concurrent with accelerated IMRT alone, or dacomitinib concurrent with bolus cisplatin and standard radiation
	NCT02113878	46	1b	BKM120 with weekly cisplatin concurrent with IMRT
	NCT01154920	128	2	Cetuximab-TPF → carboplatin-radiation vs PCC → weekly cisplatin-radiation
	NCT00736944[30,a]	30	2	APF-cetuximab → CRT (nab-paclitaxel 100 mg/m^2/wk; cisplatin 75 mg/m^2 on day 1; cetuximab 250 mg/m^2/wk; 5-FU 750 mg/m^2/d on days 1–3) every 21 d for 3 cycles followed by CRT (cisplatin 100 mg/m^2 on days 1, 22, and 43 of RT)
	GORTEC trial (NCT02216617)	22	1b	Afatinib-docetaxel/cisplatin induction: docetaxel 75 mg/m^2 at day 1, cisplatin 75 mg/m^2 at day 1; afatinib x mg/d day 2–21 by level (level 1 = 20 mg/d; level 2 = 30 mg/d; level 3 = 40 mg/d)
	NCT01732640	71	1–2	Afatinib-carboplatin/paclitaxel → weekly cisplatin-IMRT (afatinib, carboplatin AUC 6 and paclitaxel 175 mg/m^2 every 21 × 2 cycles followed by weekly cisplatin [40 mg/m^2] concurrent with radiation)
	NCT01133678	80	1–2	Everolimus-cisplatin/paclitaxel/cetuximab induction

Abbreviation: PCC, paclitaxel-cetuximab-carboplatin; PR, Partial response.
[a] Trial completed.

to TPF include substituting docetaxel with nab-paclitaxel, to enhance transport of drug into cells. A phase II trial of 30 patients treated with induction nab-paclitaxel, cisplatin, 5-FU, and cetuximab (APF-C) followed by bolus cisplatin-radiation showed a complete response rate of 53% and PFS of 65% at 2 years.[30] APF-C may have promising clinical activity compared with cetuximab-TPF but has not been compared in a clinical trial.[31] Nab-paclitaxel in combination with carboplatin-paclitaxel induction is also feasible,[32] and a phase II study of nab-paclitaxel with carboplatin-cetuximab induction in poor-prognosis LAHNC is ongoing (NCT01412229). Targeted agents, including afatinib, a second-generation oral EGFR kinase inhibitor, are being tested in induction regimens combined with carboplatin-paclitaxel in HPV-negative LAHNC (NCT01732640), or combined with docetaxel-cisplatin induction (NCT02216617). A phase I/II trial of everolimus combined with cisplatin/paclitaxel/cetuximab induction is also underway (NCT01133678).

SUMMARY

ST and CRT are valid, definitive, nonsurgical management options for LAHNC. Controversy remains regarding the superiority of one regimen compared with another because recent phase III randomized controlled trials have had limited statistical power to detect a survival difference.[8–10] Only 1 adequately powered randomized phase III trial has recently shown a survival benefit favoring ST compared with CRT.[11] Definitive management of LAHNC continues to evolve with increasing efforts to investigate deintensification of therapy for HPV-positive low-risk LAHNC, and to pursue therapeutic intensification for high-risk LAHNC. Both ST and CRT serve as potential modalities to achieve these goals. Deintensification strategies currently under investigation include chemosparing CRT with bioradiation regimens, and the use of induction chemotherapy to select patients for subsequent reduced-dose radiation as part of ST. In contrast, therapeutic intensification is being explored with the addition of novel agents to the CRT backbone, and novel induction regimens as part of ST. Therefore ST and CRT may both play critical roles in shaping treatment paradigms and future progress.

REFERENCES

1. Ferlay J, Soerjomatarm I, Ervik M, et al. Cancer incidence and mortality worldwide: IARC CancerBase No. 11. Lyon (France): International Agency for Research On Cancer; 2012. v1.0. Accessed March 31, 2015. Available at: http://globocan.iarc.fr/Default.aspx.
2. Blanchard P, Baujat B, Holostenco V, et al. Meta-analysis of Chemotherapy in Head and Neck Cancer (MACH-NC): a comprehensive analysis by tumour site. Radiother Oncol 2011;100:33–40.
3. Pignon JP, le Maitre A, Maillard E, et al. Meta-analysis of Chemotherapy in Head and Neck Cancer (MACH-NC): an update on 93 randomised trials and 17,346 patients. Radiother Oncol 2009;92:4–14.
4. Pignon JP, Bourhis J, Domenge C, et al. Chemotherapy added to locoregional treatment for head and neck squamous-cell carcinoma: three meta-analyses of updated individual data. MACH-NC Collaborative Group. Meta-Analysis of Chemotherapy on Head and Neck Cancer. Lancet 2000;355:949–55.
5. Posner MR, Hershock DM, Blajman CR, et al. Cisplatin and fluorouracil alone or with docetaxel in head and neck cancer. N Engl J Med 2007;357:1705–15.
6. Vermorken JB, Remenar E, van Herpen C, et al. Cisplatin, fluorouracil, and docetaxel in unresectable head and neck cancer. N Engl J Med 2007;357: 1695–704.

7. Pointreau Y, Garaud P, Chapet S, et al. Randomized trial of induction chemotherapy with cisplatin and 5-fluorouracil with or without docetaxel for larynx preservation. J Natl Cancer Inst 2009;101:498–506.
8. Haddad R, O'Neill A, Rabinowits G, et al. Induction chemotherapy followed by concurrent chemoradiotherapy (sequential chemoradiotherapy) versus concurrent chemoradiotherapy alone in locally advanced head and neck cancer (PARADIGM): a randomised phase 3 trial. Lancet Oncol 2013;14:257–64.
9. Cohen EE, Karrison TG, Kocherginsky M, et al. Phase III randomized trial of induction chemotherapy in patients with N2 or N3 locally advanced head and neck cancer. J Clin Oncol 2014;32:2735–43.
10. Hitt R, Grau JJ, Lopez-Pousa A, et al. A randomized phase III trial comparing induction chemotherapy followed by chemoradiotherapy versus chemoradiotherapy alone as treatment of unresectable head and neck cancer. Ann Oncol 2014;25:216–25.
11. Ghi MG, Paccagnella A, Ferrari D, et al. Concomitant CRT or Cetuximab/RT Versus Induction Docetaxel/Cisplatin/5-FU (TPF) followed by CRT or Cetuximab/RT in patients with LASCCHN: A randomized phase III factorial study - efficacy results (NCT01086826). J Clin Oncol 2014;32:5s [abstract: 6004].
12. Haddad RI, Tishler RB, Norris C, et al. Phase I study of C-TPF in patients with locally advanced squamous cell carcinoma of the head and neck. J Clin Oncol 2009;27:4448–53.
13. Induction chemotherapy plus radiation compared with surgery plus radiation in patients with advanced laryngeal cancer. The Department of Veterans Affairs Laryngeal Cancer Study Group. N Engl J Medicine 1991;324:1685–90.
14. Forastiere AA, Goepfert H, Maor M, et al. Concurrent chemotherapy and radiotherapy for organ preservation in advanced laryngeal cancer. N Engl J Med 2003;349:2091–8.
15. Forastiere AA, Zhang Q, Weber RS, et al. Long-term results of RTOG 91-11: a comparison of three nonsurgical treatment strategies to preserve the larynx in patients with locally advanced larynx cancer. J Clin Oncol 2013;31:845–52.
16. Lefebvre JL, Pointreau Y, Rolland F, et al. Induction chemotherapy followed by either chemoradiotherapy or bioradiotherapy for larynx preservation: the TREMPLIN randomized phase II study. J Clin Oncol 2013;31:853–9.
17. Posner MR, Lorch JH, Goloubeva O, et al. Survival and human papillomavirus in oropharynx cancer in TAX 324: a subset analysis from an international phase III trial. Ann Oncol 2011;22:1071–7.
18. Ang KK, Harris J, Wheeler R, et al. Human papillomavirus and survival of patients with oropharyngeal cancer. N Engl J Med 2010;363:24–35.
19. O'Sullivan B, Huang SH, Siu LL, et al. Deintensification candidate subgroups in human papillomavirus-related oropharyngeal cancer according to minimal risk of distant metastasis. J Clin Oncol 2013;31:543–50.
20. Seiwert TY, Zuo Z, Keck MK, et al. Integrative and comparative genomic analysis of HPV-positive and HPV-negative head and neck squamous cell carcinomas. Clin Cancer Res 2015;21:632–41.
21. Das LC, Karrison TG, Witt ME, et al. Comparison of outcomes of locoregionally advanced oropharyngeal and non-oropharyngeal squamous cell carcinoma over two decades. Ann Oncol 2015;26:198–205.
22. Nguyen-Tan PF, Zhang Q, Ang KK, et al. Randomized phase III trial to test accelerated versus standard fractionation in combination with concurrent cisplatin for head and neck carcinomas in the Radiation Therapy Oncology Group 0129 trial: long-term report of efficacy and toxicity. J Clin Oncol 2014;32:3858–66.

23. Giralt J, Trigo J, Nuyts S, et al. Panitumumab plus radiotherapy versus chemora-diotherapy in patients with unresected, locally advanced squamous-cell carcinoma of the head and neck (CONCERT-2): a randomised, controlled, open-label phase 2 trial. Lancet Oncol 2015;16:221–32.
24. Cmelak A, Li S, Marur S, et al. E1308: Reduced-dose IMRT in HPV-associated resectable oropharyngeal squamous cell carcinomas after complete clinical response to induction chemotherapy. J Clin Oncol 2014;32:5s [abstract: 6006].
25. Adkins D, Ley J, Wildes TM, et al. RTOG 0522: huge investment in patients and resources and no benefit with addition of cetuximab to radiotherapy-why did this occur? J Clin Oncol 2015;33:1223–4.
26. Ang KK, Zhang Q, Rosenthal DI, et al. Randomized phase III trial of concurrent accelerated radiation plus cisplatin with or without cetuximab for stage III to IV head and neck carcinoma: RTOG 0522. J Clin Oncol 2014;32:2940–50.
27. Mesia R, Henke M, Fortin A, et al. Chemoradiotherapy with or without panitumu-mab in patients with unresected, locally advanced squamous-cell carcinoma of the head and neck (CONCERT-1): a randomised, controlled, open-label phase 2 trial. Lancet Oncol 2015;16:208–20.
28. Charalambakis N, Kouloulias V, Vaja H, et al. Feasibility of Induction docetaxel, cisplatin, 5-fluorouracil, cetuximab (TPF-C) followed by concurrent cetuximab radiotherapy for locally advanced head and neck squamous cell carcinoma. Front Oncol 2013;3:5.
29. Kies MS, Holsinger FC, Lee JJ, et al. Induction chemotherapy and cetuximab for locally advanced squamous cell carcinoma of the head and neck: results from a phase II prospective trial. J Clin Oncol 2010;28:8–14.
30. Adkins D, Ley J, Trinkaus K, et al. A phase 2 trial of induction nab-paclitaxel and cetuximab given with cisplatin and 5-fluorouracil followed by concurrent cisplatin and radiation for locally advanced squamous cell carcinoma of the head and neck. Cancer 2013;119:766–73.
31. Schell A, Ley J, Wu N, et al. Nab-paclitaxel-based compared to docetaxel-based induction chemotherapy regimens for locally advanced squamous cell carcinoma of the head and neck. Cancer Med 2015;4:481–9.
32. Loong HH, Winquist E, Waldron J, et al. Phase 1 study of nab-paclitaxel, cisplatin and 5-fluorouracil as induction chemotherapy followed by concurrent chemora-diotherapy in locoregionally advanced squamous cell carcinoma of the oropharynx. Eur J Cancer 2014;50:2263–70.

Transoral Endoscopic Head and Neck Surgery

The Contemporary Treatment of Head and Neck Cancer

Gil Chai Lim, MD[a], Floyd Christopher Holsinger, MD[b], Ryan J. Li, MD[b],*

KEYWORDS

- Transoral endoscopic head and neck surgery • Transoral robotic surgery
- Head and neck neoplasms • Transoral laser microsurgery • Oropharynx
- Human papillomavirus

KEY POINTS

- Quality of life in patients with head and neck cancer can be largely affected by posttreatment preservation of laryngeal function.
- Comprehensive radiation therapy usually creates a significant swallowing dysfunction that may be potentiated by chemotherapy.
- Transoral endoscopic head and neck surgeries with or without adjuvant therapy show survival rates comparable with those of nonsurgical organ-preservation therapy in head and neck cancer, and may result in less swallow impairment for select patients.

BACKGROUND AND INTRODUCTION
The Multidisciplinary Care of Head and Neck Cancer

Head and neck cancer (HNC) is a significant public health problem worldwide, with more than 500,000 new cases per year.[1] India, the United States, and western Europe have the highest incidences of HNC worldwide with age-standardized incidence rates of 10.5 to 14.1 per 100,000 persons in 2012.[2] Tobacco use and alcohol consumption are major causes of HNC, showing a multiplicative effect on cancer risk when used

The authors have nothing to disclose.
[a] Department of Otolaryngology-Head and Neck Surgery, Jeju National University School of Medicine, 102 Jejudaehak-ro, Jeju Special Self-Governing Province 63243, Republic of Korea;
[b] Department of Otolaryngology – Head and Neck Surgery, Stanford University School of Medicine, 875 Blake Wilbur Drive, Palo Alto, CA 94305-5820, USA
* Corresponding author. Head and Neck Surgery, Department of Otolaryngology – Head and Neck Surgery, Stanford University, 875 Blake Wilbur Drive, Palo Alto, CA 94305-5820.
E-mail address: rli@ohns.stanford.edu

Hematol Oncol Clin N Am 29 (2015) 1075–1092
http://dx.doi.org/10.1016/j.hoc.2015.08.001
0889-8588/15/$ – see front matter © 2015 Elsevier Inc. All rights reserved.

hemonc.theclinics.com

together.[3] In the last 2 decades, human papillomavirus (HPV) has been identified as an important risk factor for developing HNC. Chaturvedi and colleagues[4] described the striking new association between oropharyngeal cancer (OPC) and high-risk strains of HPV, elucidating a new epidemiology in a subset of HNC patients. This study estimated population-based incidence of HPV-positive and HPV-negative OPC in the United States using the Surveillance, Epidemiology, and End Results (SEER) database from 1988 to 2004. During this period, HPV-positive OPC increased by 225% (95% confidence interval [CI] 208%–242%; from 0.8 per 100,000 to 2.6 per 100,000), whereas the incidence of HPV-negative cancers declined by 50% (95% CI[5] 47%–53%; from 2.0 per 100,000 to 1.0 per 100,000). Patients with HPV-associated OPC are more likely to be nonsmokers, male, and younger than "traditional" patients with HNC[6] (**Table 1**).

In the past, OPCs were often treated with disfiguring transfacial, transmandibular approaches,[7] yet many patients still required extensive adjuvant therapy postoperatively. Poor posttreatment function led multidisciplinary teams worldwide to explore alternative options, such as concurrent chemotherapy with radiation therapy (CCRT).[8]

The Radiation Therapy Oncology Group (RTOG) trial 0129 provided strong evidence that HPV status is an independent prognostic factor for overall survival (OS) and progression-free survival (PFS) among patients with OPC.[9] Furthermore, HPV-positive tumors were exquisitely responsive to CCRT. Locoregional failure at 3 years was 21% lower in patients with HPV-positive tumors, at 13.6% (95% CI 8.9%–18.3%) versus 35.1% (95% CI 26.4–43.8) for HPV-negative tumors ($P<.001$).[9] The 3-year OS for HPV-positive patients treated with CCRT was 83%, including T3-T4 patients and those with advanced staged regional disease.

The treatment of advanced-stage laryngeal and hypopharyngeal cancers historically required radical surgery, most often a total laryngectomy with partial or total pharyngectomy, followed by adjuvant radiation therapy. Although radical surgery can achieve oncologic control, the functional sacrifices to voice, swallowing, and

Table 1
Comparison of HPV-positive and HPV-negative oropharyngeal carcinoma

	HPV-Positive	HPV-Negative
Incidence	Increasing	Decreasing
Age	Younger	Older
Gender	3:1 (M/F)	3:1 (M/F)
Risk factors	Sexual behavior	Tobacco, alcohol
Cofactors	Marijuana, immunosuppression	Diet, oral hygiene
Molecular genetics	p16 ↑ Rb ↓ p53 wild-type	p16 ↓ Rb ↑ p53 mutated
Anatomic site	Lingual and palatine tonsils	All sites
Pathologic findings		
Primary	Basaloid	Keratinized
Lymphatic metastasis	Cystic, mixed	Solid
Survival	Better	Worse

From Westra WH. The changing face of head and neck cancer in the 21st century: the impact of HPV on the epidemiology and pathology of oral cancer. Head Neck Pathol 2009;3:79.

cosmesis can be devastating for patients. In 1991 the Veterans Affairs Laryngeal Cancer Study Group (VALCSG) reported the first randomized comparison between laryngectomy with or without radiation therapy, and induction chemotherapy followed by radiation therapy for the treatment of advanced laryngeal cancer. This study demonstrated the role of induction chemotherapy (cisplatin and 5-fluorouracil) followed by radiation therapy[10] in laryngeal preservation. Equivalent survival rates were achieved in the surgical and nonsurgical treatment arms. Of the patients receiving induction chemotherapy, 64% ultimately preserved their larynges, a major development in functional preservation that led to widespread adoption of nonsurgical treatment protocols. Subsequent important randomized trials demonstrated a significant potential for laryngeal preservation in the nonsurgical treatment of laryngeal and hypopharyngeal cancers.[11–14]

Despite enthusiasm for CCRT and induction chemotherapy protocols, significant delayed toxicity and functional morbidity can still result, even with anatomic larynx preservation. Dysphagia related to chronic xerostomia and impaired laryngeal function may be the most debilitating of functional impairments in HNC survivors.[15] In a pooled analysis of 3 RTOG trials of concomitant chemoradiotherapy,[16] late onset of RTOG grade 3 and 4 laryngeal toxicity was reported in 35% of 101 OPC survivors. The 3-year prevalence of dysphagia approaches 50% in population-level data from OPC survivors in the SEER-Medicare database.[17] As the landscape of HNC continues to evolve, in particular with the growing incidence of HPV-associated OPC patients achieving long-term survival, a renewed interest in the role of surgery as a function-preserving treatment is being investigated.[18]

TRANSORAL ENDOSCOPIC HEAD AND NECK SURGERY

Transoral endoscopic head and neck surgery (eHNS)[19] has emerged as a vital part of multidisciplinary HNC care. In comparison with open surgical approaches, eHNS minimizes the extent of soft-tissue dissection that may potentially disrupt organs of speech, voice, and swallowing. For this reason eHNS has received increasing attention for the primary treatment of select HNCs. When performed with elective neck dissection, the ability to obtain pathologic staging information by primary surgical treatment is an important advantage that may direct adjuvant therapy or negate its need. The ability to determine the presence or absence of perineural invasion (PNI) or lymphovascular invasion (LVI) at the primary site, in addition to the regional lymph node burden and presence of extracapsular extension, can dictate whether to intensify or de-intensify adjuvant therapy. Walvekar and colleagues[20] reported a series of 49 patients with clinically early-stage OPC, treated with primary surgery. Clinical staging was modified in 20 of 49 (40%) patients after surgery, with 12 of these patients pathologically downstaged. The additional information provided by eHNS staging may allow select patients to minimize treatment morbidity when adjuvant therapy can be de-intensified or avoided.

The role of eHNS in HPV-positive OPC patients is currently being studied in the phase II randomized clinical trial ECOG 3311. This trial examines the role of transoral surgical resection in p16-positive oropharyngeal cancers, for the de-escalation of the overall treatment regimen. In particular, p16-positive, locally advanced (stage III/IV: cT1–2, N1-N2b, M0) OPC patients are eligible for participation. There are essentially 4 treatment arms:

- All patients undergo transoral surgical resection of the primary tumor, with a neck dissection of cervical levels II through IV.
- Treatment arm 1 (low risk: pT1–2, N0–1) patients are subsequently observed.

- Treatment arms 2 and 3 (intermediate risk: including clear but close margins; perineural or lymphovascular invasion; <1 mm of nodal extracapsular extension; or 2–4 metastatic lymph nodes)
  - These patients are randomized to either arm 2: intensity-modulated radiation therapy (IMRT) of 50 Gy in 25 fractionated doses; or arm 3: IMRT of 60 Gy in 30 fractionated doses.
- Treatment arm 4 (high risk: positive margins; >1 mm of nodal extracapsular extension; or at least 5 metastatic lymph nodes)
  - These patients receive IMRT of 66 Gy in 33 fractionated doses and cisplatin 40 mg/mm^2 weekly.

This trial primarily aims to compare 2-year PFS in patients receiving low-dose adjuvant radiation (treatment arm 2) versus current standard adjuvant dosing at 60 Gy (treatment arm 3). Secondarily the trial will evaluate treatment toxicity, functional outcomes, and patients' quality of life. Patients at intermediate risk for disease progression are the primary interest: in these patients full adjuvant dosing of radiation therapy may be reduced to lessen toxicity. Transoral surgery may play a role in determining which patients are at intermediate risk for disease progression, and whether de-escalation of therapy is oncologically feasible.

The 2 most commonly used eHNS techniques for HNC are transoral laser microsurgery (TLM)[21] and transoral robotic surgery (TORS).[22] In contrast to open surgical approaches, TLM and TORS approach mucosal tumors via direct, magnified visualization. Whether using a binocular microscope and carbon dioxide laser for TLM or the da Vinci Surgical System (Intuitive Surgical, Sunnyvale, CA, USA) for TORS, the successful resection of select laryngeal and pharyngeal tumors relies on both adequate visualization of the tumor and adequate exposure for surgical ablative instruments. There are several differences between these 2 eHNS techniques.

TLM is performed under direct suspension laryngoscopy (or in OPC, pharyngoscopy), using a binocular operating microscope, microsurgical instruments, and a carbon dioxide laser. TLM relies on the surgeon's understanding of the 3-dimensional anatomy of the tumor's extent and surrounding anatomy. Described first in the late 1960s and early 1970s,[23] the technique of TLM has being progressively refined. Steiner[21] first described division of the tumor as a means to understand the full depth and extent of the lesion, before systematically performing circumferential resection with appropriate surgical margins. TLM requires a direct line-of-sight approach to tumors, which was a limitation to its use in the treatment of tongue-base tumors. The development of curved and angled fiberoptic lasers has facilitated operations around the curvature of the tongue base. In tongue-base TLM, tumor resection may require piecemeal excision rather than en bloc excision. Although this may seem oncologically contentious, several studies have reported equivalent negative margins achieved during piecemeal and en bloc resection.[24,25]

In 2009, the US Food and Drug Administration (FDA) approved the use of the da Vinci Surgical System for transoral surgical treatment of OPC and sleep apnea procedures. TORS for HNC is performed using a central endoscopic camera arm and 2 surgical arms. All 3 arms are controlled by a surgeon sitting at a remote console. After appropriate dental protection, an oral retractor is positioned within the mouth, and a 0° or 30° endoscopic camera is introduced into the oropharynx followed by 2 surgical arms carrying interchangeable 5-mm or 8-mm wide working instruments (eg, grasping forceps, electrocautery, CO_2 or thulium laser).[26,27] The instruments have 540° of wristed range of motion. At the remote console, the surgeon views a 3-dimensional display of the surgical site, with finger-control handpieces directing movements of the robot's instruments and camera. In tongue-base cancer surgery, the use of a 30° scope may offer improved visual exposure in comparison with the line-of-sight microscope views of TLM, and can facilitate en bloc tumor resection.

Numerous retrospective single-institution studies have examined the oncologic and functional outcomes of TLM and TORS in HNC treatment, in addition to 2 larger multicenter retrospective studies reporting outcomes comparable with those after radiation-based primary treatment protocols.[19,22,28,29] As described earlier, important initiatives to prospectively study the role of eHNS techniques in multidisciplinary HNC care are under way.[30] In many cases of primary HNC surgery, eHNS has replaced open surgical approaches with reduced acute morbidity, shorter hospital stay, and quicker functional recovery.[22,28,31,32] Defining which HNC patients are appropriate candidates for eHNS is challenging; oncologic principles for resection margins must be achievable.[33] Studies consistently report TLM and TORS achieving negative surgical margins at rates greater than 88%.[34–39] The American Joint Committee on Cancer tumor staging system alone does not sufficiently identify which patients will benefit from eHNS. For example, a T1 midline tongue-base tumor may be small in absolute volume, but have a broad-based, sessile shape requiring extensive bilateral tongue-base resection to obtain negative margins. Conversely, a 4.5-cm T3 tonsillar primary may have a pedunculated, narrow-stalked shape, making negative margins attainable with less sacrifice of normal tissue. In the former scenario, primary radiation therapy may offer the least morbidity. In the latter, if transoral surgery can achieve negative margins and both PNI and LVI are absent, this situation may argue for dose reduction or deferral of adjuvant radiation.

Role of Endoscopic Head and Neck Surgery in Oropharyngeal Cancer

Traditional open surgical approaches to the oropharynx have included lateral or supraglottic pharyngotomy, and mandibular osteotomy and swing.[40] Transoral access without specialized instrumentation is difficult for both tumor visualization and maneuverability of surgical instruments. Therefore the open approaches were the most accepted surgical techniques, despite requiring dissection through supporting oral cavity musculature and/or disrupting mandibular integrity. Complex reconstruction was often indicated after open surgical approaches to the oropharynx given the resultant extensive tissue loss. Although no prospective, randomized controlled studies exist to directly compare oncologic outcomes in surgical and nonsurgical approaches, primary radiation or chemoradiation protocols have largely superseded open approaches in previously untreated oropharyngeal cancers. Proponents of TLM and TORS have led a renewed interest in eHNS for the treatment of OPC. As already discussed, both techniques provide excellent access to select tonsillar primaries, whereas the line-of-sight limitations of TLM in tongue-base surgery may be overcome in part by flexible fiberoptic lasers, or avoided by using TORS in these cases.[41,42]

While currently available oncologic outcomes research that evaluates eHNS in OPC has been retrospective, reported disease-free survival (DFS) and OS rates have been greater than 90% in advanced disease, a finding comparable with historical data for nonsurgical primary treatments.[22,43–45] Negative margins at the time of eHNS are critical for obtaining local control.[16]

As previously discussed, the rising epidemic of HPV-associated OPC is a driving force for close scrutiny of primary treatment protocols. These patients tend to be younger with less medical comorbidity relative to HPV-negative OPC. HPV-associated OPC seems to show a greater response to both surgical and nonsurgical treatment modalities.[46–49] With longer-term survival comes increased susceptibility to late-onset adverse effects of treatment: osteoradionecrosis (in the case of radiation therapy), fibrosis and trismus, dental deterioration, xerostomia with dysphagia, and aspiration. With these considerations the prospective randomized trial ECOG 3311 specifically focuses on HPV-associated OPC, attempting to answer the question whether eHNS may be used to lower the dosage of adjuvant radiation therapy these patients receive, with lower morbidity than open oropharyngeal procedures, and accurate pathologic staging. From this trial it may become evident that eHNS and nonsurgical treatment protocols will frequently be complementary in the treatment of HPV-associated OPC, with the former facilitating reduced radiation dosages.

Role of Endoscopic Head and Neck Surgery in Laryngeal Cancer

TLM is a valuable technique in the treatment of laryngeal cancer, wherein preservation of the uninvolved laryngeal subsites can significantly contribute to posttreatment quality of life. Many centers have adopted TLM for primary treatment of early-stage tumors. Morbidity is reduced and duration of treatment is shorter in TLM when compared with open surgical approaches and radiation therapy, respectively. Even with T1b lesions involving both true vocal folds,[43] unilateral TLM resection followed by a staged contralateral TLM has been advocated, so that anterior commissural webbing is avoided. Although the indications for TLM in more advanced tumors (eg, T3 with preepiglottic invasion) become contentious, local control can be achieved in select cases.[42,50,51] Determination of the appropriate T3 patients for TLM must consider whether exposure of the tumor site is attainable, whether the patient can tolerate temporary aspiration, whether the tumor truly is free from cartilage involvement, or whether there is extension into soft tissue of the neck beyond the preepiglottic space. Although the use of TORS in supraglottic and even total laryngectomy has been described previously,[52,53] significant access limitations exist for sites caudal to the oropharynx, both in visualization and ability to maneuver surgical instruments.

Role of Endoscopic Head and Neck Surgery in Hypopharyngeal Cancer

Hypopharyngeal cancers are often localized to the apical or medial pyriform wall, or postcricoid area, necessitating sacrifice of the adjacent larynx for adequate margins. Often these tumors remain asymptomatic until the advanced stage, another reason why open total laryngectomy with partial or complete pharyngectomy becomes the only surgical option. Primary chemoradiation protocols are widely advocated for hypopharyngeal primaries, given their propensity for submucosal spread that is difficult to surgically clear, and because there is a high risk for regional and distant metastatic disease. Unfortunately pharyngeal strictures, fibrosis, and chondronecrosis of the adjacent larynx do occur in 21% to 37% of chemoradiated patients.[54,55] The access limitations of eHNS in hypopharyngeal surgery is analogous to the challenges encountered in laryngeal procedures. In the case of hypopharyngeal cancer, however, endoscopic resection of lesions (eg, T1/T2 lesions of the lateral pyriform sinus or posterior hypopharyngeal wall) may mitigate the risk of pharyngocutaneous fistula formation inherent to open pharyngectomy techniques. Although some retrospective studies have described similar DFS and OS rates in TLM or TORS for select cases when compared with open pharyngectomy or concurrent chemoradiation, the biology of this disease is far more aggressive than most oropharyngeal and glottic tumors, and a stronger argument for aggressive multimodality treatment from the onset may be made.[56–58]

ONCOLOGIC OUTCOMES OF ENDOSCOPIC HEAD AND NECK SURGERY

Although no prospective studies of oncologic outcomes in TLM or TORS have been reported, several large retrospective studies have been published from multi-institutional collaborations, in addition to a series of informative, but smaller, single-center reports.

Endoscopic Head and Neck Surgery Outcomes for Oropharyngeal Cancer

In one multi-institutional study, Haughey and colleagues[34] reported on 204 patients with stage III and IV OPC who underwent primary TLM with or without adjuvant radiation or chemoradiation. The 5-year OS, disease-specific survival (DSS), and DFS rates were 78%, 84%, and 74%, respectively. HPV and p16 testing was available in 174 of 204 (85%) and 185 of 204 (91%) of patients, respectively. Of those with available testing, 74% and 90% of patients were HPV-positive and p16-positive, respectively. Both p16 and HPV positivity were associated with a significant decrease in risk of death by any cause (hazard ratio 0.11–0.12 and 0.3–0.4) on multivariate analysis, a finding consistent with primary radiation protocol data.

The past decade saw a rapid growth in the application of TORS for the treatment of select OPCs.[43–45,59] Oncologic outcomes were comparable with those obtained historically in nonsurgical treatment protocols. Weinstein and colleagues[45] reviewed 47 OPC patients who had undergone TORS, observing a 90% 2-year DSS. In this study local recurrence occurred in 2% of patients. Similarly, White and colleagues studied[60] HNC patients who had undergone TORS, 77 of whom had oropharyngeal primaries (87%). In this study, 3 of 89 (3.3%) patients experienced a local recurrence. Overall recurrence-free survival (RFS) was 86.5% at 2 years. Weinstein and colleagues[22] more recently investigated surgical margin status in a multicenter series of 177 TORS patients, finding 7 of 161 (4.3%) patients with available margin data being positive on final analysis. For historical comparison, in 1978 Byers and colleagues[61] published a series of 216 patients with oral cavity, oropharyngeal, and hypopharyngeal cancers treated with open surgery, achieving negative margins in nearly 90% of cases.

In the largest retrospective multicenter study of oncologic outcomes in TORS to date, 13 institutions collaborated for a pooled analysis of 410 patients, 364 (89%) of whom had OPC.[29] HPV tumor status was available in 229 of 410 (55.9%) patients, of whom 159 (69.4%) were HPV positive. In this series, 43 of 410 (10.5%) patients experienced a locoregional recurrence, and 10 of 410 (2.4%) developed distant metastases. The 2-year and 3-year locoregional control (LRC) rates were 91.8% and 88.8%, respectively. OS at 2 and 3 years was 91% and 87.1%, respectively, with DSS of 94.5% and 92.5%. On multivariate analysis only tobacco use predicted worse OS, whereas tonsillar primary site predicted improved OS. The results of this multicenter study compared favorably with studies of primary radiation therapy in the treatment of OPC, in which LRC ranged from 91% to 97%. No differences in outcomes were observed between HPV-positive and HPV-negative patients, although only 56% of patients had data on HPV status. Furthermore, 91% of patients in this study had early T stage (T2 or less), which could explain in part why no observable differences in survival and I was found between HPV-positive and HPV-negative tumors. In this series early T stage may have been a strong driving force for favorable survival, irrespective of HPV status.

Endoscopic Head and Neck Surgery Outcomes for Laryngeal Cancer

As discussed earlier, TLM has a clear role in early and select advanced laryngeal cancers. A retrospective review of 404 patients with T1 glottic cancers showed a 5-year local control (LC) rate of 86.8%, OS of 87.8%, DSS of 98%, and RFS of 76.1%.[62] In a systematic review of TLM versus primary radiation therapy, Yoo and colleagues[63] found no data in support of one modality over the other, although some studies suggested a higher rate of long-term laryngeal preservation in the TLM group.

Table 2
Oncologic outcomes of endoscopic head and neck surgery in oropharynx

	Primary	eHNS	Stage	No of Patients	LRC	5-Year DFS	5-Year DSS	5-Year OS
Canis et al,[90] 2013	Oropharynx	TLM	T1, T2	46	78	64	74	59
			T3, T4	56	75	60	68	56
Grant et al,[41] 2009	Oropharynx	TLM	All patients	69	82	—	—	86
			I, II	25			88	79
			III, IV	44			86	86
Haughey et al,[34] 2011	Oropharynx	TLM	III, IV	204	93.2	74	84	78
Rich et al,[36] 2009	Oropharynx	TLM	III, IV	84	94	—	92	88
Patel et al,[91] 2014	Oropharynx	TLM	III, IV	80	98.6	91.1 (3-y)	—	93.7 (3-y)
van Loon et al,[44] 2015	Oropharynx	TORS	I, II	18	—	86 (2-y)	—	100 (2-y)
Weinstein et al,[45] 2010	Oropharynx	TORS	III, IV	47	96	79 (2-y)	90 (2-y)	82 (2-y)
Park et al,[92] 2013	Oropharynx	TORS	I, II, III, IV	39	—	92 (2-y)	—	96 (2-y)
Moore et al,[32] 2012	Oropharynx	TORS	I, II, III, IV	66	94 (3-y)	92.4 (3-y)	95.1 (3-y)	—
Dabas et al,[59] 2014	Oropharynx	TORS	I, II, III (salvage included)	60	—	64 (18-mo)	—	93 (18-mo)
de Almeida et al,[29] 2015	Oropharynx (89% of patients)	TORS	T1, T2 (91% of patients)	410	91.8 (2-y) 88.8 (3-y)	—	94.5 (2-y) 92.5 (3-y)	91 (2-y) 87.1 (3-y)

Study	Subsite	Approach	Stage	n				
Hartl et al,[42] 2011	Glottis	TLM	I (T1)	79	86	89 (RFS)	97.3	—
Peretti et al,[93] 2010	Glottis	TLM	I, II (Tis-T3)	595	92.7 (LC)	81.3	99	87.5
Canis et al,[62] 2015;	Glottis	TLM	I (T1a)	404	86.8 (LC)	76.1	98	87.8
Canis et al,[64] 2013;	Glottis	TLM	II, III (T3)	122	71.5 (LC)	57.8 (RFS)	84.1	58.6
Canis et al,[66] 2014	Supraglottis	TLM	I, II, III, IV	277	87.5 (stage I/II, LC) 81.1 (stage III/IV, LC)	81 (stage I/II, RFS) 65 (stage III/IV, RFS)	92 (stage I/II) 81 (stage III/IV)	76 (stage I/II) 59 (stage III/IV)
Roh,[81] 2008	Supraglottis	TLM	I, II, III	21	81	71	—	79
Caicedo-Granados et al,[65] 2013	Larynx	TLM	II, III	32	—	39.6 (RFS)	—	53.8
Hinni et al,[50] 2007	Larynx	TLM	III, IV	117	68	58	—	55
Steiner et al,[57] 2001	Piriform sinus	TLM	I, II, III, IV	129	82 (stage I/II, LC) 69 (stage III/IV, LC)	95 (stage I/II, RFS) 69 (stage III/IV, RFS)	—	71 (stage I/II) 47 (stage III/IV)
Rudert & Höft,[68] 2003	Hypopharynx	TLM	I, II, III, IV	29	72.4	82	58	78 (stage I/II) 35 (stage III/IV)
Martin et al,[67] 2008	Hypopharynx	TLM	I, II, III, IV	172	84 (pT1) 70 (pT2) 75 (pT3) 57 (pT4)	73 (stage I/II, RFS) 59 (stage III, RFS) 47 (stage IV, RFS)	96 (stage I/II) 86 (stage III) 57 (stage IV)	68 (stage I/II) 64 (stage III) 41 (stage IV)
Karatzanis et al,[69] 2010	Hypopharynx	TLM	I, II, III	119	85.4	—	72.6	—
Park et al,[56] 2013	Hypopharynx	TORS	I, II, III, IV	30	—	—	81 (3-y)	85 (3-y)

Abbreviations: DFS, disease-free survival; DSS, disease-specific survival; eHNS, endoscopic head and neck surgery; LC, local control; LRC, locoregional control; OS, overall survival; RFS, recurrence-free survival; TLM, transoral laser microsurgery; TORS, transoral robotic surgery.
Data from Refs.[29,32,34,36,41,42,44,45,50,56,57,59,62,64–69,81,90–93]

When treating supraglottic cancers with TLM, Canis and colleagues[64] achieved a 5-year LC of 85% for T1/T2, 82% for T3, and 76% for T4 tumors, similar to historical rates after open partial laryngectomy. Numerous additional studies have corroborated similar LC in the treatment of T3 laryngeal cancers compared with open partial laryngectomy.[63,65,66]

Endoscopic Head and Neck Surgery Outcomes for Hypopharyngeal Cancer

Oncologic results of eHNS for hypopharyngeal cancer have been reported to be comparable with those of open conventional approaches. Martin and colleagues[67] reported the results of TLM in 172 patients with hypopharyngeal carcinoma. Five-year LC was 84% for T1, 70% for T2, 75% for T3, and 57% for T4a tumors. The 5-year RFS for stage I/II, III, and IVa were 73%, 59%, and 47%, respectively. Rudert and Höft reported the outcomes of 29 patients with hypopharyngeal cancer with 5-year OS and DSS of 58% and 48%, respectively. The 5-year OS in stage I/II disease was 71% and in stage III/IV disease 47%.[68] Results of TLM were reported by Karatzanis and colleagues[69] in 119 patients with T1 and T2 cancer of the hypopharynx. The LC was 90% and 5-year DSS 77.8% for T1. In T2 stage disease the LC and 5-year DSS were 83.1% and 70%, respectively. Park and colleagues[70] reported the results of TORS in 23 patients with hypopharyngeal cancer: 3-year OS was 89% and DFS 84%.

Table 2 summarizes the results of the eHNS studies.

FUNCTIONAL OUTCOMES OF ENDOSCOPIC HEAD AND NECK SURGERY

In OPC patients, the preservation of swallow may be the most important functional determinant of long-term quality of life.[71] Unlike open approaches to the pharynx, eHNS does not generally risk injury to the pharyngeal constrictors of the neck, and the primary-site defect is healed by soft-tissue contraction and covered with oral mucosa. Dysphagia may occur as an immediate complication during radiation therapy, or as a late manifestation of fibrosis. Mucositis, xerostomia, constrictor muscle dysfunction, and pharyngeal/esophageal stricture are other reasons for radiation-induced dysphagia. Radiation dosage to the pharyngeal area is a major determinant for the development of dysphagia that could be enhanced by concurrent chemotherapy.[72] Al-Khudari and colleagues[73] reported 50% to 70% rates of severe swallowing dysfunction following CCRT. Fifteen percent to 20% of patients required gastrostomies for their nutritional support after radiation treatment, and concurrent chemoradiation raised enteral tube rates to between 18.1% and 51%.[73] Adjuvant radiation therapy may be avoided in early-stage oropharyngeal cancer when negative tumor margins are achieved after surgery. Moreover, as previously mentioned, the total dosage of adjuvant radiotherapy may be decreased by primary surgery. Therefore, the rates of gastrostomy may be lower in eHNS. Published dependency on gastrostomy related to TLM treatment of oropharyngeal cancer ranges from 0% to 18.8%.[32,34,41,74] Weinstein and colleagues[22] reported good functional results after TORS in carefully selected patients, particularly when adjuvant therapy was avoided. In this study, 124 of 153 (81%) patients had T1 or T2 oropharyngeal squamous cell carcinoma; it is primarily these patients with early-stage disease who are the best candidates to avoid radiation therapy with eHNS. Overall 2.3% of patients remained tracheostomy-tube dependent at the last follow-up, and 5.0% of patients who had no treatment before TORS remained gastrostomy-tube dependent.

Investigators have also evaluated the difference in voice quality after both TLM and radiation therapy in early glottic cancer. In several studies, there were no significant differences in objective measurements (acoustic and spectrographic analyses) and subjective reports of voice quality between TLM and radiation.[75–78] In addition, Preuss and colleagues[79] reported a low frequency of intraoperative tracheostomy after TLM, at less than 2% of cases. eHNS also provided better posttreatment swallowing function and a shorter duration of feeding-tube dependency.[80,81]

In the treatment of hypopharyngeal cancer, eHNS may potentially facilitate preservation of the larynx and swallow function. Vilaseca and colleagues[82] reported laryngeal preservation in 78.5% of patients. A nasogastric feeding tube was not required in 32.1% of patients, and for the others the mean duration of tube dependency was 15.3 days. Kutter and colleagues[83] suggested in their series that TLM resulted in earlier restoration of oral feeding; 37 of 55 (67%) patients temporarily required a feeding tube. When the investigators compared this TLM cohort with a prior series of their open surgery experience, the median duration of feeding-tube dependency was shorter (7 vs 18 days). Karatzanis and colleagues[69] reported a series of 119 patients with T1/T2 hypopharyngeal cancers treated with TLM, wherein 3 of 119 (2.5%) patients developed severe postoperative aspiration requiring placement of a gastrostomy tube.

Table 3 summarizes the results of these published articles.

ROLE OF ENDOSCOPIC HEAD AND NECK SURGERY IN RECURRENT OROPHARYNGEAL CANCER

There are few published studies reporting results of eHNS in salvage treatment for recurrent OPC (rOPC). Salvage treatment for rOPC is traditionally an open radical procedure, with extensive transcervical dissection necessary to gain exposure to a previously treated site. Complication rates after open surgical salvage of previously irradiated patients with HNC range from 37% to 74%, with pharyngocutaneous fistula among the most common problems.[84–87] If prior radiation has been given, trismus and fibrosis may severely limit pliability of the pharynx, which is necessary for eHNS instrumentation. Grant and colleagues[88] reported 2-year DSS of 75% after salvage TLM for 15 rOPC patients (recurrent T1–T4). There were no severe complications such as fistula formation, infection, or surgery-related mortality. TORS has also been used in salvage oropharyngeal surgery. White and colleagues[60] retrospectively compared a series of TORS salvage patients with matched open oropharyngectomy controls. These investigators reported higher 2-year RFS rates in their TORS salvage group compared with open surgery (74% vs 43%, $P = .01$) with a lower incidence of treatment-related complications. Also, the incidence of positive margins was lower in the TORS group (9% vs 29.7%, $P = .007$). Although an endoscopic salvage approach may reduce the risk of pharyngocutaneous fistula, limited surgical exposure must be carefully considered, as salvage surgery often is the final opportunity to gain oncologic control.

FUTURE PERSPECTIVE AND SUMMARY

There are currently no clinical data from randomized controlled trials providing a comparison between eHNS and nonsurgical protocols. As of 2014, the National Cancer Institute–funded prospective, randomized clinical trial ECOG 3311 has been enrolling patients to specifically define the role of TORS in HPV-associated OPC, but even this trial is not a direct comparison of TORS with an initial nonsurgical approach.

eHNS has undergone a rapid evolution with improved laser delivery devices and robotic technology, providing a surgical platform analogous to conformal and intensity-modulated variants of external beam radiation therapy for maximally

Table 3
Functional outcomes of endoscopic head and neck surgery

	Primary	eHNS	Stage	Tracheostomy		Gastrostomy	
				Temporary (%)	Permanent (%)	Temporary (%)	Permanent (%)
Canis et al,[90] 2013	Oropharynx	TLM	I, II, III, IV	1	0	4	2
Grant et al,[41] 2009	Oropharynx	TLM	I, II, III, IV	16	0	7.3	0
Rich et al,[36] 2009	Oropharynx	TLM	III, IV	0	0	18.8	9.3 (at 2 y)
Patel et al,[91] 2014	Oropharynx	TLM	III, IV	—	—	38.8	6.3 (at 1 y)
Steiner et al,[94] 2003	Oropharynx	TLM	I, II, III, IV	0	0	15 (semisolid food only) 4 (aspiration without pneumonia)	6
Sumer et al,[37] 2013	Oropharynx	TLM	I, II, III, IV	6	0	38	0
Chen et al,[95] 2015	Oropharynx	TORS	I, II, III	—	—	13 (at adjuvant RT) 29 (at adjuvant CCRT)	3 (at adjuvant RT) 10 (at adjuvant CCRT)
Iseli et al,[96] 2009	Oropharynx	TORS	I, II, III, IV	12.1	0	—	6 (at 1 y)
Moore et al,[32] 2012	Oropharynx	TORS	I, II, III, IV	25.8	1.5	27.3	4.5
Sumer et al,[37] 2013	Oropharynx	TORS	I, II, III, IV	0	0	24	0
Weinstein et al,[45] 2010	Oropharynx	TORS	III, IV	10.6	—	—	2.4 (at 1 y)
Davas et al,[59] 2014	Oropharynx	TORS	I, II, III (salvage included)	—	—	3.3	0
Canis et al,[62] 2015; Canis et al,[64] 2013; Canis et al,[66] 2014	Glottis Supraglottis Larynx	TLM TLM TLM	I (T1a) I, II, III, IV II, III (T3)	No tracheostomy 77 (7 d median duration) 2.7	0 0.9	No gastrostomy 5 2.7	— 2 1
Roh,[81] 2008	Supraglottis	TLM	I, II, III	14.3	0	0	0
Hinni et al,[50] 2007	Larynx	TLM	III, IV	—	3	—	7
Caicedo-Granados[65]	Larynx	TLM	II, III	6	0	6	3
Steiner et al,[57] 2001	Piriform sinus	TLM	I, II, III, IV	—	0.8	—	1.6
Martin et al,[67] 2008	Hypopharynx	TLM	I, II, III, IV	—	3.5	4.1	3.5
Karatzanis et al,[69] 2010	Hypopharynx	TLM	I, II, III, IV	—	2.5	—	2.5
Park[56]	Hypopharynx	TORS	I, II, III, IV	100 (preventive purpose)	0	3.3	3.3

Abbreviations: CCRT, concurrent chemotherapy with radiation therapy; RT, radiation therapy.

preserving healthy tissue. Transoral eHNS has been included in the most recent National Comprehensive Cancer Network guidelines for patients with HNC, although its ultimate role, particularly in OPCs, is yet to be determined.[89] The results of ECOG 3311 are anticipated to shed light on the indications for eHNS within the multidisciplinary approach to a growing subgroup of patients with head and neck cancer.

REFERENCES

1. Ferlay J, Soerjomataram I, Dikshit R, et al. Cancer incidence and mortality worldwide: sources, methods and major patterns in GLOBOCAN 2012. Int J Cancer 2015;136:E359–86.
2. Pezzuto F, Buonaguro L, Caponigro F, et al. Update on head and neck cancer: current knowledge on epidemiology, risk factors, molecular features and novel therapies. Oncology 2015;89(3):125–36.
3. Hashibe M, Brennan P, Chuang SC, et al. Interaction between tobacco and alcohol use and the risk of head and neck cancer: pooled analysis in the International Head and Neck Cancer Epidemiology Consortium. Cancer Epidemiol Biomarkers Prev 2009;18:541–50.
4. Chaturvedi AK, Engels EA, Pfeiffer RM, et al. Human papillomavirus and rising oropharyngeal cancer incidence in the United States. J Clin Oncol 2011;29:4294–301.
5. Chaturvedi AK, Anderson WF, Lortet-Tieulent J, et al. Worldwide trends in incidence rates for oral cavity and oropharyngeal cancers. J Clin Oncol 2013;31:4550–9.
6. Westra WH. The changing face of head and neck cancer in the 21st century: the impact of HPV on the epidemiology and pathology of oral cancer. Head Neck Pathol 2009;3:78–81.
7. Sugarbaker ED, Gilford J. Combined jaw resection neck dissection for metastatic carcinoma of cervical lymph nodes secondarily involving the mandible. Surg Gynecol Obstet 1946;83:767–77.
8. Calais G, Alfonsi M, Bardet E, et al. Randomized trial of radiation therapy versus concomitant chemotherapy and radiation therapy for advanced-stage oropharynx carcinoma. J Natl Cancer Inst 1999;91:2081–6.
9. Ang KK, Harris J, Wheeler R, et al. Human papillomavirus and survival of patients with oropharyngeal cancer. N Engl J Med 2010;363:24–35.
10. Induction chemotherapy plus radiation compared with surgery plus radiation in patients with advanced laryngeal cancer. The Department of Veterans Affairs Laryngeal Cancer Study Group. N Engl J Med 1991;324:1685–90.
11. Forastiere AA, Goepfert H, Maor M, et al. Concurrent chemotherapy and radiotherapy for organ preservation in advanced laryngeal cancer. N Engl J Med 2003;349:2091–8.
12. Forastiere AA, Zhang Q, Weber RS, et al. Long-term results of RTOG 91-11: a comparison of three nonsurgical treatment strategies to preserve the larynx in patients with locally advanced larynx cancer. J Clin Oncol 2013;31:845–52.
13. Lefebvre JL, Andry G, Chevalier D, et al. Laryngeal preservation with induction chemotherapy for hypopharyngeal squamous cell carcinoma: 10-year results of EORTC trial 24891. Ann Oncol 2012;23:2708–14.
14. Lefebvre JL, Rolland F, Tesselaar M, et al. Phase 3 randomized trial on larynx preservation comparing sequential vs alternating chemotherapy and radiotherapy. J Natl Cancer Inst 2009;101:142–52.
15. Wilson JA, Carding PN, Patterson JM. Dysphagia after nonsurgical head and neck cancer treatment: patients' perspectives. Otolaryngol Head Neck Surg 2011;145:767–71.

16. Machtay M, Moughan J, Trotti A, et al. Factors associated with severe late toxicity after concurrent chemoradiation for locally advanced head and neck cancer: an RTOG analysis. J Clin Oncol 2008;26:3582–9.

17. Francis DO, Weymuller EA Jr, Parvathaneni U, et al. Dysphagia, stricture, and pneumonia in head and neck cancer patients: does treatment modality matter? Ann Otol Rhinol Laryngol 2010;119:391–7.

18. Holsinger FC, Weber RS. Swing of the surgical pendulum: a return to surgery for treatment of head and neck cancer in the 21st century? Int J Radiat Oncol Biol Phys 2007;69:S129–31.

19. Holsinger FC, Sweeney AD, Jantharapattana K, et al. The emergence of endoscopic head and neck surgery. Curr Oncol Rep 2010;12:216–22.

20. Walvekar RR, Li RJ, Gooding WE, et al. Role of surgery in limited (T1-2, N0-1) cancers of the oropharynx. Laryngoscope 2008;118:2129–34.

21. Steiner W. Experience in endoscopic laser surgery of malignant tumours of the upper aero-digestive tract. Adv Otorhinolaryngol 1988;39:135–44.

22. Weinstein GS, O'Malley BW Jr, Magnuson JS, et al. Transoral robotic surgery: a multicenter study to assess feasibility, safety, and surgical margins. Laryngoscope 2012;122:1701–7.

23. Strong MS, Jako GJ. Laser surgery in the larynx. Early clinical experience with continuous CO 2 laser. Ann Otol Rhinol Laryngol 1972;81:791–8.

24. Davis RK, Kriskovich MD, Galloway EB 3rd, et al. Endoscopic supraglottic laryngectomy with postoperative irradiation. Ann Otol Rhinol Laryngol 2004;113:132–8.

25. Peretti G, Nicolai P, Piazza C, et al. Oncological results of endoscopic resections of Tis and T1 glottic carcinomas by carbon dioxide laser. Ann Otol Rhinol Laryngol 2001;110:820–6.

26. Desai SC, Sung CK, Jang DW, et al. Transoral robotic surgery using a carbon dioxide flexible laser for tumors of the upper aerodigestive tract. Laryngoscope 2008;118:2187–9.

27. Solares CA, Strome M. Transoral robot-assisted CO2 laser supraglottic laryngectomy: experimental and clinical data. Laryngoscope 2007;117:817–20.

28. Hutcheson KA, Holsinger FC, Kupferman ME, et al. Functional outcomes after TORS for oropharyngeal cancer: a systematic review. Eur Arch Otorhinolaryngol 2015;272:463–71.

29. de Almeida JR, Li RJ, Duvvuri U, et al. Oncologic outcomes following transoral robotic surgery (TORS): a multi-institutional study. 2015.

30. Adelstein DJ, Ridge JA, Brizel DM, et al. Transoral resection of pharyngeal cancer: summary of a National Cancer Institute Head and Neck Cancer Steering Committee Clinical Trials Planning Meeting, November 6-7, 2011, Arlington, Virginia. Head Neck 2012;34:1681–703.

31. Hurtuk AM, Marcinow A, Agrawal A, et al. Quality-of-life outcomes in transoral robotic surgery. Otolaryngol Head Neck Surg 2012;146:68–73.

32. Moore EJ, Olsen SM, Laborde RR, et al. Long-term functional and oncologic results of transoral robotic surgery for oropharyngeal squamous cell carcinoma. Mayo Clin Proc 2012;87:219–25.

33. Garden AS, Kies MS, Weber RS. To TORS or Not to TORS: but is that the question? Comment on "transoral robotic surgery for advanced oropharyngeal carcinoma". Arch Otolaryngol Head Neck Surg 2010;136:1085–7.

34. Haughey BH, Hinni ML, Salassa JR, et al. Transoral laser microsurgery as primary treatment for advanced-stage oropharyngeal cancer: a United States multicenter study. Head Neck 2011;33:1683–94.

35. Hurtuk A, Agrawal A, Old M, et al. Outcomes of transoral robotic surgery: a preliminary clinical experience. Otolaryngol Head Neck Surg 2011;145:248–53.
36. Rich JT, Milov S, Lewis JS Jr, et al. Transoral laser microsurgery (TLM) +/- adjuvant therapy for advanced stage oropharyngeal cancer: outcomes and prognostic factors. Laryngoscope 2009;119:1709–19.
37. Sumer BD, Goyal V, Truelson JM, et al. Transoral robotic surgery and transoral laser microsurgery for oropharyngeal squamous cell cancer. J Robot Surg 2013;7:377–83.
38. Hinni ML, Zarka MA, Hoxworth JM. Margin mapping in transoral surgery for head and neck cancer. Laryngoscope 2013;123:1190–8.
39. Sansoni ER, Gross ND. The role of transoral robotic surgery in the management of oropharyngeal squamous cell carcinoma: a current review. Curr Oncol Rep 2015; 17:432.
40. Holsinger FC, Laccoureye O, Weber RS. Surgical approaches for cancer of the oropharynx. Operative Techniques in Otolaryngology-Head and Neck Surgery 2005;16:40–8.
41. Grant DG, Hinni ML, Salassa JR, et al. Oropharyngeal cancer: a case for single modality treatment with transoral laser microsurgery. Arch Otolaryngol Head Neck Surg 2009;135:1225–30.
42. Hartl DM, Ferlito A, Silver CE, et al. Minimally invasive techniques for head and neck malignancies: current indications, outcomes and future directions. Eur Arch Otorhinolaryngol 2011;268:1249–57.
43. de Almeida JR, Byrd JK, Wu R, et al. A systematic review of transoral robotic surgery and radiotherapy for early oropharynx cancer: a systematic review. Laryngoscope 2014;124:2096–102.
44. van Loon JW, Smeele LE, Hilgers FJ, et al. Outcome of transoral robotic surgery for stage I-II oropharyngeal cancer. Eur Arch Otorhinolaryngol 2015;272:175–83.
45. Weinstein GS, O'Malley BW Jr, Cohen MA, et al. Transoral robotic surgery for advanced oropharyngeal carcinoma. Arch Otolaryngol Head Neck Surg 2010; 136:1079–85.
46. Fakhry C, Westra WH, Li S, et al. Improved survival of patients with human papillomavirus-positive head and neck squamous cell carcinoma in a prospective clinical trial. J Natl Cancer Inst 2008;100:261–9.
47. Gillison M. HPV and its effect on head and neck cancer prognosis. Clin Adv Hematol Oncol 2010;8:680–2.
48. Gillison ML. HPV and prognosis for patients with oropharynx cancer. Eur J Cancer 2009;45(Suppl 1):383–5.
49. Licitra L, Perrone F, Bossi P, et al. High-risk human papillomavirus affects prognosis in patients with surgically treated oropharyngeal squamous cell carcinoma. J Clin Oncol 2006;24:5630–6.
50. Hinni ML, Salassa JR, Grant DG, et al. Transoral laser microsurgery for advanced laryngeal cancer. Arch Otolaryngol Head Neck Surg 2007;133:1198–204.
51. Silver CE, Beitler JJ, Shaha AR, et al. Current trends in initial management of laryngeal cancer: the declining use of open surgery. Eur Arch Otorhinolaryngol 2009;266:1333–52.
52. Dowthwaite S, Nichols AC, Yoo J, et al. Transoral robotic total laryngectomy: report of 3 cases. Head Neck 2013;35:E338–42.
53. Weinstein GS, O'Malley BW Jr, Snyder W, et al. Transoral robotic surgery: supraglottic partial laryngectomy. Ann Otol Rhinol Laryngol 2007;116:19–23.
54. Abdel-Wahab M, Abitbol A, Lewin A, et al. Quality-of-life assessment after hyperfractionated radiation therapy and 5-fluorouracil, cisplatin, and paclitaxel (Taxol)

in inoperable and/or unresectable head and neck squamous cell carcinoma. Am J Clin Oncol 2005;28:359–66.

55. Lee WT, Akst LM, Adelstein DJ, et al. Risk factors for hypopharyngeal/upper esophageal stricture formation after concurrent chemoradiation. Head Neck 2006;28:808–12.

56. Park YM, Byeon HK, Chung HP, et al. Comparison study of transoral robotic surgery and radical open surgery for hypopharyngeal cancer. Acta Otolaryngol 2013;133:641–8.

57. Steiner W, Ambrosch P, Hess CF, et al. Organ preservation by transoral laser microsurgery in piriform sinus carcinoma. Otolaryngol Head Neck Surg 2001;124:58–67.

58. Takes RP, Strojan P, Silver CE, et al. Current trends in initial management of hypopharyngeal cancer: the declining use of open surgery. Head Neck 2012;34:270–81.

59. Dabas S, Dewan A, Ranjan R, et al. Transoral robotic surgery in management of oropharyngeal cancers: a preliminary experience at a tertiary cancer centre in India. Int J Clin Oncol 2014;20(4):693–700.

60. White H, Ford S, Bush B, et al. Salvage surgery for recurrent cancers of the oropharynx: comparing TORS with standard open surgical approaches. JAMA Otolaryngol Head Neck Surg 2013;139:773–8.

61. Byers RM, Bland KI, Borlase B, et al. The prognostic and therapeutic value of frozen section determinations in the surgical treatment of squamous carcinoma of the head and neck. Am J Surg 1978;136:525–8.

62. Canis M, Ihler F, Martin A, et al. Transoral laser microsurgery for T1a glottic cancer: review of 404 cases. Head Neck 2015;37:889–95.

63. Yoo J, Lacchetti C, Hammond JA, et al. Role of endolaryngeal surgery (with or without laser) versus radiotherapy in the management of early (T1) glottic cancer: a systematic review. Head Neck 2014;36:1807–19.

64. Canis M, Martin A, Ihler F, et al. Results of transoral laser microsurgery for supraglottic carcinoma in 277 patients. Eur Arch Otorhinolaryngol 2013;270:2315–26.

65. Caicedo-Granados E, Beswick DM, Christopoulos A, et al. Oncologic and functional outcomes of partial laryngeal surgery for intermediate-stage laryngeal cancer. Otolaryngol Head Neck Surg 2013;148:235–42.

66. Canis M, Ihler F, Martin A, et al. Results of 226 patients with T3 laryngeal carcinoma after treatment with transoral laser microsurgery. Head Neck 2014;36:652–9.

67. Martin A, Jackel MC, Christiansen H, et al. Organ preserving transoral laser microsurgery for cancer of the hypopharynx. Laryngoscope 2008;118:398–402.

68. Rudert HH, Höft S. Transoral carbon-dioxide laser resection of hypopharyngeal carcinoma. Eur Arch Otorhinolaryngol 2003;260:198–206.

69. Karatzanis AD, Psychogios G, Waldfahrer F, et al. T1 and T2 hypopharyngeal cancer treatment with laser microsurgery. J Surg Oncol 2010;102:27–33.

70. Park YM, Kim WS, De Virgilio A, et al. Transoral robotic surgery for hypopharyngeal squamous cell carcinoma: 3-year oncologic and functional analysis. Oral Oncol 2012;48:560–6.

71. Koyfman SA, Adelstein DJ. Enteral feeding tubes in patients undergoing definitive chemoradiation therapy for head-and-neck cancer: a critical review. Int J Radiat Oncol Biol Phys 2012;84:581–9.

72. Sinclair CF, McColloch NL, Carroll WR, et al. Patient-perceived and objective functional outcomes following transoral robotic surgery for early oropharyngeal carcinoma. Arch Otolaryngol Head Neck Surg 2011;137:1112–6.

73. Al-Khudari S, Bendix S, Lindholm J, et al. Gastrostomy tube use after transoral robotic surgery for oropharyngeal cancer. ISRN Otolaryngol 2013;2013:190364.

74. Rich JT, Liu J, Haughey BH. Swallowing function after transoral laser microsurgery (TLM) +/- adjuvant therapy for advanced-stage oropharyngeal cancer. Laryngoscope 2011;121:2381–90.
75. Cohen SM, Garrett CG, Dupont WD, et al. Voice-related quality of life in T1 glottic cancer: irradiation versus endoscopic excision. Ann Otol Rhinol Laryngol 2006; 115:581–6.
76. Goor KM, Peeters AJ, Mahieu HF, et al. Cordectomy by CO_2 laser or radiotherapy for small T1a glottic carcinomas: costs, local control, survival, quality of life, and voice quality. Head Neck 2007;29:128–36.
77. Nunez Batalla F, Caminero Cueva MJ, Senaris Gonzalez B, et al. Voice quality after endoscopic laser surgery and radiotherapy for early glottic cancer: objective measurements emphasizing the voice handicap index. Eur Arch Otorhinolaryngol 2008;265:543–8.
78. Sjogren EV, van Rossum MA, Langeveld TP, et al. Voice outcome in T1a midcord glottic carcinoma: laser surgery vs radiotherapy. Arch Otolaryngol Head Neck Surg 2008;134:965–72.
79. Preuss SF, Cramer K, Klussmann JP, et al. Transoral laser surgery for laryngeal cancer: outcome, complications and prognostic factors in 275 patients. Eur J Surg Oncol 2009;35:235–40.
80. Cabanillas R, Rodrigo JP, Llorente JL, et al. Functional outcomes of transoral laser surgery of supraglottic carcinoma compared with a transcervical approach. Head Neck 2004;26:653–9.
81. Roh JL, Kim DH, Park CI. Voice, swallowing and quality of life in patients after transoral laser surgery for supraglottic carcinoma. J Surg Oncol 2008;98:184–9.
82. Vilaseca I, Blanch JL, Bernal-Sprekelsen M, et al. CO_2 laser surgery: a larynx preservation alternative for selected hypopharyngeal carcinomas. Head Neck 2004;26:953–9.
83. Kutter J, Lang F, Monnier P, et al. Transoral laser surgery for pharyngeal and pharyngolaryngeal carcinomas. Arch Otolaryngol Head Neck Surg 2007;133: 139–44.
84. Goodwin WJ Jr. Salvage surgery for patients with recurrent squamous cell carcinoma of the upper aerodigestive tract: when do the ends justify the means? Laryngoscope 2000;110:1–18.
85. Lavertu P, Bonafede JP, Adelstein DJ, et al. Comparison of surgical complications after organ-preservation therapy in patients with stage III or IV squamous cell head and neck cancer. Arch Otolaryngol Head Neck Surg 1998;124:401–6.
86. Sassler AM, Esclamado RM, Wolf GT. Surgery after organ preservation therapy. Analysis of wound complications. Arch Otolaryngol Head Neck Surg 1995;121: 162–5.
87. Weber RS, Berkey BA, Forastiere A, et al. Outcome of salvage total laryngectomy following organ preservation therapy: the Radiation Therapy Oncology Group trial 91-11. Arch Otolaryngol Head Neck Surg 2003;129:44–9.
88. Grant DG, Salassa JR, Hinni ML, et al. Transoral laser microsurgery for recurrent laryngeal and pharyngeal cancer. Otolaryngol Head Neck Surg 2008;138:606–13.
89. National Comprehensive Cancer Network. Clinical practice guidelines in oncology (NCCN guidelines®) head and neck cancers. Version 1 2015. Available at: http://www.nccn.org/professionals/physician_gls/PDF/head-and-neck.pdf. Accessed July 3, 2015.
90. Canis M, Martin A, Kron M, et al. Results of transoral laser microsurgery in 102 patients with squamous cell carcinoma of the tonsil. Eur Arch Otorhinolaryngol 2013;270:2299–306.

91. Patel SH, Hinni ML, Hayden RE, et al. Transoral laser microsurgery followed by radiation therapy for oropharyngeal tumors: the Mayo Clinic Arizona experience. Head Neck 2014;36:220–5.

92. Park YM, Kim WS, Byeon HK, et al. Oncological and functional outcomes of transoral robotic surgery for oropharyngeal cancer. Br J Oral Maxillofac Surg 2013;51:408–12.

93. Peretti G, Piazza C, Cocco D, et al. Transoral CO(2) laser treatment for T(is)-T(3) glottic cancer: the University of Brescia experience on 595 patients. Head Neck 2010;32:977–83.

94. Steiner W, Fierek O, Ambrosch P, et al. Transoral laser microsurgery for squamous cell carcinoma of the base of the tongue. Arch Otolaryngol Head Neck Surg 2003;129:36–43.

95. Chen AM, Daly ME, Luu Q, et al. Comparison of functional outcomes and quality of life between transoral surgery and definitive chemoradiotherapy for oropharyngeal cancer. Head Neck 2015;37:381–5.

96. Iseli TA, Kulbersh BD, Iseli CE, et al. Functional outcomes after transoral robotic surgery for head and neck cancer. Otolaryngol Head Neck Surg 2009;141:166–71.

Radiation Oncology—New Approaches in Squamous Cell Cancer of the Head and Neck

CrossMark

Danielle N. Margalit, MD, MPH, Jonathon D. Schoenfeld, MD, MPH, Roy B. Tishler, MD, PhD*

KEYWORDS

- Squamous cancer • Head and neck • Intensity modulated radiation therapy
- Radiation planning • Adaptive replanning • Image guided

KEY POINTS

- Changes in the use and implementation of multiple types of imaging can lead to improvements in the targeting of radiation therapy for head and neck cancers.
- Therapeutic radiation for head and neck cancers is improving based on the use of image guidance and different techniques for treatment delivery.
- The unique biology of human papilloma virus (HPV)-related cancers opens up the possibility of delivering less radiation to less tissue while maintaining efficacy.

INTRODUCTION

The field of radiation therapy for squamous cell cancer of the head and neck (SCCHN) has been transformed over the past decade, but the basic elements of radiotherapy remain the same: determining the appropriate dose to deliver, accurately identifying the targets, and delivering treatment with minimal normal tissue toxicity. The current standard of care, intensity modulated radiation therapy (IMRT), delivers improved tumor doses compared with the historical 3-field/3-dimensional conformal approaches, which were both effective in treating SCCHN. Current studies assessing the efficacy of IMRT demonstrate excellent outcomes,[1–3] while acknowledging a contribution from the changing nature of oropharynx cancers and the use of retrospective data. Much of the benefit derived from IMRT has been in the area of normal tissue sparing. The treating physician exercises substantial control over where the dose is (and is not) directed; thus IMRT has led to significant improvements in obtaining a differential

---

Department of Radiation Oncology, Dana-Farber Cancer Institute, Harvard Medical School, 450 Brookline Avenue, Boston, MA 02115, USA
* Corresponding author.
E-mail address: roy_tishler@dfci.harvard.edu

Hematol Oncol Clin N Am 29 (2015) 1093–1106
http://dx.doi.org/10.1016/j.hoc.2015.07.008
0889-8588/15/$ – see front matter © 2015 Elsevier Inc. All rights reserved.

between the doses delivered to the tumor related targets and normal tissue structures. These improvements were first clearly demonstrated in nasopharynx cancer where, because of anatomic considerations, the benefits are potentially the most significant. Results were derived from a combination of phase 2, 3, and retrospective studies.[4–7] A phase 3 study that included oropharynx and hypopharynx compared IMRT and lateral opposed fields using 3-dimensional conformal methods and demonstrated similar results.[8] For these sites, there is also a significant body of retrospective data highlighting the excellent normal tissue outcomes resulting from IMRT-based improved dose distributions.[9,10] In order to achieve these distributions, one must precisely determine which structures need to be treated. This determination requires optimal imaging data and also requires a detailed knowledge of the disease behavior. The imaging component will be addressed in this article, while the second item emphasizes the importance of treatment at a high-volume center, which was demonstrated for 3-field treatment[11]; IMRT potentially increases the benefit expected from the expertise of the individual practitioner. The concept used to describe the balance between tumor control and normal tissue effects is the therapeutic ratio (TR), and improving the TR has been a longstanding goal of radiation therapy. Further improvements in TR have taken on increased importance, as it is known that there are myriad effective treatments for SCCHN occurring in a younger and healthier population.

Overview

Multiple pathways to improving the TR for radiation therapy SCCHN patients will be addressed in this article. Advances in imaging allow the physician to more accurately identify tumor and adjacent tissues that are at risk of containing microscopic disease. The approaches addressed here include improvements of existing technologies (eg, MRI, positron emission tomography [PET]) as well as the use of other modalities. A second approach for improving TR is to improve the methods used for delivering radiation to the patient. The topics included in this paradigm are modifying how standard IMRT—photon based—is given, as well as the use of proton therapy. Underlying the designation of appropriate targets is the understanding of the disease being treated and how that disease may be changing. Specifically, there is the ever-present influence of HPV-related disease and the questions it raises in radiation therapy, such as how much radiation is necessary and how big a volume needs to be treated.

This article focuses on radiation therapy alone and cannot address the many important relationships with surgery and systemic therapy.

IMAGING ADVANCES

As head and neck radiation treatments have become more targeted, accurate target delineation has become more critical to avoid missing tumor and identifying areas at highest risk for microscopic tumor spread.[12,13] Additionally, the steep dose gradients and high doses delivered in close proximity to critical organs such as the spinal cord and brainstem necessitate millimeter-level accuracy in the definition of these normal structures. Thus, it is crucial to incorporate all anatomic information available during the radiation treatment-planning process. In many cases, the clinical examination is the cornerstone of this process; however, diagnostic imaging modalities such as computed tomography (CT), PET, and MRI provide complimentary information and have been increasingly incorporated into clinical practice.[14]

Computed Tomography Scans

Diagnostic CT imaging with intravenous contrast is recommended by national guidelines for the majority of SCCHN patients (Network 2015) and can aid in identifying primary lesions and pathologically involved lymph nodes. For subsites in close proximity to bone (eg, the mandible or clivus), CT can help determine the extent of tumor spread. In patients who do not undergo primary surgical treatment, diagnostic CT represents a significant improvement over clinical examination alone to identify pathologically involved lymph nodes. These radiographically positive nodes can then be irradiated to higher doses appropriate for gross disease. Similarly, diagnostic CT is commonly used to follow responses after the completion of radiation of involved lymph nodes to help determine whether a post-treatment neck dissection is warranted.

In addition to diagnostic CT scans, CT is also typically incorporated directly into the modern radiotherapy treatment planning process using CT simulators, which can produce images that approach diagnostic quality. The treating clinician uses these images, reformatted in the axial, coronal, and sagittal planes, to better identify areas either involved by disease or at risk of harboring microscopic disease spread. Ideally, images from multiple planes are used in tandem during the radiation treatment-planning process; over-reliance on axial images, for example, can lead to inadequate superior and inferior treatment margins.

PET, PET–Computed Tomography Imaging

The use of PET/PET-CT scans has increased dramatically over the last few decades, largely as a result of their utilization in oncology.[15] For head and neck cancers, PET can be used alongside or in place of chest CT to evaluate for metastatic disease, with the benefit that PET also identifies metastases to unusual sites such as bone or soft tissue. PET can also serve as a useful adjunct in radiation target delineation. PET performed in addition to CT may have improved sensitivity and specificity for identifying pathologically involved lymph nodes[16–19] and is also likely more cost-effective.[20] Similarly, PET may help delineate the extent of primary disease; indeed, PET/CT-derived target volumes were the most reproducible in a study that compared various imaging modalities,[21] and also the most accurate.[22] However, caution is warranted, as the spatial resolution of PET scans is larger than the margins typically used in head and neck radiation treatment planning.[21,23] Additionally, the absolute standard uptake values (SUVs) or other criteria such as adaptive thresholding best suited to identify malignancy has yet to be determined and can lead to large variability in tumor volume.[24]

In order to best utilize the biologic information provided by diagnostic PET scans, PET images can be viewed alongside treatment-planning CT scans, or fused to these CT scans so the 2 scans can be viewed simultaneously.[25] A potential issue when incorporating PET scans into the radiation-planning process is the variability in position that occurs between diagnostic PET and treatment-planning CT scans. Deformable registration is one technique that can help address this limitation by more accurately mapping the diagnostic PET scan using adjustable landmarks.[26] Deformable registration may also be helpful for addressing changes in anatomy that occur following induction chemotherapy or surgery,[26,27] because current guidelines specify treatment fields should be based on the pretreatment disease extent.[28]

MRI Imaging

Similar to PET, MRI is being increasingly incorporated into radiation treatment planning,[15] using fusion or deformable registration techniques.[29] MRI can be particularly useful for identification of pathologic retropharyngeal lymph nodes or defining the extent of primary disease in critical areas such as the nasopharynx, sinuses, oral tongue, or parotid. MRI can also provide better resolution for targeting tumor-invading cranial nerves or critical structures such as the brainstem, optic nerves, and optic chiasm. Finally, MRI can aid in target delineation when CT scans are limited by dental artifact. In head and neck treatment planning, evidence suggests that MRI may be complimentary with PET and CT for target volume delineation.[14]

Recent advances are expanding the ways various imaging modalities can be incorporated into radiation treatment planning. SUVs or metabolic tumor volumes (MTVs) obtained by PET may be prognostic, with higher initial SUV or larger MTV associated with local recurrence in patients treated with standard radiation with or without chemotherapy.[30,31] Therefore, next-generation dose-painting approaches could attempt to incorporate this information to escalate radiation dose to biologically active or bulky regions within a tumor and perhaps decrease the radiation dose delivered to those areas of a tumor that are less active. PET is also increasingly used to follow treatment response of SCCHN. For example, patients with PET-negative lymph nodes following radiotherapy may not benefit from a neck dissection, even if they remain visible on CT.[32,33]

MRI scans also have the potential to change the practice of head and neck oncology. Conventional T1 or T2 weighted MRI sequences provide high-quality imaging of areas of the head and neck that were previously difficult to assess, such as the maxillary and sphenoid sinuses.

Additional MRI sequences have been investigated for their ability to identify tumors and monitor response, with promising early results.[34] For example, diffusion weighted MRI (DWI) can help differentiate involved lymph nodes from benign reactive lymphadenopathy because of the increased cellularity of lymph nodes with tumor infiltration, and have demonstrated superior sensitivity and specificity for this purpose when compared with CT or traditional MRI sequences in small studies.[18,35] Dynamic contrast-enhanced (DCE)-MRI provides information on vascular perfusion and permeability that could also add complimentary information in the identification of regions in head and neck tumors at risk for relapse because of poor baseline functional vasculature.[34]

Future developments will likely further integrate diagnostic imaging and radiation treatment planning. MRI- and PET-based simulators and simulation techniques are increasingly being developed and refined for radiation oncology practice.[24,36] These range from careful use of the same immobilization devices for both radiation simulation and diagnostic scan to fully integrated treatment-planning devices that offer the capabilities for multiparametric imaging. PET-based delineation of treatment volumes can also potentially be automated[37]; however, this technique would remain dependent on the validity of parameters used to define PET positivity.[38]

Novel functional imaging techniques allow physicians and researchers to better identify disease at the onset of treatment and track parameters that may be important predictors of treatment response.[39,40] Areas of hypoxia in head and neck cancers may promote radioresistance.[34] Therefore, identifying these regions could allow for tailoring of radiation plans and monitoring the effects of radiation on this aspect of tumor response. Fluorine-18-labeled fluoromisonidazole PET (18F-FMISO-PET) is one potential imaging modality capable of identifying hypoxic areas within a tumor. Early studies have incorporated 18F-FMISO-PET based treatment planning for SCCHN to show the feasibility of dose escalation to the hypoxic component of tumor volumes.[41] 18F-FMISO-PET is somewhat limited by relatively slow diffusion and uptake; therefore, other next-generation nitroimidizaole derivatives are also being explored for their ability to identify hypoxic tumor regions.[38] In addition to hypoxia, other potential PET tracers that may eventually be useful for radiation target delineation are being explored for their ability to detect tumor cell proliferation (18FLT), protein synthesis (18FET, 11C-MET), or anabolic pathway metabolism in cancer tissues (11C-ACE).[38]

ADVANCES IN RADIATION DELIVERY

Appropriately identifying clinical targets via physical examination and imaging represents an important element in treating SCCHN. It is also essential to deliver radiation therapy in as accurate and conformal a manner as possible to those targets.

Image Guidance

The sharp dose gradients present in IMRT dose distributions can be significantly altered by small variations in the day–to-day patient position/setup[42,43]; thus, it is essential to minimize the variation. This is achieved by several means:

- With reliable, reproducible daily positioning
- By building in an additional margin of uncertainty for setup variability (the planning target volume, PTV), typically a 3 to 5 mm volumetric expansion of the target volume
- Using image guidance

   Image guided radiation therapy (IGRT) refers to the use of images acquired during treatment to guide delivery of RT principally by ensuring patient positioning prior to treatment.[44] Major advancements in 2-dimensional and 3-dimensional image guidance occurred when kilovoltage (kV) X-ray units and image detectors were built into newer linear accelerators. Other forms of setup verification include the use the megavoltage (MV) treatment beam itself to construct an image, although these have inferior image quality to diagnostic kV beams. Once the patient is setup, kV images are taken in orthogonal planes and compared with the digitally reconstructed radiographs from the initial planning CT. The patient is then shifted in order to align bone landmarks, with the assumption that the soft tissues will track with the bone. The positioning of both soft tissue and bone can be assessed using cone beam CT (CBCT), which provides 3-dimensional IGRT. In kV CBCT, the gantry makes a single rotation around the patient and provides 3-dimensional images, although several factors contribute to the CBCT image quality being inferior to diagnostic-quality CT images.[45,46] One of the challenges in utilizing IGRT in SCCHN is that different regions within the treated area have different daily variability in positioning.[47] Therefore, the clinicians must decide upon the critical areas to use for any shifts in the treatment positioning during IGRT.

Adaptive Replanning

In addition to setup variability, there are also changes in patient and tumor anatomy that occur as tumors respond, patients gain or lose weight, or postoperative anatomy evolves. The changes can lead to reduced tumor dose and increased normal structures dose.[48] These changes have led to the growing recognition of the importance of adaptive replanning (AR), which refers to adapting the plan to anatomic changes that occur during treatment.

   The AR concept seems straightforward, yet the practical application is complex. One issue is that gross tumor volumes generally do not shrink symmetrically and may change position over time.[49] One approach is deformable image registration, which uses the original delineated tumor and normal tissue volumes deformed onto the new image set. However, the most common method of deformable registration does not consistently capture the change in tumor over time, even though it does well in capturing changes in normal tissue positioning.[50]

There are additional challenges to clinically implementing AR:

- There are no clear-cut criteria to select patients for AR; an important line of research is to use the 3-dimensional CBCT images to reconstruct the radiation dose distribution for that day[51,52]
- AR has the potential to be prohibitively resource intensive, with contouring a standard IMRT case taking an average of 144 minutes,[53] without factoring in the time for IMRT planning and quality assurance

Therefore, AR algorithms are essential to facilitate routine RT replanning.

Alternative Photon Delivery

Standard IMRT delivers radiation through static fields at different angles around the patient, either using fixed multileaf collimators (MLCs) or dynamic MLC that move during treatment. Two new approaches to photon delivery involve radiation that is delivered in a 360° rotation or in smaller arcs around the patient: helical tomotherapy (HT) and volumetric modulated arc therapy (VMAT). Despite being advertised as superior,[54] there are no randomized prospective data showing a clinically significant difference in oncologic or toxicity outcomes.[55] Multiple dosimetric studies have compared the different methods of delivering photons with variable claims of superiority.[56–58] These studies need to be interpreted with care due to bias introduced by variation in planner experience with the different planning strategies, limitations in different optimization software packages, and different emphasis on which metrics are to be used in assessing clinically significant differences (eg, homogeneity index, conformality index, and dose to a specific organ at risk).

Helical Tomotherapy

Helical tomogherapy (HT), first used at the University of Wisconsin,[59] combines the properties of a helical CT scanner with a megavoltage photon linear accelerator that delivers RT by rotating around the ring gantry while the patient moves through the bore of the machine. There are distinguishing features of HT:

- Image guidance is built into the treatment itself as exiting radiation is detected for image reconstruction
- The delivery is given over the full 360° and can provide homogeneous tumor dose while providing steep gradients between tumor and critical organs[55]

Limitations of HT are that noncoplanar treatment angles are typically not used, and it results in more low-dose irradiated tissue than some IMRT plans, although the clinical significance of this is unknown.

VMAT[60] currently includes 2 major delivery units, the Elekta VMAT (Stockholm, Sweden) and Varian RapidArc (Palo Alto, CA). Unlike HT, where the beam of radiation is a fan and the volume is treated slice by slice, VMAT uses a cone beam, and apertures are designed to account for the entire treated volume. Challenges of arc therapy include the relative complexity of the plan optimization software, which can make treatment planning more tedious than for static field IMRT. VMAT provides the fastest treatment time and the lowest number of monitor units, which may theoretically lead to a decreased risk of second malignancy. However, there are no supportive clinical data at this point. The high dose rate to the tumor provided by both forms of rotational therapy (VMAT and HT), compared with static-field IMRT, has led some researchers to postulate an increase in tumor control probability.[61]

Proton Therapy

Proton therapy holds promise for maximizing the TR in SCCHN. Protons and photons have similar biologic properties, but the difference in physical dose distribution distinguishes them and may have an effect on clinical outcomes. The dose from a photon beam decreases exponentially with depth in tissue resulting in nonessential radiation beyond the target. In contrast, a proton beam delivers most of its dose at a specified range in tissue with essentially no dose beyond the point of maximum dose deposition, known as the Bragg Peak,[62,63] which can be specified through the treatment planning process.

Over the last 10 years there has been dramatic expansion of the number of proton facilities worldwide. For example, there were only 29 operational facilities in 2008 compared with 46 facilities as of November 2014. This number will likely continue to increase due to the development of smaller and less costly delivery units.

Clinical Experience

There are no completed randomized trials comparing proton and photon radiotherapy for SCCHN. Currently, a phase 2/3 randomized trial sponsored by the University of Texas MD Anderson Cancer Center (UTMDACC) is accruing and will compare intensity-modulated proton beam therapy (IMPT) with IMRT for oropharyngeal cancer with a primary outcome of toxicity (NCT01893307).

Sinonasal malignancies

The Massachusetts General Hospital treated 102 patients with advanced sinonasal cancers and a range of histologies using proton therapy from 1991 to 2002. The 5-year local control (LC) was 86%, which is impressive considering the advanced stages and inherent challenge of treating cancers so close to the brain, brainstem, and optic structures.[64,65] Researchers from Japan published outcomes with hypofractionated proton therapy for unresectable T4 nasal cavity tumors with favorable 1-year LC of 77%, with 1 treatment-related death and 12.8% grade 3–5 toxicity.[66]

Nasopharyngeal cancer

Early prospective data suggest that proton therapy for nasopharyngeal carcinoma may result in a meaningful reduction in acute and possibly late toxicity. The first prospective phase 2 study of proton therapy for nasopharyngeal carcinoma showed that swallowing function compared favorably with historical outcomes, especially given the advanced nature of the tumors.[67] A recent case–control study of patients treated with IMPT and IMRT at UTMDACC and Linkou Chang-Gung Memorial Hospital, Taiwan, showed a significantly lower proportion of gastrostomy tube insertion in the IMPT group (23.1% vs 57.7%).[68]

Oropharyngeal cancer

Loma Linda University used protons as a boost after a predominantly photon-based treatment for stage 2 to 4 oropharyngeal cancer.[69] The 2-year LC was 93%, and the 2-year RTOG grade 3 toxicity was 16%; it was difficult to interpret the relative contribution of protons, because most doses were given with photons. A UTMDACC abstract of a case–control study comparing 26 IMPT cases and 26 IMRT cases showed a lower rate of grade 3 dysphagia for IMPT.[70]

Intensity Modulated Proton Therapy

The true potential for proton therapy to spare uninvolved tissue has not yet been realized, but there is promise in the form of optimized IMPT. Therapeutic proton beams are generated using passive scattering of a mono-energetic beam or with pencil beam scanning where magnets are used to steer the positively charged proton beam.[71] IMPT, based on this scanning technology, has the potential to provide superior dose conformality and normal tissue sparing than other forms of proton or photon delivery. In IMPT, a small circular proton beam, characterized by the beam spot size, is scanned across the defined treatment field with varying beam energy and intensity. The conformality of an IMPT treatment plan has a direct dependence on the spot size and also on the strategy of how spots are placed within the patient.[72] Current research is aimed at optimizing the ability to deliver proton therapy by accurate manipulation of the pencil beam, and in minimizing the effective spot size of the beam to increase the dose conformality and minimize the amount of normal tissue receiving radiation.[73,74]

CLINICALLY BASED ADVANCES

In addition to the technical areas of progress in radiation oncology, clinical changes are influencing its practice, primarily related to the increasing prevalence of HPV-related SCCHN. Multiple studies have demonstrated the improved outcome for patients with HPV-related oropharynx cancer treated with a variety of treatment models, ranging from surgery to combined chemoradiotherapy.[75,76] It remains to be determined what the best way is to translate the favorable clinical behavior into decreased treatment intensity. Chemoradiotherapy is the standard treatment for intermediate to locally advanced oropharynx cancer, and the approaches to dose de-escalation have addressed all aspects of the combined modality treatment model.

The most commonly used chemotherapy/radiotherapy combination is concurrent chemoradiotherapy. Within this paradigm, a joint University of North Carolina/University of Florida trial study is examining a decrease in radiation dose for definitive treatment. Patients were treated with a reduced dose of radiotherapy (60 Gy in 2 Gy fractions) with concurrent weekly cisplatin (30 mg/M^2). All patients underwent a dissection of involved lymph node regions and primary site biopsy following treatment in order to assess for (and possibly treat) residual disease. The preliminary data from ASCO 2015[77] demonstrated the following: 37 of 43 patients with pathologic complete response (CRs) and 6 patients with residual microscopic disease. All patients were alive without evidence of disease at a median follow-up of 15 months. These encouraging results suggest this approach has potential for maintaining treatment efficacy using a 14% decrease in radiotherapy dose. In this study, patients were selected solely on the basis of favorable upfront characteristics including HPV status, nonsmoking status, and stage. A recently activated NRG trial (HN002) will examine a similar model of decreasing radiation dose with or without concurrent systemic therapy, using a radiation dose of 60 Gy. Decreasing chemoradiotherapy dose intensity (but with radiation therapy held constant) was also examined in RTOG (Radiation Therapy Oncology Group) study 1016 where the standard of care, 70 Gy IMRT over 6 weeks with 2 doses of bolus cisplatin, was compared with what is presumed to be less intensive treatment using weekly cetuximab for cisplatin. This trial is closed to accrual, but outcomes have yet to be reported.

An alternative model for decreasing chemoradiotherapy dose intensity employs induction chemotherapy (IC) prior to definitive radiation-based therapy. This approach allows radiation treatment to be modified based on the chemotherapy response, which has been proposed as 1 rationale for IC. For reference, the standard radiotherapy in postinduction patients is 70 Gy to the pre-chemotherapy tumor volumes, regardless of treatment response,[28] and (2) the overall dose intensity of chemoradiotherapy is a function of the dose of radiation and the volume treated. In a completed phase 1 trial, ECOG has examined a reduction in radiation dose (but not target volume) from 70 Gy to 54 Gy in patients having clinical CRs to induction chemotherapy with paclitaxel/carboplatin.[78] Patients treated with reduced dose radiation therapy demonstrated a progression-free survival (PFS) of 80%, which was encouraging, although it was slightly outside the goal of 85%. In retrospect, adjusting the entry criteria to better reflect current understanding of prognostic factors (particularly smoking) could have increased the PFS to over 90%. These data clearly identify dose reduction based on IC response as a viable approach in terms of early treatment outcome. A recent update of the study[79] demonstrated improved quality-of-life metrics, indicating that this treatment warrants further investigation. Radiation treatment deintensification can also be achieved by decreasing the extent of the treatment volume. In a study using the University of Chicago DHFX (Docetaxol, continuous infusion 5-fuorouracil, hydroxyurea) regimen,[80] Villaflor and colleagues[81] investigated shrinking the target volume in postinduction patients and treating only the extent of residual disease. The definition of target volume was in sharp contrast with the standard of treating the pre-IC tumor volume. In a preliminary presentation, their data suggest that this is also a safe method for radiation-based deintensification. The quality-of-life consequences of this approach are expected to be an important benefit, as decreased target volumes will allow less dose to be delivered to the normal tissue. This aspect of the study has yet to be reported.

SUMMARY

The many advances in radiotherapy for SCCHN described in this article will have significant effects on the ultimate outcomes of patients who receive either definitive or postoperative treatment. The technological and clinical advances should allow one to maintain or improve disease control, while moderating the toxicity associated with head and neck radiation therapy.

REFERENCES

1. Setton J, Caria N, Romanyshyn J, et al. Intensity-modulated radiotherapy in the treatment of oropharyngeal cancer: an update of the Memorial Sloan-Kettering Cancer Center experience. Int J Radiat Oncol Biol Phys 2012;82:291–8.
2. Garden AS, Dong L, Morrison WH, et al. Patterns of disease recurrence following treatment of oropharyngeal cancer with intensity modulated radiation therapy. Int J Radiat Oncol Biol Phys 2013;85:941–7.
3. Sher DJ, Thotakura V, Balboni TA, et al. Treatment of oropharyngeal squamous cell carcinoma with IMRT: patterns of failure after concurrent chemoradiotherapy and sequential therapy. Ann Oncol 2012;23:2391–8.
4. Kam MK, Leung SF, Zee B, et al. Prospective randomized study of intensity-modulated radiotherapy on salivary gland function in early-stage nasopharyngeal carcinoma patients. J Clin Oncol 2007;25:4873–9.
5. Fang FM, Chien CY, Tsai WL, et al. Quality of life and survival outcome for patients with nasopharyngeal carcinoma receiving three-dimensional conformal radiotherapy vs intensity-modulated radiotherapy-a longitudinal study. Int J Radiat Oncol Biol Phys 2008;72:356–64.
6. Zeng L, Tian YM, Sun XM, et al. Late toxicities after intensity-modulated radiotherapy for nasopharyngeal carcinoma: patient and treatment-related risk factors. Br J Cancer 2014;110:49–54.

7. Huang TL, Chien CY, Tsai WL, et al. Long-term late toxicities and quality of life for survivors of nasopharyngeal carcinoma treated by intensity modulated radiotherapy (IMRT) vs non-IMRT. Head Neck 2015. [Epub ahead of print].

8. Nutting CM, Morden JP, Harrington KJ, et al. Parotid-sparing intensity modulated versus conventional radiotherapy in head and neck cancer (PARSPORT): a phase 3 multicentre randomised controlled trial. Lancet Oncol 2011;12:127–36.

9. Graff P, Lapeyre M, Desandes E, et al. Impact of intensity-modulated radiotherapy on health-related quality of life for head and neck cancer patients: matched-pair comparison with conventional radiotherapy. Int J Radiat Oncol Biol Phys 2007;67:1309–17.

10. Kohler RE, Sheets NC, Wheeler SB, et al. Two-year and lifetime cost-effectiveness of intensity modulated radiation therapy versus 3-dimensional conformal radiation therapy for head-and-neck cancer. Int J Radiat Oncol Biol Phys 2013;87:683–9.

11. Peters LJ, O'Sullivan B, Giralt J, et al. Critical impact of radiotherapy protocol compliance and quality in the treatment of advanced head and neck cancer: results from TROG 02.02. J Clin Oncol 2010;28:2996–3001.

12. Dawson LA, Anzai Y, Marsh L, et al. Patterns of local-regional recurrence following parotid-sparing conformal and segmental intensity-modulated radiotherapy for head and neck cancer. Int J Radiat Oncol Biol Phys 2000;46:1117–26.

13. Eisbruch A, Marsh LH, Dawson LA, et al. Recurrences near base of skull after IMRT for head-and-neck cancer: implications for target delineation in high neck and for parotid gland sparing. Int J Radiat Oncol Biol Phys 2004;59:28–42.

14. Thiagarajan A, Caria N, Schöder H, et al. Target volume delineation in oropharyngeal cancer: impact of PET, MRI, and physical examination. Int J Radiat Oncol Biol Phys 2012;83:220–7.

15. Smith-Bindman R, Miglioretti DL, Johnson E, et al. Use of diagnostic imaging studies and associated radiation exposure for patients enrolled in large integrated health care systems, 1996-2010. JAMA 2012;307:2400–9.

16. Schwartz DL, Ford E, Rajendran J, et al. FDG-PET/CT imaging for preradiotherapy staging of head-and-neck squamous cell carcinoma. Int J Radiat Oncol Biol Phys 2005;61:129–36.

17. Murakami R, Uozumi H, Hirai T, et al. Impact of FDG-PET/CT imaging on nodal staging for head-and-neck squamous cell carcinoma. Int J Radiat Oncol Biol Phys 2007;68:377–82.

18. Bryson TC, Shah GV, Srinivasan A, et al. Cervical lymph node evaluation and diagnosis. Otolaryngol Clin North Am 2012;45:1363–83.

19. Kastrinidis N, Kuhn FP, Hany TF, et al. 18F-FDG-PET/CT for the assessment of the contralateral neck in patients with head and neck squamous cell carcinoma. Laryngoscope 2013;123:1210–5.

20. Sher DJ, Tishler RB, Annino D, et al. Cost-effectiveness of CT and PET-CT for determining the need for adjuvant neck dissection in locally advanced head and neck cancer. Ann Oncol 2010;21:1072–7.

21. Anderson CM, Sun W, Buatti JM, et al. Interobserver and intermodality variability in GTV delineation on simulation CT, FDG-PET, and MR Images of head and neck cancer. Jacobs J Radiat Oncol 2014;1:6.

22. Daisne J-F, Duprez T, Weynand B, et al. Tumor volume in pharyngolaryngeal squamous cell carcinoma: comparison at CT, MR imaging, and FDG PET and validation with surgical specimen. Radiology 2004;233:93–100.

23. Ng S-H, Yen T-C, Liao C-T, et al. 18F-FDG PET and CT/MRI in oral cavity squamous cell carcinoma: a prospective study of 124 patients with histologic correlation. J Nucl Med 2005;46:1136–43.

24. Speirs CK, Grigsby PW, Huang J, et al. PET-based radiation therapy planning. PET Clin 2015;10:27–44.
25. Hwang AB, Bacharach SL, Yom SS, et al. Can positron emission tomography (PET) or PET/computed tomography (CT) acquired in a nontreatment position be accurately registered to a head-and-neck radiotherapy planning CT? Int J Radiat Oncol Biol Phys 2009;73:578–84.
26. Ireland RH, Dyker KE, Barber DC, et al. Nonrigid image registration for head and neck cancer radiotherapy treatment planning with PET/CT. Int J Radiat Oncol Biol Phys 2007;68:952–7.
27. Schoenfeld JD, Kovalchuk N, Subramaniam RM, et al. PET/CT of cancer patients: part 2, deformable registration imaging before and after chemotherapy for radiation treatment planning in head and neck cancer. AJR Am J Roentgenol 2012;199:968–74.
28. Salama JK, Haddad RI, Kies MS, et al. Clinical practice guidance for radiotherapy planning after induction chemotherapy in locoregionally advanced head-and-neck cancer. Int J Radiat Oncol Biol Phys 2009;75:725–33.
29. Fortunati V, Verhaart RF, Angeloni F, et al. Feasibility of multimodal deformable registration for head and neck tumor treatment planning. Int J Radiat Oncol Biol Phys 2014;90:85–93.
30. Allal AS, Dulguerov P, Allaoua M, et al. Standardized uptake value of 2-[(18)F] fluoro-2-deoxy-D-glucose in predicting outcome in head and neck carcinomas treated by radiotherapy with or without chemotherapy. J Clin Oncol 2002;20: 1398–404.
31. Schwartz DL, Harris J, Yao M, et al. Metabolic tumor volume as a prognostic imaging-based biomarker for head-and-neck cancer: pilot results from Radiation Therapy Oncology Group protocol 0522. Int J Radiat Oncol Biol Phys 2015;91: 721–9.
32. Khodayari B, Daly ME, Bobinski M, et al. Observation versus neck dissection for positron-emission tomography-negative lymphadenopathy after chemoradiotherapy. Laryngoscope 2014;124:902–6.
33. Sjövall J, Chua B, Pryor D, et al. Long-term results of positron emission tomography-directed management of the neck in node-positive head and neck cancer after organ preservation therapy. Oral Oncol 2015;51:260–6.
34. Quon H, Brizel DM. Predictive and prognostic role of functional imaging of head and neck squamous cell carcinomas. Semin Radiat Oncol 2012;22: 220–32.
35. Dirix P, Vandecaveye V, De Keyzer F, et al. Diffusion-weighted MRI for nodal staging of head and neck squamous cell carcinoma: impact on radiotherapy planning. Int J Radiat Oncol Biol Phys 2010;76:761–6.
36. Paulson ES, Erickson B, Schultz C, et al. Comprehensive MRI simulation methodology using a dedicated MRI scanner in radiation oncology for external beam radiation treatment planning. Med Phys 2015;42:28–39.
37. Schinagl DAX, Vogel WV, Hoffmann AL, et al. Comparison of five segmentation tools for 18F-fluoro-deoxy-glucose-positron emission tomography-based target volume definition in head and neck cancer. Int J Radiat Oncol Biol Phys 2007; 69:1282–9.
38. Troost EGC, Schinagl DAX, Bussink J, et al. Clinical evidence on PET-CT for radiation therapy planning in head and neck tumours. Radiother Oncol 2010;96: 328–34.
39. Nyflot MJ, Kruser TJ, Traynor AM, et al. Phase 1 trial of bevacizumab with concurrent chemoradiation therapy for squamous cell carcinoma of the head and neck

with exploratory functional imaging of tumor hypoxia, proliferation, and perfusion. Int J Radiat Oncol Biol Phys 2015;91:942–51.

40. Schaefferkoetter JD, Carlson ER, Heidel RE. Can 3'-Deoxy-3'-((18)F) Fluorothymidine Out Perform 2-Deoxy-2-((18)F) Fluoro-d-Glucose positron emission tomography/computed tomography in the diagnosis of cervical lymphadenopathy in patients with oral/head and neck cancer? J Oral Maxillofac Surg 2015;73(7):1420–8.

41. Choi W, Lee S-W, Park SH, et al. Planning study for available dose of hypoxic tumor volume using fluorine-18-labeled fluoromisonidazole positron emission tomography for treatment of the head and neck cancer. Radiother Oncol 2010; 97:176–82.

42. Hong TS, Tome WA, Chappell RJ, et al. The impact of daily setup variations on head-and-neck intensity-modulated radiation therapy. Int J Radiat Oncol Biol Phys 2005;61:779–88.

43. Manning MA, Wu Q, Cardinale RM, et al. The effect of setup uncertainty on normal tissue sparing with IMRT for head-and-neck cancer. Int J Radiat Oncol Biol Phys 2001;51:1400–9.

44. Dawson LA, Jaffray DA. Advances in image-guided radiation therapy. J Clin Oncol 2007;25:938–46.

45. Boda-Heggemann J, Lohr F, Wenz F, et al. kV cone-beam CT-based IGRT: a clinical review. Strahlenther Onkol 2011;187:284–91.

46. Scarfe WC, Farman AG. What is cone-beam CT and how does it work? Dent Clin North Am 2008;52:707–30, v.

47. Zhang L, Garden AS, Lo J, et al. Multiple regions-of-interest analysis of setup uncertainties for head-and-neck cancer radiotherapy. Int J Radiat Oncol Biol Phys 2006;64:1559–69.

48. Hansen EK, Bucci MK, Quivey JM, et al. Repeat CT imaging and replanning during the course of IMRT for head-and-neck cancer. Int J Radiat Oncol Biol Phys 2006;64:355–62.

49. Barker JL Jr, Garden AS, Ang KK, et al. Quantification of volumetric and geometric changes occurring during fractionated radiotherapy for head-and-neck cancer using an integrated CT/linear accelerator system. Int J Radiat Oncol Biol Phys 2004;59:960–70.

50. Mencarelli A, van Kranen SR, Hamming-Vrieze O, et al. Deformable image registration for adaptive radiation therapy of head and neck cancer: accuracy and precision in the presence of tumor changes. Int J Radiat Oncol Biol Phys 2014; 90:680–7.

51. Richter A, Hu Q, Steglich D, et al. Investigation of the usability of conebeam CT data sets for dose calculation. Radiat Oncol 2008;3:42.

52. van Zijtveld M, Dirkx M, Breuers M, et al. Evaluation of the 'dose of the day' for IMRT prostate cancer patients derived from portal dose measurements and cone-beam CT. Radiother Oncol 2010;96:172–7.

53. Hong TS, Tome WA, Harari PM. Heterogeneity in head and neck IMRT target design and clinical practice. Radiother Oncol 2012;103:92–8.

54. Bice W. Medical physicists should actively discourage institutions from advertising technologies such as IMRT and HDR brachytherapy in order to recruit patients. Against the proposition. Med Phys 2005;32:308–10.

55. Van Gestel D, Verellen D, Van De Voorde L, et al. The potential of helical tomotherapy in the treatment of head and neck cancer. Oncologist 2013;18:697–706.

56. Wiezorek T, Brachwitz T, Georg D, et al. Rotational IMRT techniques compared to fixed gantry IMRT and tomotherapy: multi-institutional planning study for head-and-neck cases. Radiat Oncol 2011;6:20.

57. Van Gestel D, van Vliet-Vroegindeweij C, Van den Heuvel F, et al. RapidArc, Smar-tArc and TomoHD compared with classical step and shoot and sliding window intensity modulated radiotherapy in an oropharyngeal cancer treatment plan comparison. Radiat Oncol 2013;8:37.

58. Lu SH, Cheng JC, Kuo SH, et al. Volumetric modulated arc therapy for nasopharyn-geal carcinoma: a dosimetric comparison with TomoTherapy and step-and-shoot IMRT. Radiother Oncol 2012;104:324–30.

59. Mackie TR, Kapatoes J, Ruchala K, et al. Image guidance for precise conformal radiotherapy. Int J Radiat Oncol Biol Phys 2003;56:89–105.

60. Yu CX. Intensity-modulated arc therapy with dynamic multileaf collimation: an alternative to tomotherapy. Phys Med Biol 1995;40:1435–49.

61. Shaikh M, Burmeister J, Joiner M, et al. Biological effect of different IMRT delivery techniques: SMLC, DMLC, and helical tomotherapy. Med Phys 2010;37:762–70.

62. Suit HD. Protons to replace photons in external beam radiation therapy? Clin Oncol (R Coll Radiol) 2003;15:S29–31.

63. Suit H, Goldberg S, Niemierko A, et al. Proton beams to replace photon beams in radical dose treatments. Acta Oncol 2003;42:800–8.

64. Chan AW. Change in patterns of relapse after combined proton and photon irra-diation for locally advanced paranasal sinus cancer. Int J Radiat Oncol Biol Phys 2004;60:320.

65. Pommier P, Liebsch NJ, Deschler DG, et al. Proton beam radiation therapy for skull base adenoid cystic carcinoma. Arch Otolaryngol Head Neck Surg 2006; 132:1242–9.

66. Zenda S, Kohno R, Kawashima M, et al. Proton beam therapy for unresectable malignancies of the nasal cavity and paranasal sinuses. Int J Radiat Oncol Biol Phys 2011;81:1473–8.

67. Goldsmith T, Holman AS, Parambi RG, et al. Swallowing function after proton beam therapy for nasopharyngeal cancer: a prospective study. Int J Radiat Oncol Biol Phys 2012;84:S62–3.

68. Holliday E, Garden AS, Fuller CD, et al. Gastrostomy tube rates decrease by over 50% in patients with nasopharyngeal cancer treated with intensity modulated proton therapy (IMPT): a case–control study. Int J Radiat Oncol Biol Phys 2014; 90:S528.

69. Slater JD, Yonemoto LT, Mantik DW, et al. Proton radiation for treatment of cancer of the oropharynx: early experience at Loma Linda University Medical Center using a concomitant boost technique. Int J Radiat Oncol Biol Phys 2005;62: 494–500.

70. Frank SJ, Rosenthal D, Ang KK, et al. Gastrostomy tubes decrease by over 50% with intensity modulated proton therapy (IMPT) during the treatment of oropha-ryngeal cancer patients: a case–control study. Int J Radiat Oncol Biol Phys 2013;87:S144.

71. Kanai T, Kawachi K, Kumamoto Y, et al. Spot scanning system for proton radio-therapy. Med Phys 1980;7:365–9.

72. Kooy HM, Grassberger C. Intensity modulated proton therapy. Br J Radiol 2015; 88:20150195.

73. Hyer DE, Hill PM, Wang D, et al. Effects of spot size and spot spacing on lateral penumbra reduction when using a dynamic collimation system for spot scanning proton therapy. Phys Med Biol 2014;59:N187–96.

74. Margalit DN, Adams JA, Kooy H, et al. Proton beam therapy for head and neck cancer. In: Bernier J, editor. Head and Neck Cancer: Multimodality Management. 2 edition. New York: Springer; 2015.

75. Ang KK, Harris J, Wheeler R, et al. Human papillomavirus and survival of patients with oropharyngeal cancer. N Engl J Med 2010;363:24–35.

76. Fischer CA, Zlobec I, Green E, et al. Is the improved prognosis of p16 positive oropharyngeal squamous cell carcinoma dependent of the treatment modality? Int J Cancer 2010;126:1256–62.

77. Chera BS, Amdur RJ, Tepper JE, et al. A prospective phase II trail of de-intensified chemoradiotherapy for low-risk HPV-associated oropharyngeal squamous cell carcinoma. ASCO Meet Abstr 2015;33(Suppl 15):6004.

78. Cmelak A, Li S, Marur S, et al. E1308: reduced-dose IMRT in human papilloma virus (HPV)-associated resectable oropharyngeal squamous carcinomas (OPSCC) after clinical complete response (cCR) to induction chemotherapy (IC). ASCO Meet Abstr 2014;32(Suppl 5):LBA6006.

79. Cmelak A, Li S, Marur S, et al. Symptom reduction from IMRT dose deintensification: results from ECOG 1308 using the vanderbilt head and neck symptom survey version 2 (VHNSS V2). ASCO Meet Abstr 2015;33(Suppl 15):6021.

80. Brockstein B, Haraf DJ, Stenson K, et al. A phase I-II study of concomitant chemoradiotherapy with paclitaxel (one-hour infusion), 5-fluorouracil and hydroxyurea with granulocyte colony stimulating factor support for patients with poor prognosis head and neck cancer. Ann Oncol 2000;11:721–8.

81. Villaflor VM, Cohen EEW, Melotek JM, et al. Response-adapted volume de-escalation (RAVD) of radiotherapy (RT) using induction chemotherapy (IC) in locally advanced head and neck squamous cell cancer (LA-HNSCC). ASCO Meet Abstr 2015;33(Suppl 15):6050.

Chemotherapy for Nasopharyngeal Carcinoma – Current Recommendation and Controversies

Henry Sze, FRCR[a,b], Pierre Blanchard, MD, PhD[c],
Wai Tong Ng, MD, FRCR[d], Jean-Pierre Pignon, MD, PhD[e],
Anne W.M. Lee, MD, FRCR[a,b],*

KEYWORDS

- Nasopharyngeal carcinoma • Chemoradiotherapy • Therapeutic benefit
- Randomized trial • Meta-analysis

KEY POINTS

- Although chemotherapy has a major role in enhancing treatment outcomes, there is a wide variation in clinical practice and the best way to deliver chemotherapy is still clouded with controversies.
- Although timely and flexible modification of treatment strategy is necessary, whether it is time to move away from the established standard of care and what defines the highest level of evidence need to be asked.
- There are concerted efforts worldwide in promoting further advances in this important area and, with stronger global collaboration, it is hoped that future trials can address the current controversial issues.

The Meta-Analysis of Chemotherapy in Nasopharyngeal Carcinoma (MAC-NPC) was funded by grants from French Ministry of Health (Programme d'actions intégrées de recherche [VADS]) and Ligue Nationale Contre le Cancer and support for the investigator meeting from Sanofi-Aventis.
[a] Department of Clinical Oncology, Li Ka Shing Faculty of Medicine, The University of Hong Kong, Queen Mary Hospital, 102 Pokfulam Road, Hong Kong, China; [b] Department of Clinical Oncology, The University of Hong Kong – Shenzhen Hospital, 1 Haiyuan First Road, Futian District, Shenzhen, Guangdong 518053, China; [c] Department of Radiation Oncology, Research in Epidemiology and Population Health, INSERM U1018, Paris-Saclay University, Gustave-Roussy, 114 rue Edouard Vaillant, 94 805 Villejuif Cedex, France; [d] Department of Clinical Oncology, Pamela Youde Nethersole Eastern Hospital, 3 Lock Man Road, Chai Wan, Hong Kong, China; [e] Department of Biostatistics and Epidemiology, Ligue National Contre le Cancer Platform of Meta-analyses in Oncology, Research in Epidemiology and Population Health, INSERM U1018, Paris-Saclay University, Gustave-Roussy, 114 rue Edouard Vaillant, 94 805 Villejuif Cedex, France
* Corresponding author.
E-mail address: annelee@hku-szh.org

Hematol Oncol Clin N Am 29 (2015) 1107–1122
http://dx.doi.org/10.1016/j.hoc.2015.07.004
0889-8588/15/$ – see front matter © 2015 Elsevier Inc. All rights reserved.

hemonc.theclinics.com

INTRODUCTION

Nasopharyngeal carcinoma (NPC) has a peculiarly skewed distribution; this is a rare cancer in North America but highly prevalent in Southeast Asia. The classical nonkeratinizing type is unanimously associated with Epstein-Barr virus (EBV). This cancer is notorious not only for its extensive local infiltration and early lymphatic spread but also its high propensity for hematogenous dissemination. A majority of patients present with advanced locoregional disease. It is important to understand the behavior and management of this unique cancer because it is highly treatable.

There is little controversy that radiotherapy (RT) is the mainstay of primary treatment. Locoregional control is steadily improving with advances in technology. A key problem to overcome is distant failure. For patients with locoregionally advanced disease, addition of chemotherapy serves dual purposes of potentiating RT for better locoregional control (especially for tumors infiltrating/abutting critical neurologic structures) and eradicating subclinical micrometastasis.

BACKGROUND FOR THE CURRENT GUIDELINES

Randomized phase III trials to evaluate the therapeutic benefit of various chemotherapy approaches have been initiated since 1979. It was not until 1998 that achievement of significant benefit in overall survival (OS) was first reported: this landmark was achieved by an Intergroup 0099 study (n = 193) using concurrent chemotherapy (cisplatin, 100 mg/m^2, every 3 weeks for 3 cycles) followed by adjuvant chemotherapy (cisplatin, 80 mg/m^2, and fluorouracil, 4000 mg/m^2, in 96 hours every 4 weeks for 3 cycles) during the post-RT period.[1,2] There was initial skepticism about the benefit of this regimen because the result of the RT-alone arm was substantially poorer than that achieved by major centers. Four confirmatory trials have subsequently been conducted[3–10]; although the magnitude of benefit was smaller, all concurred that concurrent-adjuvant chemotherapy could improve event-free survival compared with RT alone; all but one also reported significant improvement in OS.[11] This regimen has hence become one of the standard recommendations since the late 1990s.

The first patient-data Meta-Analysis of Chemotherapy in Nasopharyngeal Carcinoma (MAC-NPC), with 1753 patients from 8 trials, confirmed that addition of chemotherapy achieved a significant survival benefit compared with RT alone (absolute gain of 6% at 5 years).[12] Timing of chemotherapy was important. Only trials including a concurrent +/– adjuvant component achieved significant survival benefit; trials of adjuvant chemotherapy alone did not show significant benefit in any endpoint. This raised doubt about the exact magnitude of contribution by the adjuvant component in the Intergroup 0099 regimen. Furthermore, tolerance is often poor during the post-RT period, for only approximately 60% of patients can complete all 3 cycles of adjuvant chemotherapy after definitive concurrent cisplatin and radiation. It is desirable to eliminate adjuvant chemotherapy if its contribution above concurrent chemoradiation is minimal.

The concurrent regimen most commonly recommended is cisplatin, 40 mg/m^2 weekly, as used in the trial by Chan and colleagues[13] (n = 350). In the preliminary report, progression-free survival (PFS) was not significantly different between the concurrent arm and the RT-alone arm in the overall comparison (76% vs 69% at 2 years; P = .10), but PFS was significantly prolonged in the subgroup of patients with advanced T stage (P = .0075). In the subsequent report,[14] unadjusted analysis showed borderline significance in OS (70% vs 59%; P = .065); but the difference reached significance when adjusted for T stage, age, and overall stage (P = .049) for the whole series, particularly in the subgroup with advanced T stage (P = .013).

Another approach that has been extensively studied is induction chemotherapy followed by concurrent chemotherapy with radiation. Changing the timing from adjuvant to induction is potentially advantageous because the tolerance to chemotherapy is substantially better and up-front use of potent combinations of drugs can be more effective in eradicating micrometastasis. Furthermore, shrinkage of bulky tumor could lead to better tumor coverage by subsequent RT, which is especially important for tumors abutting critical neurologic structures. Since the first report by Rischin and colleagues,[15] more than 18 single-arm phase II studies using various duplet or triplet combinations have been conducted and all reported encouraging results. The first randomized study by Hui and colleagues[16] (n = 65) showed that the addition of induction chemotherapy using cisplatin-docetaxel had significantly better 3-year OS compared with concurrent cisplatin alone. This benefit became insignificant, however, with longer follow-up (HR = 0.64 [0.69–1.39]).[11] Furthermore, 2 other randomized studies showed negative results: both Fountzilas and colleagues[17] (n = 141), using cisplatin-epirubicin-paclitaxel, and Tan and colleagues[18] (n = 172), using carboplatin-gemcitabine-paclitaxel, reported that addition of induction chemotherapy did not achieve significant benefit beyond concurrent cisplatin alone.

CURRENT INTERNATIONAL GUIDELINES

Both the Clinical Practice Guidelines in Oncology by the National Comprehensive Cancer Network (NCCN) on Head and Neck Cancers (2015, version 1)[19] in North America and the European Head & Neck Society, European Society for Medical Oncology, European Society for Radiotherapy and Oncology (EHNS-ESMO-ESTRO) Clinical Practice Guidelines[20] in Europe recommended RT alone for stage I and the use of chemotherapy in combination with RT for all other stages of nondisseminated NPC. There are subtle differences, however, in their recommendations on the timing of chemotherapy. The NCCN guidelines list concurrent-adjuvant, concurrent-alone (category 2B), and induction-concurrent (category 3) chemotherapy as their recommendation for stages II–IVB. The EHNS-ESMO-ESTRO guidelines give more-specific recommendation based on stage: concurrent-alone for stage II (category 1B); concurrent +/– adjuvant for stages III–IVB (category 1A); and induction-concurrent chemotherapy for stages IVA–B with problematic RT (category 2B).

These guidelines reflect subtle differences in beliefs and preferences. Although there is little controversy that addition of chemotherapy is needed for patients with advanced locoregional disease, there is yet no consensus on which is the best regimen and how to optimize treatment based on individual risk. Many unanswered questions warrant critical review.

UNANSWERED QUESTIONS AND RECENT STUDIES
Is Chemotherapy Necessary for All Stage II?

All except one clinical trial comparing chemo-RT versus RT alone were initially planned for patients with advanced locoregional disease. Due to the major change in staging criteria with the introduction of the *AJCC Cancer Staging Manual, 5th Edition*,[21] however, the trials started before 1997 included patients who were recategorized as stage II by current criteria. Hence, the recommendations on chemo-RT by the 2 major international guidelines included stage II–IVB diseases. Detailed review of the past trials that achieved significant benefit showed, however, that only the Intergroup 0099 study did include stage II patients and there were only 5 such early cases.

The only randomized study that was designed to evaluate the benefit in early cases was that by Chen and colleagues.[22] In this study, 230 patients with stage II disease by the Chinese 1992 staging system were randomized to radical RT with or without concurrent cisplatin, 30 mg/m^2 weekly. Due to difference in staging criteria, 87% of the series were stage II and 13% stage III by the current American Joint Committee on Cancer (AJCC) system. The study reported significant improvement in the 5-year OS (95% versus 86%, HR = 0.30 [0.12–0.76]; P = .007) by chemo-RT, due mainly to improvement in distant control. All patients in this trial were treated, however, by conventional 2-D RT. A retrospective study by Lee and colleagues[23] showed that patients with stage II irradiated by 3-D conformal or intensity-modulated RT (IMRT) technique could achieve 5-year disease-specific survival of 95% without addition of chemotherapy. Another retrospective study by Su and colleagues[24] of patients with stage I–II disease treated by IMRT alone showed that 5-year distant failure-free rate (D-FFR) of 94% could be achieved even the worst subgroup with T2N1 disease. Data on the magnitude of benefit by concurrent chemotherapy for patients treated in the era of IMRT, with improved RT technique and staging modalities (MRI and PET/CT), are still lacking.

In the updated individual patient data meta-analysis by the MAC-NPC Collaborative Group (MAC-NPC2),[11] a study of the variation of chemotherapy effect according to stage showed that the HR (95% CI) was 0.95 (0.65–1.44) for stage I–II (mostly stage II), 0.75 (0.59–0.94) for stage III, and 0.72 (0.58–0.89) for stage IVA–B (test for trend P = .24). The corresponding absolute benefits at 5-year OS were 3.6%, 6.0%, and 8.1%, respectively. The meta-analysis results, considering in particular the nonsignificant HR and small magnitude of absolute OS benefit at 5 years, are not in favor of addition of chemotherapy in early stage. Furthermore, addition of chemotherapy incurs not only medical costs but also significant increase in hearing impairment.[11]

The current indiscriminant recommendation of chemo-RT for all patients with stage II should be revisited. A more personalized approach to confine chemotherapy to high-risk patients should be considered. Factors, including the volume of the primary tumor[25,26] and pretreatment EBV DNA level,[27] are promising candidates to be considered. Trials to evaluate the benefit of concurrent chemotherapy in patients with high-risk, early-stage disease treated by modern RT techniques are warranted.

Which Is the Best Treatment of Stage III–IVB?

Although the role of combined RT and chemotherapy is well established for locoregionally advanced disease and concurrent sequence is the most potent timing, there is yet no consensus on whether concurrent alone is adequate and, if more chemotherapy is needed, whether adjuvant or induction timing is more advantageous.

Concurrent versus concurrent-adjuvant chemoradiotherapy

An exploratory study in patients irradiated with conventional fractionation from NPC-9901 and NPC-9902 trials[28] showed that although the concurrent phase and dose of concurrent cisplatin were important for locoregional control and survival, the adjuvant phase and dose of fluorouracil had significant impact on distant control. Further analysis on correlation with the number of chemotherapy cycles suggested that 2 concurrent cycles (total cisplatin, 200 mg/m^2) might be adequate. For the adjuvant phase, patients who received 3 or more cycles achieved significantly better D-FFR than those with 0 to 1 adjuvant cycles.

A phase III randomized trial by Chen and colleagues[29] randomized 508 patients with stage III–IVB disease (except T3-4N0) to concurrent versus concurrent-adjuvant chemo-RT. Preliminary results showed that the arm with addition of adjuvant cisplatin-fluorouracil did not achieve significant difference in failure-free survival rates at 2 year (86% vs 84%) compared with those treated by concurrent cisplatin alone. The investigators stated that concurrent-adjuvant chemotherapy should not be used outside well-designed clinical trials. The results must be interpreted, however, with caution. Compliance with adjuvant chemotherapy was poor: 18% of patients allocated to the concurrent-adjuvant arm were actually treated by concurrent chemo-RT alone; another 20% discontinued after starting adjuvant chemotherapy; 49% had dose reduction; and 69% had delays in treatment. Despite this poor compliance, the concurrent-adjuvant arm showed a favorable trend in locoregional failure-free rate (LR-FFR) (HR 0.50 [0.21–1.16]; P = .10), D-FFR (HR 0.71 [0.46–1.10]; P = .12), and failure-free survival (HR 0·74 [0.49–1.10]; P = .13). Furthermore, the median follow-up was only 38 months. Longer observation is needed for definitive conclusion.

In a literature-based meta-analysis by Chen and colleagues[30] of 2144 patients in 8 trials that evaluated the benefit of concurrent chemo-RT over RT alone, bayesian network analysis showed that the effect of concurrent adjuvant was statistically insignificant compared with concurrent alone (HR for OS was 0.86 [0.60–1.16]) by a fixed effects model. However, the probability of each treatment being ranked the best, second and third best, and the cumulative probabilities for the most efficacious treatments were as follows (OS, LR-FFR, D-FFR): concurrent-adjuvant (84%, 90%, 85%), concurrent alone (16%, 10%, 15%) and RT alone (0%, 0%, 0%). The study did have limitations because information extracted from published data may have resulted in publication and reporting bias.

The MAC-NPC2, with 4806 patients from 19 valid trials and a median follow-up of 7.7 years, provides further insights.[11] **Table 1** shows the updated results of trials that evaluated the benefit of chemotherapy added to RT over RT alone. In this update, concurrent adjuvant and concurrent alone were analyzed as distinct groups. This study reconfirmed a small but significant benefit in OS by adding chemotherapy (6% absolute gain for OS at 5 years and 8% at 10 years). A significant interaction between treatment effect on OS and the timing of chemotherapy was again observed: the HR by concurrent-adjuvant chemotherapy was 0.65 (0.56–0.76) and concurrent-alone chemotherapy was 0.79 (0.68–0.92) compared with induction (HR 0.96 [0.80–1.16]) and adjuvant-alone chemotherapy (HR 0.93 [0.70–1.24]).

In the concurrent-adjuvant chemotherapy group, all (except 5 patients from the Intergroup 0099 study) had stage III–IVB disease by current staging system. All used concurrent cisplatin followed by adjuvant cisplatin-fluorouracil and the standard arm was RT alone. The outcome was consistent: all (except part of the NPC-9902 trial) confirmed significant survival benefit. Even the NPC-9901 trial, which initially reported no significant differences in OS at 3 and 5 years,[5,6] became significant with longer follow-up: HR was 0.73 (0.54–0.99).[11]

The concurrent-alone group was more heterogeneous: 20% of the patients had stage II disease, and various chemotherapy regimens had been used. Among the trials that used RT alone as the standard arm, only the trial by Chen and colleagues[22] (n = 230), using cisplatin 30 mg/m^2 weekly for stage II (as discussed previously), and the trial by Zhang and colleagues[36] (n = 115), using oxaliplatin 70 mg/m^2 weekly for stage III–IVB disease,[37] achieved significant improvement in OS.

A recent individual patient-data network meta-analysis by the MAC-NPC Collaborative Group[38] attempted to provide more data for selecting the best treatment. The effect by concurrent-adjuvant chemotherapy showed favorable trend in terms of OS (HR 0.84 [0.67–1.03]) and D-FFR (HR 0.90 [0.69–1.17]) and significant advantage in terms of LR-FFR (HR 0.67 [0.46–0.95]) compared with concurrent alone. The probability for being ranked as the most efficacious treatment of OS was highest by concurrent-adjuvant chemotherapy (84%) compared with only 3% by concurrent alone. In terms of D-FFR, the probability for being the most efficacious treatment was highest by induction-concurrent chemotherapy (83%), followed by concurrent-adjuvant chemotherapy

Table 1
Updated results on hazard ratios for overall survival of trials that evaluated the benefit of chemotherapy added to radiotherapy over radiotherapy alone according to the updated Meta-Analysis of Chemotherapy in Nasopharyngeal Carcinoma

Trial	Stage	Regimen	Overall Survival Hazard Ratio (95% CI)
Induction alone			
Chua[31]	II–IVB	Cisplatin 60 mg/m² + epirubicin 110 mg/m² every 3 wk × 2–3	0.99 (0.68–1.44)
VUMCA I[32]	III–IVB	Bleomycin, 15 mg IV day 1, followed by 12 mg/m²/d, days 1–5, + epirubicin, 70 mg/m² day 1 + cisplatin 100 mg/m² day 1 every 3 wk × 3	1.00 (0.75–1.33)
Hareyama[33]	I–IVB	Cisplatin 80 mg/m² day 1 + fluorouracil 800 mg/m²/d, days 2–5, every 3 wk × 2	0.77 (0.40–1.46)
Adjuvant alone			
Chi[34]	II–IVB	Cisplatin 20 mg/m² + fluorouracil 2200 mg/m² + leucovorin 120 mg/m² in a 24-h infusion weekly × 9	0.95 (0.65–1.40)
Kwong[35]	II–IVB	Alternating cisplatin 100 mg/m² day 1 + fluorouracil 1000 mg/m²/d, days 1–3 (PF), and vincristine 2 mg day 1 + bleomycin 30 mg day 1 + methotrexate 150 mg/m² day 1 (VBM) every 3 wk × 6	1.07 (0.66–1.88)
Concurrent alone			
Cha[13]	II–IVB	Cisplatin 40 mg/m² weekly	0.81 (0.61–1.07)
Kwong[35]	II–IVB	Oral uracil + tegafur (UFT) 200 mg 3 times/d, 7 d/wk	1.00 (0.57–1.75)
Zhang[36]	III–IVB	Oxaliplatin 70 mg/m² weekly × 6	0.54 (0.31–0.93)
Chen[22]	II–III	Cisplatin 30 mg/m² weekly	0.34 (0.18–0.66)
Concurrent adjuvant			
Al-Sarraf[1]	II–IVB	C: cisplatin 100 mg/m² every 3 wk × 3 A: cisplatin 80 mg/m² day 1 + fluorouracil 1000 mg/m²/d, days 1–4, every 4 wk × 3	0.50 (0.36–0.71)
Wee[3]	III–IVB	C: cisplatin 25 mg/m²/d, days 1–4, every 3 wk × 3 A: cisplatin 20 mg/m²/d, days 1–4, + fluorouracil 1000 mg/m²/d, days 1–4, every 4 wk × 3	0.66 (0.48–0.96)
Lee[5]	N2–3	C: cisplatin 100 mg/m² every 3 wk × 3 A: cisplatin 80 mg/m² day 1 + fluorouracil 1000 mg/m²/d, days 1–4, every 4 wk × 3	0.73 (0.54–0.99)
Lee[7] (conventional)	T3–4 N0–1	C: cisplatin 100 mg/m² every 3 wk × 3 A: cisplatin 80 mg/m² day 1 + fluorouracil 1000 mg/m²/d, days 1–4, every 4 wk × 3	0.97 (0.52–1.82)
Lee[7] (accelerated)	T3–4 N0–1	C: cisplatin 100 mg/m² every 3 wk × 3 A: cisplatin 80 mg/m² day 1 + fluorouracil 1000 mg/m²/d, days 1–4, every 4 wk × 3	0.50 (0.28–0.90)

Abbreviations: A, adjuvant; C, concurrent.
Data from Refs.[1,3,5,7,13,16,22,31–36]

(8%), compared with only 1% by concurrent alone. These findings showed that although pairwise HRs are not significant except for LR-FFR, concurrent alone never ranked first for all endpoints; more chemotherapy seems to provide an additional benefit.

Omitting additional adjuvant chemotherapy would be justifiable if it incurs excessive toxicity and minimal to no benefit. Although this addition inevitably causes more acute toxicity, analyses in MAC-NPC2[11] showed that there were no differences in noncancer deaths between concurrent adjuvant and RT alone (HR 1.19 [0.77–1.85]) as well as concurrent alone and RT alone (HR 1.20 [0.77–1.87]). Furthermore, if concurrent alone is to be used, it is unclear which regimen to recommend, because the most commonly used regimen of weekly cisplatin, 40 mg/m^2, did not achieve significant benefit of OS (HR 0.81 [0.61–1.07]). The only regimen that achieved significance was weekly oxaliplatin based on a small trial with 115 patients.[36,37] Therefore, further validation of specific concurrent chemotherapy drugs and doses is still needed.

The authors conclude that concurrent cisplatin and adjuvant cisplatin-fluorouracil may be considered the first option for patients with stage III–IVB disease. Nevertheless, the adjuvant phase is not easy to tolerate. Identifying a subgroup of low-risk patients for whom this adjuvant chemotherapy can be safely omitted without jeopardizing the chance of survival is a priority. One attractive marker is the postradiation plasma EBV-DNA level.[39–41] The NRG (NSABP [National Surgical Adjuvant Breast and Bowel Project]- N, RTOG [Radiation Therapy Oncology Group]- R, GOG [Gynecologic Oncology Group]- G) is now conducting a randomized phase II and III study of individualized treatment of NPC based on using the plasma EBV-DNA level as a biomarker (the NRG-HN001 study [NCT02135042]). Patients with stage II–IVB disease are to be treated with IMRT and concurrent cisplatin. Those without detectable plasma EBV-DNA 1-week post-RT, thought to be the low-risk patients, are randomized to either adjuvant chemotherapy using standard cisplatin-fluorouracil or observation, whereas those with detectable plasma EBV-DNA after radiation, thought to be the high-risk patients, are given adjuvant chemotherapy with randomization to either standard cisplatin-fluorouracil or a new regimen using gemcitabine-paclitaxel. The results of this study will help to explore the possibility of more personalized treatment of patients with locoregionally advanced disease.

Concurrent versus induction-concurrent chemoradiotherapy

Updated results from MAC-NPC2[11] confirmed that induction chemotherapy significantly improved D-FFR (HR 0.62 [0.48–0.79]), although this did not translate into significant reduction of cancer deaths (HR 0.89 [0.73–1.09]). It did not distinguish, however, between trials on induction chemotherapy versus none and those of addition of induction chemotherapy to concurrent chemo-RT.

Table 2 shows the 5 trials comparing concurrent versus induction-concurrent chemo-RT. As discussed previously, the first 3 randomized studies[16–18] did not achieve statistically significant survival benefit. The sample sizes in all these studies, however, were small (range, 65–172). The preliminary results from 2 additional trials,[42,43] recently released at an academic conference, reported more encouraging results. Both used a triplet combination of docetaxel-cisplatin-fluorouracil (TPF). The French Head and Neck Oncology and Radiotherapy Group (GORTEC) 2006-01 trial (NCT00828386),[42] initially designed to study 260 stage II–IVB patients, was prematurely terminated due to slow accrual. Only 83 patients had been randomized; early results showed significant improvement in OS, PFS, and LR-FFR. A trial from China (NCT01245959),[43] which accrued 480 stage III–IVB patients, demonstrated significant improvement in 2-year failure-free survival and D-FFR. The median follow-up, however, was only 21 months; longer follow-up is needed to evaluate the efficacy and late toxicity.

Table 2
Trials comparing induction-concurrent versus concurrent chemoradiotherapy

Trial	Stage	Regimen	Results HR (95% CI)
Hui[16]	III–IVB	I: docetaxel 75 mg/m² + cisplatin 75 mg/m² every 3 wk × 2 C: cisplatin 40 mg/m² weekly × 8	OS: 0.64 (0.29–1.40) PFS: 0.63 (0.29–1.38) DMFS: 0.37 (0.12–1.10) (according to MAC-NPC2[11])
Fountzilas[17]	IIB–IVB	I: epirubicin 75 mg/m² + paclitaxel 175 mg/m² + cisplatin 75 mg/m² every 3 wk × 3 C: cisplatin 40 mg/m² weekly	OS: 0.99 (0.59–1.66) PFS: 0.86 (0.53–1.39) DMFS: 0.47 (0.22–1.01) (according to MAC-NPC2[11])
Tan[18]	III–IVB	I: paclitaxel 70 mg/m² + carboplatin AUC 2.5 + gemcitabine 1000 mg/m², day 1 and day 8, every 3 wk × 3 C: cisplatin 40 mg/m² weekly × 8	OS: 1.05 (0–2.19) DFS: 0.77 (0.44–1.35) DMFS: 0.80 (0.38–1.67)
Daoud[42]	II–IVA	I: docetaxel + cisplatin + fluorouracil × 2–3 cycles C: cisplatin 40 mg/m² weekly	OS: 0.37 (0.14–0.96) PFS: 0.43 (0.19–0.95)
Sun[43]	III–IVB	I: docetaxel 60 mg/m² day 1 + cisplatin 60 mg/m² day 1 + fluorouracil 600 mg/m²/d, days 1–5, every 3 wk × 3 cycles C: cisplatin 100 mg/m² every 3 wk × 3	FFS: 0.60 (0.39–0.94) DMFS: 0.51 (0.29–0.90)

Abbreviations: AUC, area under the curve; C, concurrent; DFS, disease-free survival; DMFS, distant metastases-free survival; FFS, failure-free survival; I, induction.
  Data from Refs.[16–18,42,43]

Concurrent-adjuvant versus induction-concurrent chemoradiotherapy

The NPC-0501 trial by the Hong Kong Nasopharyngeal Cancer Study Group[44] used the Intergroup 0099 regimen as the standard arm to evaluate the therapeutic benefit by changing the timing of chemotherapy from concurrent adjuvant to induction concurrent, replacing fluorouracil with oral capecitabine and changing RT from conventional to accelerated fractionation. A total of 803 patients were randomized. The study showed that induction chemotherapy was much better tolerated than adjuvant chemotherapy: a significantly higher proportion of patients in the induction group completed 3 nonconcurrent cycles compared with the adjuvant group (88% vs 64%, P<.001); however, a lower proportion had greater than or equal to 2 concurrent doses in the induction arm (90% vs 95%; P = .009). Preliminary results (median follow-up 3.3 years) showed that changing the timing alone did not achieve significant improvement in PFS, but more encouraging results were achieved by changing both the sequence and the induction regime: unadjusted comparison of induction cisplatin-capecitabine versus adjuvant cisplatin-fluorouracil showed favorable trend when given with conventionally fractionated RT (81% vs 75% at 3 years; P = .045); reduction in hazard of progression (hazard ratio [HR] = 0.54 [0.36–0.80]) and death (HR 0.42 [0.25–0.70]) reached significance when adjusted for other significant factors and fractionation. For comparison of induction using cisplatin-capecitabine versus cisplatin-fluorouracil, unadjusted comparisons did not show significant difference, but adjusted analyses showed lower hazard of death (HR 0.57 [0.34–0.97]); in addition, induction cisplatin-capecitabine incurred less toxicity (neutropenia and electrolyte disturbance). Longer follow-up is needed to confirm the current findings, but in view of convenience, favorable toxicity profile, and at least equivalent (if not better) efficacy, this regimen of induction cisplatin-capecitabine and concurrent cisplatin warrants further validation. In addition, this study confirmed that accelerated fractionation is not recommended for patients treated with chemo-RT. This concurs with the findings from other head and neck cancers. Both the GORTEC 99-02 trial[45] and the RTOG 0129 study[46] demonstrated that acceleration is not beneficial for patients who receive concurrent chemo-RT.

Can the Current Regimen Be Replaced by More Potent and/or Less Toxic Drugs?

Replacing cisplatin with other platinum

Cisplatin is one of the most potent cytotoxic drugs for NPC, but it is desirable if this can be replaced by other drugs with less toxicity, particularly in terms of ototoxicity, nephrotoxicity, and nausea/vomiting. Carboplatin has been evaluated as a substitute for cisplatin. A retrospective study by Yau and colleagues[47] cautioned that patients with concurrent cycles replaced by carboplatin had significantly inferior LR-FFR, PFS, and OS at 3 years.

A randomized noninferiority trial by Chitapanarux and colleagues[48] (n = 206) compared concurrent carboplatin and adjuvant carboplatin-fluorouracil versus concurrent cisplatin and adjuvant cisplatin-fluorouracil. They demonstrated that the carboplatin group had better tolerance than the cisplatin group. There was a higher rate of completion of concurrent chemo-RT (73% vs 59%) and adjuvant chemotherapy (70% vs 42%). Carboplatin was associated with less renal toxicity, leukopenia, and anemia but more thrombocytopenia. Preliminary results showed similar disease-free survival at 3 years (61% vs 63%). There are serious concerns, however, about the validity of this study due to short follow-up (26 months), large number of patients excluded for the per-protocol analysis, and exceptionally poor tolerance of the cisplatin group (only 26% completed all 6 cycles). In the intention-to-treat analysis, a better survival was demonstrated in the cisplatin arm but the HR was not reported. Due to lack of confirmatory study, the use of carboplatin to replace cisplatin has yet to become a standard option.

Oxaliplatin is another potential candidate to substitute for cisplatin. As discussed previously, the small randomized trial by Zhang and Wu and colleagues[36,37] using concurrent oxaliplatin showed significant survival benefit compared with RT alone. The tolerance was excellent, with 97% of patients completing all planned doses of oxaliplatin and RT. Unfortunately there is no confirmatory study and no direct comparison of oxaliplatin versus cisplatin. The value of oxaliplatin needs further validation.

Nedaplatin, a second-generation cisplatin analog, is also an attractive candidate. A randomized trial by Cao and colleagues[49] (n = 100) comparing nedaplatin-fluorouracil and cisplatin-fluorouracil (PF) showed that the nedaplatin group had significantly less nausea and vomiting (56% vs 88.0%, $P<.001$) but similar rates of leukopenia, thrombocytopenia, and hepatic and renal impairment. No long-term data on the treatment outcome were available; further studies are needed to compare disease control and long-term toxicities.

Replacing fluorouracil with other drugs

Fluorouracil is a potent drug for NPC, particularly in terms of distant failure,[28] but intravenous infusion over 96 to 120 hours causes substantial inconvenience and additional medical expense. The trial by Kwong and colleagues[35] using concurrent oral uracil-tegafur and the VUMCA-95 trial using hydroxyurea (unpublished results shown in NPC-MAC2[11]) both demonstrated no advantage to these agents when added concurrently to radiation.

Capecitabine (given orally) is an attractive candidate to replace fluorouracil. This comparison has been extensively studies for other solid cancers. Studies comparing capecitabine versus fluorouracil in gastrointestinal cancers consistently confirmed that capecitabine is a favorable alternative with at least equivalent efficacy, lower toxicities, and better patient acceptance. A meta-analysis comparing capecitabine- versus fluorouracil-containing chemotherapy for colorectal and gastric cancers[50] showed that unadjusted HR for OS was 0.94 (0.89–1.00; P = .0489). This drug has not been extensively studied, however, for head and neck cancers.

Promising efficacy of capecitabine has been reported in a phase II study of patients with recurrent and metastatic NPC[51]: 24% showed overall response with significant tumor regression after 3 cycles despite heavy pretreatment with cisplatin-based chemotherapy. As discussed previously, preliminary results from the NPC-0501 trial[44] showed that induction using cisplatin-capecitabine had equivalent (if not superior) efficacy compared with cisplatin-fluorouracil and favorable toxicity profile. Further validation is warranted.

The value of taxanes and gemcitabine combination

A retrospective study by Yau and colleagues[47] comparing induction with platinum-gemcitabine versus platinum-fluorouracil in patients with stage IVA–B showed that there were no significant differences in 3-year LR-FFR, D-FFR, PFS, or OS between the regimens.

Unlike other head and neck cancers, for which docetaxel-cisplatin-fluorouracil (TPF) regimen has proved more effective than cisplatin-fluorouracil as induction chemotherapy,[52–56] the exact magnitude of benefit for NPC had not yet been tested by randomized studies. The only available data are from a retrospective study by Jin and colleagues[57] that studied the toxicity and efficacy of 5 commonly used regimens in 822 patients with distant metastasis from a single institute. The results showed that TPF and gemcitabine-cisplatin regimens achieved higher response rates than cisplatin-fluorouracil (P = .033 and P = <0.001, respectively). There were no statistically significant differences in time, however, to progression (P = .247) and OS (P = .127) among the 5 groups. Furthermore, there were significant differences in toxicity grade 3 or above. Neutropenia was the most common toxicity; the proportion of patients requiring growth factors support was 73% by TPF, 64% by gemcitabine-cisplatin, 58% by bleomycin-cisplatin-fluorouracil, and 45% by paclitaxel-cisplatin compared with 31% by cisplatin-fluorouracil. Furthermore, 3% treatment-related mortalities occurred in the TPF group and none in other groups. The exact benefit of TPF over the standard cisplatin-fluorouracil should be studied further in NPC before substitution of PF by TPF is recommended.

What Is the Implication on the Use of Chemotherapy by Modern Radiotherapy Technique?

RT technique has evolved from 2-D RT to 3-D conformal technique (3-D RT) and then IMRT, which leads to substantial improvement in physical radiation dose distribution, thus increasing conformity of tumor coverage with better sparing of normal structures. The early reports using IMRT all showed excellent locoregional control.[58–66] In a retrospective review by Lee and colleagues[67] of 1593 patients spanning 15 years, it was shown that significant improvement in survival rates and reduction of serious toxicity could be achieved as 2-D RT evolved to 3-D RT and IMRT. In a prospective, randomized trial by Peng and colleagues,[68] 616 patients with stage I–IVb NPC were randomly assigned to receive 2-D RT or IMRT. After a median follow-up of 42 months, the 5-year OS rate was significantly improved by IMRT (79.6% vs 67.1%; P = .001). Patients in

IMRT group also had significantly lower radiation-induced toxicities than those in 2-D RT group.

With the use of IMRT, further benefit of adding chemotherapy and its magnitude become less certain because a majority of the clinical trials were conducted before the modern IMRT era. In a retrospective study by Sun and colleagues,[69] the long-term outcome and toxicities of 868 nonmetastatic NPC patients treated with IMRT were evaluated. Among them, 602 patients had stage III–IVb disease (according to 2002 Union for International Cancer Control stage system) and concurrent chemotherapy was given to 217 patients. The addition of concurrent chemotherapy to IMRT failed to demonstrate any benefit in 5-year disease-specific survival, LR-FFR, D-FFR, and PFS and only caused higher incidence of acute toxicity, such as severe mucositis, xerostomia, and tympanitis as well as late ototoxicities. In another retrospective study by Lin and colleagues,[70] 370 patients with locoregionally advanced NPC were treated with IMRT after induction chemotherapy, with or without concomitant chemotherapy. With a median follow-up of 31 months, subgroup analysis revealed that concurrent chemotherapy provided no significant benefit to IMRT in locoregionally advanced NPC but was associated with higher rates of acute toxicities. Further studies are warranted to re-evaluate the role of combination chemotherapy when it is incorporated into IMRT.

SUMMARY

This review summarizes the latest clinical data on the use of chemotherapy in combination with RT in the management of NPC. Although chemotherapy has a major role in enhancing the treatment outcome, there is a wide variation in clinical practice and the best way to deliver chemotherapy is still clouded with controversies. It depends a lot on the interpretation of the currently available clinical data. Although timely and flexible modification of treatment strategy is necessary, whether it is time to move away from the established standard of care and what defines the highest level of evidence need to be asked. Fortunately, there are concerted efforts worldwide in promoting further advances in this important area and, with stronger global collaboration, it is hoped that future trials can address the current controversial issues.

REFERENCES

1. Al-Sarraf M, LeBlanc M, Giri PGS, et al. Chemoradiotherapy versus radiotherapy in patients with advanced nasopharyngeal cancer: phase III randomized Intergroup study 0099. J Clin Oncol 1998;16(4):1310–7.
2. Al-Sarraf M, LeBlanc M, Giri PGS, et al. Superiority of five year survival with chemoradiotherapy (CT-RT) vs radiotherapy in patients (pts) with locally advanced nasopharyngeal cancer (NPC). Intergroup (0099) (SWOG 8892, RTOG 8817, ECOG 2388) phase III study: final report [abstract]. Proc Annu Meet Am Soc Clin Oncol 2001;20:905.
3. Wee J, Tan EH, Tai BC, et al. Randomized trial of radiotherapy versus concurrent chemoradiotherapy followed by adjuvant chemotherapy in patients with American Joint Committee on Cancer/International Union against cancer stage III and IV nasopharyngeal cancer of the endemic variety. J Clin Oncol 2005;23:6730–8.
4. Wee J. 4th FY Khoo Memorial Lecture 2008: Nasopharyngeal Cancer Workgroup–the past, the present and the future. Ann Acad Med Singapore 2008; 37(7):606–14.
5. Lee AW, Lau WH, Tung SY, et al. Preliminary results of a randomized study on therapeutic gain by concurrent chemotherapy for regionally-advanced

nasopharyngeal carcinoma: NPC-9901 Trial by the Hong Kong Nasopharyngeal Cancer Study Group. J Clin Oncol 2005;23:6966–75.

6. Lee AW, Tung SY, Chua DT, et al. Randomized trial of radiotherapy plus concurrent-adjuvant chemotherapy vs radiotherapy alone for regionally advanced nasopharyngeal carcinoma. J Natl Cancer Inst 2010;102:1188–98.

7. Lee AW, Tung SY, Chan AT, et al. Preliminary results of a randomized study (NPC-9902 Trial) on therapeutic gain by concurrent chemotherapy and/or accelerated fractionation for locally advanced nasopharyngeal carcinoma. Int J Radiat Oncol Biol Phys 2006;66:142–51.

8. Lee AWM, Tung Y, Chan ATC, et al. A randomized trial on addition of concurrent-adjuvant chemotherapy and/or accelerated fractionation for locally-advanced nasopharyngeal carcinoma. Radiother Oncol 2011;98:15–22.

9. Chen Y, Liu MZ, Liang SB, et al. Preliminary results of a prospective randomized trial comparing concurrent chemoradiotherapy plus adjuvant chemotherapy with radiotherapy alone in patients with locoregionally advanced nasopharyngeal carcinoma in endemic regions of china. Int J Radiat Oncol Biol Phys 2008;71:1356–64.

10. Chen Y, Sun Y, Liang SB, et al. Progress report of a randomized trial comparing long-term survival and late toxicity of concurrent chemoradiotherapy with adjuvant chemotherapy versus radiotherapy alone in patients with stage III to IVB nasopharyngeal carcinoma from endemic regions of China. Cancer 2013;119(12):2230–8.

11. Blanchard P, Lee A, Marguet S, et al. MAC-NPC Collaborative Group. Chemotherapy and radiotherapy in nasopharyngeal carcinoma: an update of the MAC-NPC meta-analysis. Lancet Oncol 2015;16(6):645–55.

12. Baujat B, Audry H, Bourhis J, et al, MAC-NPC Collaborative Group. Chemotherapy in locally advanced nasopharyngeal carcinoma: an individual patient data meta-analysis of eight randomized trials and 1753 patients. Int J Radiat Oncol Biol Phys 2006;64(1):47–56.

13. Chan AT, Teo PM, Ngan RK, et al. Concurrent chemotherapy-radiotherapy compared with radiotherapy alone in locoregionally advanced nasopharyngeal carcinoma: progression-free survival analysis of a phase III randomized trial. J Clin Oncol 2002;20(8):2038–44.

14. Chan AT, Leung SF, Ngan RK, et al. Overall survival after concurrent cisplatin-radiotherapy compared with radiotherapy alone in locoregionally advanced nasopharyngeal carcinoma. J Natl Cancer Inst 2005;97(7):536–9.

15. Rischin D, Corry J, Smith J, et al. Excellent disease control and survival in patients with advanced nasopharyngeal cancer treated with chemoradiation. J Clin Oncol 2002;20(7):1845–52.

16. Hui EP, Ma BB, Leung SF, et al. Randomized phase II trial of concurrent cisplatin-radiotherapy with or without neoadjuvant docetaxel and cisplatin in advanced nasopharyngeal carcinoma. J Clin Oncol 2009;27(2):242–9.

17. Fountzilas G, Ciuleanu E, Bobos M, et al. Induction chemotherapy followed by concomitant radiotherapy and weekly cisplatin versus the same concomitant chemoradiotherapy in patients with nasopharyngeal carcinoma: a randomized phase II study conducted by the Hellenic Cooperative Oncology Group (HeCOG) with biomarker evaluation. Ann Oncol 2012;23(2):427–35.

18. Tan T, Lim WT, Fong KW, et al. Concurrent chemo-radiation with or without induction gemcitabine, carboplatin, and paclitaxel: a randomized, phase 2/3 trial in locally advanced nasopharyngeal carcinoma. Int J Radiat Oncol Biol Phys 2015;91(5):952–60.

19. National Comprehensive Cancer Network Treatment Guidelines in Oncology: Head and Neck Cancers, 2014. Available at: http://www.nccn.org/professionals/physician_gls/pdf/head-and-neck.pdf. Accessed August 14, 2015.
20. Chan AT, Gregoire V, Lefebvre JL, et al. Nasopharyngeal cancer: EHNS-ESMO-ESTRO Clinical Practice Guidelines for diagnosis, treatment and follow-up. Ann Oncol 2012;23(Suppl 7):83–5.
21. American Joint Committee On Cancer. Manual for Staging of Cancer. 5th edition. Philadelphia: J.B. Lippincott; 1997.
22. Chen QY, Wen YF, Guo L, et al. Concurrent chemoradiotherapy vs radiotherapy alone in stage II nasopharyngeal carcinoma: phase III randomized trial. J Natl Cancer Inst 2011;103(23):1761–70.
23. Lee AWM, Ng WT, Chan LK, et al. The Strength/Weakness of the AJCC/UICC Staging System (7th edition) for Nasopharyngeal Cancer and Suggestions for Future Improvement. Oral Oncol 2012;48(10):1007–13.
24. Su SF, Han F, Zhao C, et al. Long-term outcomes of early-stage nasopharyngeal carcinoma patients treated with intensity-modulated radiotherapy alone. Int J Radiat Oncol Biol Phys 2012;82(1):327–33.
25. Sze WM, Lee AW, Yau TK, et al. Primary tumor volume of nasopharyngeal carcinoma: prognostic significance for local control. Int J Radiat Oncol Biol Phys 2004; 59(1):21–7.
26. Chua DT, Sham JS, Leung LH, et al. Tumor volume is not an independent prognostic factor in early-stage nasopharyngeal carcinoma treated by radiotherapy alone. Int J Radiat Oncol Biol Phys 2004;58(5):1437–44.
27. Leung SF, Chan AT, Zee B, et al. Pretherapy quantitative measurement of circulating Epstein-Barr virus DNA is predictive of posttherapy distant failure in patients with early-stage nasopharyngeal carcinoma of undifferentiated type. Cancer 2003;98(2):288–91.
28. Lee AW, Tung SY, Ngan RK, et al. Factors contributing to the efficacy of concurrent-adjuvant chemotherapy for locoregionally advanced nasopharyngeal carcinoma: combined analyses of NPC-9901 and NPC-9902 Trials. Eur J Cancer 2011;47(5):656–66.
29. Chen L, Hu CS, Chen XZ, et al. Concurrent chemoradiotherapy plus adjuvant chemotherapy versus concurrent chemoradiotherapy alone in patients with locoregionally advanced nasopharyngeal carcinoma: a phase 3 multicentre randomised controlled trial. Lancet Oncol 2012;13(2):163–71.
30. Chen YP, Wang ZX, Chen L, et al. A Bayesian network meta-analysis comparing concurrent chemoradiotherapy followed by adjuvant chemotherapy, concurrent chemoradiotherapy alone and radiotherapy alone in patients with locoregionally advanced nasopharyngeal carcinoma. Ann Oncol 2015;26(1): 205–11.
31. Chua DT, Sham JS, Choy D, et al. Preliminary report of the Asian-Oceanian Clinical Oncology Association randomized trial comparing cisplatin and epirubicin followed by radiotherapy versus radiotherapy alone in the treatment of patients with locoregionally advanced nasopharyngeal carcinoma. Asian-Oceanian Clinical Oncology Association Nasopharynx Cancer Study Group. Cancer 1998; 83(11):2270–83.
32. International Nasopharynx Cancer Study Group, VUMCA I Trial. Preliminary results of a randomized trial comparing neoadjuvant chemotherapy (cisplatin, epirubicin, bleomycin) plus radiotherapy vs radiotherapy alone in stage IV(> or = N2, M0) undifferentiated nasopharyngeal carcinoma: a positive effect on progression-free survival. Int J Radiat Oncol Biol Phys 1996;35(3):463–9.

33. Hareyama M, Sakata K, Shirato H, et al. A prospective, randomized trial comparing neoadjuvant chemotherapy with radiotherapy alone in patients with advanced nasopharyngeal carcinoma. Cancer 2002;94(8):2217–23.

34. Chi KH, Chang YC, Guo WY, et al. A phase III study of adjuvant chemotherapy in advanced nasopharyngeal carcinoma patients. Int J Radiat Oncol Biol Phys 2002;52(5):1238–44.

35. Kwong DL, Sham JS, Au GK, et al. Concurrent and adjuvant chemotherapy for nasopharyngeal carcinoma: a factorial study. J Clin Oncol 2004;22:2643–53.

36. Zhang L, Zhao C, Peng PJ, et al. Phase III study comparing standard radiotherapy with or without weekly oxaliplatin in treatment of locoregionally advanced nasopharyngeal carcinoma: preliminary results. J Clin Oncol 2005;23(33): 8461–8.

37. Wu X, Huang PY, Peng PJ, et al. Long-term follow-up of a phase III study comparing radiotherapy with or without weekly oxaliplatin for locoregionally advanced nasopharyngeal carcinoma. Ann Oncol 2013;24(8):2131–6.

38. Blanchard P, Lee A, Leclercq J, et al. On behalf of the MAC-NPC Collaborative Group. What is the best treatment in nasopharyngeal carcinoma? An individual patient data network meta-analysis. Radiother Oncol 2015;114(Suppl 1):6–7.

39. Chan AT, Lo YM, Zee B, et al. Plasma Epstein-Barr virus DNA and residual disease after radiotherapy for undifferentiated nasopharyngeal carcinoma. J Natl Cancer Inst 2002;94(21):1614–9.

40. Lin JC, Wang WY, Liang WM, et al. Long-term prognostic effects of plasma epstein-barr virus DNA by minor groove binder-probe real-time quantitative PCR on nasopharyngeal carcinoma patients receiving concurrent chemoradiotherapy. Int J Radiat Oncol Biol Phys 2007;68(5):1342–8.

41. Le QT, Jones CD, Yau TK, et al. A comparison study of different PCR assays in measuring circulating plasma epstein-barr virus DNA levels in patients with nasopharyngeal carcinoma. Clin Cancer Res 2005;11(16):5700–7.

42. Daoud J, Aupérin A, Tao YG, et al. A randomized trial of concomitant cisplatin-RT +/- induction TPF in locally advanced nasopharyngeal carcinomas. Radiother Oncol 2015;114(Suppl 1) [abstract: OC-004].

43. Sun Y, Chen NY, Zhang N, et al. Induction chemotherapy plus concurrent chemoradiotherapy versus concurrent chemoradiotherapy alone in locoregionally advanced nasopharyngeal carcinoma: preliminary results of a phase 3 multicenter randomised controlled trial. Advances in nasopharyngeal carcinoma studies. Hong Kong: The Croucher Foundation Advanced Study Institute; 2014. November 1–4.

44. Lee AW, Ngan RK, Tung SY, et al. Preliminary results of trial NPC-0501 evaluating the therapeutic gain by changing from concurrent-adjuvant to induction-concurrent chemoradiotherapy, changing from fluorouracil to capecitabine, and changing from conventional to accelerated radiotherapy fractionation in patients with locoregionally advanced nasopharyngeal carcinoma. Cancer 2015;121(8): 1328–38.

45. Bourhis J, Sire C, Graff P, et al. Concomitant chemoradiotherapy versus acceleration of radiotherapy with or without concomitant chemotherapy in locally advanced head and neck carcinoma (GORTEC 99-02): an open-label phase 3 randomised trial. Lancet Oncol 2012;13(2):145–53.

46. Ang KK, Harris J, Wheeler R, et al. Human papilloma virus and survival of patients with oropharyngeal cancer. N Engl J Med 2010;363:24–35.

47. Yau TK, Lee AWM, Wong DHM, et al. Treatment of stage IV (A-B) nasopharyngeal carcinoma by induction-concurrent chemoradiotherapy and accelerated

fractionation: impact of chemotherapy schemes. Int J Radiat Oncol Biol Phys 2006;66(4):1004–10.

48. Chitapanarux I, Lorvidhaya V, Kamnerdsupaphon P, et al. Chemoradiation comparing cisplatin versus carboplatin in locally advanced nasopharyngeal cancer: randomised, non-inferiority, open trial. Eur J Cancer 2007;43(9): 1399–406.

49. Cao KJ, Zhang AL, Ma WJ, et al. Nedaplatin or cisplatin combined with 5-fluorouracil for treatment of stage III-IVa nasopharyngeal carcinoma: a randomized controlled study. Zhonghua Zhong Liu Za Zhi 2011;33(1):50–2 [in Chinese].

50. Cassidy J, Saltz L, Twelves C, et al. Efficacy of capecitabine versus 5-fluorouracil in colorectal and gastric cancers: a meta-analysis of individual data from 6171 patients. Ann Oncol 2011;22:2604–9.

51. Chua DTT, Sham JST, Au GKH. A phase II study of capecitabine in patients with recurrent and metastatic nasopharyngeal carcinoma pretreated with platinum-based chemotherapy. Oral Oncol 2003;39:361–6.

52. Posner MR, Hershock DM, Blajman CR, et al. Cisplatin and fluorouracil alone or with docetaxel in head and neck cancer. N Engl J Med 2007;357:1705–15.

53. Vermorken JB, Remenar E, van Herpen C, et al. Cisplatin, fluorouracil, and docetaxel in unresectable head and neck cancer. N Engl J Med 2007;357: 1695–704.

54. Hitt R, Lopez-Pousa A, Martinez-Trufero J, et al. Phase III study comparing cisplatin plus fluorouracil to paclitaxel, cisplatin, and fluorouracil induction chemotherapy followed by chemoradiotherapy in locally advanced head and neck cancer. J Clin Oncol 2005;23:8636–45.

55. Hitt R, Grau JJ, Lopez-Pousa A, et al. Final results of a randomized phase III trial comparing induction chemotherapy with cisplatin/5-FU or docetaxel/cisplatin/ 5-FU follow by chemoradiotherapy (CRT) versus CRT alone as first-line treatment of unresectable locally advanced head and neck cancer (LAHNC). J Clin Oncol 2009;27:15s [abstract: 6009].

56. Blanchard P, Bourhis J, Lacas B, et al, On behalf of the MACH-NC-Induction Collaborative Group. Taxane-cisplatin-5 Fluorouracil as induction chemotherapy in locally advanced head and neck cancers: an individual patient data meta-analysis of the MACH-NC group. J Clin Oncol 2013;31:2854–60.

57. Jin Y, Cai XY, Shi YX, et al. Comparison of five cisplatin-based regimens frequently used as the first-line protocols in metastatic nasopharyngeal carcinoma. J Cancer Res Clin Oncol 2012;138:1717–25.

58. Bakst RL, Lee N, Pfister DG, et al. Hypofractionated dose-painting intensity modulated radiation therapy with chemotherapy for nasopharyngeal carcinoma: a prospective trial. Int J Radiat Oncol Biol Phys 2011;80:148–53.

59. Lee N, Xia P, Quivey JM, et al. Intensity-modulated radiotherapy in the treatment of nasopharyngeal carcinoma: an update of the UCSF experience. Int J Radiat Oncol Biol Phys 2002;53:12–22.

60. Kwong DL, Pow EH, Sham JS, et al. Intensity-modulated radiotherapy for early-stage nasopharyngeal carcinoma: a prospective study on disease control and preservation of salivary function. Cancer 2004;101:1584–93.

61. Kam MK, Teo PM, Chau RM, et al. Treatment of nasopharyngeal carcinoma with intensity-modulated radiotherapy: the Hong Kong experience. Int J Radiat Oncol Biol Phys 2004;60:1440–50.

62. Wolden SL, Chen WC, Pfister DG, et al. Intensity-modulated radiation therapy (IMRT) for nasopharynx cancer: update of the Memorial Sloan-Kettering experience. Int J Radiat Oncol Biol Phys 2006;64:57–62.

63. Lin S, Pan J, Han L, et al. Nasopharyngeal carcinoma treated with reduced-volume intensity-modulated radiation therapy: report on the 3-year outcome of a prospective series. Int J Radiat Oncol Biol Phys 2009;75:1071–8.

64. Lee N, Harris J, Garden AS, et al. Intensity-modulated radiation therapy with or without chemotherapy for nasopharyngeal carcinoma: radiation therapy oncology group phase II trial 0225. J Clin Oncol 2009;27:3684–90.

65. Wong FC, Ng AW, Lee VH, et al. Whole-field simultaneous integratedboost intensity-modulated radiotherapy for patients with nasopharyngeal carcinoma. Int J Radiat Oncol Biol Phys 2010;76:138–45.

66. Ng WT, Lee MC, Hung WM, et al. Clinical outcomes and patterns of failure after intensity-modulated radiotherapy for nasopharyngeal carcinoma. Int J Radiat Oncol Biol Phys 2011;79:420–8.

67. Lee AW, Ng WT, Chan LL, et al. Evolution of treatment for nasopharyngeal cancer–success and setback in the intensity-modulated radiotherapy era. Radiother Oncol 2014;110(3):377–84.

68. Peng G, Wang T, Yang KY, et al. A prospective, randomized study comparing outcomes and toxicities of intensity-modulated radiotherapy vs conventional two-dimensional radiotherapy for the treatment of nasopharyngeal carcinoma. Radiother Oncol 2012;104(3):286–93.

69. Sun X, Su S, Chen C, et al. Long-term outcomes of intensity-modulated radiotherapy for 868 patients with nasopharyngeal carcinoma: an analysis of survival and treatment toxicities. Radiother Oncol 2014;110(3):398–403.

70. Lin S, Lu JJ, Han L, et al. Sequential chemotherapy and intensity-modulated radiation therapy in the management of locoregionally advanced nasopharyngeal carcinoma: experience of 370 consecutive cases. BMC Cancer 2010;10:39.

Thyroid Gland Malignancies

Maria E. Cabanillas, MD[a],*, Ramona Dadu, MD[a,1], Mimi I. Hu, MD[a,1], Charles Lu, MD[b], Gary Brandon Gunn, MD[c], Elizabeth G. Grubbs, MD[d], Stephen Y. Lai, MD, PhD[e], Michelle D. Williams, MD[f]

KEYWORDS

- Anaplastic • Medullary • Differentiated • Thyroid cancer • Cabozantinib • Lenvatinib
- Sorafenib • Vandetanib

KEY POINTS

- Surgery remains the treatment of choice for differentiated thyroid cancer (DTC) and medullary thyroid cancer (MTC), with tyrosine kinase inhibitors reserved for symptomatic or rapidly progressive disease not amenable to surgery or other targeted therapies.
- Four multikinase inhibitors are US Food and Drug Administration approved for thyroid cancer: sorafenib and lenvatinib for DTC and vandetanib and cabozantinib for MTC.
- Anaplastic thyroid cancer (ATC) is a rare, highly aggressive, and lethal malignancy with median survival of less than 6 months. Initial evaluation and management require a rapid, coordinated, multidisciplinary team approach.
- Effective systemic therapies for ATC are lacking. Future improvement in outcomes will require the identification of driver genetic abnormalities or other aberrancies in the tumor microenvironment that can be targeted with novel agents.

Disclosures: M.E. Cabanillas has received grant funding from Eisai, Exelixis, and Roche. M.E. Cabanillas has received consultant fees from AstraZeneca, Exelixis, Eisai, and Bayer. M.I. Hu has received grant funding from AstraZeneca. R. Dadu, C. Lu, G.B. Gunn, E.G. Grubbs, S.Y. Lai, and M.D. Williams have nothing to disclose.

[a] Department of Endocrine Neoplasia and Hormonal Disorders, The University of Texas MD Anderson Cancer Center, 1515 Holcombe Boulevard, Unit 1461, Houston, TX 77030, USA; [b] Department of Thoracic/Head and Neck Medical Oncology, The University of Texas MD Anderson Cancer Center, 1515 Holcombe Boulevard, Unit 432, Houston, TX 77030, USA; [c] Department of Radiation Oncology, The University of Texas MD Anderson Cancer Center, 1515 Holcombe Boulevard, Unit 97, Houston, TX 77030, USA; [d] Department of Surgical Oncology, The University of Texas MD Anderson Cancer Center, 1515 Holcombe Boulevard, Unit 1484, Houston, TX 77030, USA; [e] Department of Head and Neck Surgery, The University of Texas MD Anderson Cancer Center, 1515 Holcombe Boulevard, Houston, TX 77030, USA; [f] Pathology Head and Neck Section, Department of Pathology, The University of Texas MD Anderson Cancer Center, 1515 Holcombe Boulevard, Unit 85, Houston, TX 77030, USA
[1] Dual second authorship because of equal contribution.
* Corresponding author.
E-mail address: mcabani@mdanderson.org

INTRODUCTION

Thyroid cancer is the most common endocrine malignancy. Despite an increase in incidence in thyroid cancer, death rates have not changed significantly. There are 3 major types of thyroid cancers:

- Differentiated thyroid cancer (DTC) accounts for more than 90% of all thyroid cancer cases. DTC is derived from epithelial thyroid cells and includes papillary thyroid cancer (PTC), follicular thyroid cancer, Hürthle cell and poorly differentiated thyroid cancer (PDTC; **Fig. 1**) histologies. In theory, these types of thyroid cancers should be able to concentrate iodine, thus, in contrast with the other thyroid cancers, these types are treated with radioactive iodine (RAI). The prognosis for patients with well-differentiated DTC is generally very good, with a survival rate of more than 90%. PDTC represents intermediate entities in the progression of DTC to anaplastic thyroid cancer (ATC).
- ATC is a rare type of thyroid cancer that is also derived from epithelial thyroid cells. It accounts for less than 2% of thyroid cancers and its incidence is approximately 500 cases/year in the United States. Unlike DTC and medullary thyroid cancer (MTC), ATC is one of the most aggressive malignancies in humans, with a median survival of less than 6 months.[1] Patients often present with a rapidly enlarging neck mass associated with compressive symptoms (dyspnea, dysphagia) and pain. At diagnosis, more than one-third of patients have extrathyroidal extension and/or regional nodal metastases, whereas distant metastases are present in more than 40%.[1] ATC can develop de novo or can derive from a thyroid cancer that is well differentiated. Morphologically ATC is undifferentiated, growing as sheets of cells without organization, with pleomorphism and high-grade features, including mitoses and necrosis (**Fig. 2**). Diagnosis can be difficult because the cells usually have lost thyroid and epithelial cell-specific

Epithelial-derived thyroid carcinoma

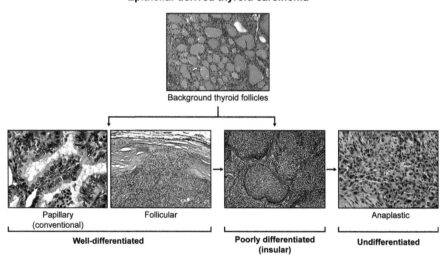

Fig. 1. Epithelial-derived thyroid cancer histologies. The most common types of thyroid cancer are derived from the epithelial thyroid cancer cells and includes papillary, follicular, poorly differentiated, and anaplastic thyroid cancers (hematoxylin-eosin, original magnification: *top panel* ×100; *bottom panel* ×400, ×100, ×100, and ×200).

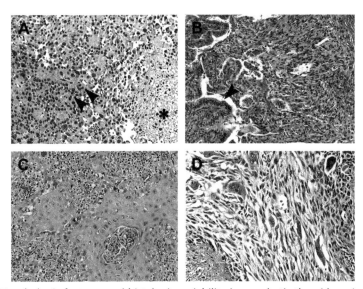

Fig. 2. Morphologic features and histologic variability in anaplastic thyroid carcinoma. (*A*) Discohesive, pleomorphic, and mitotically active tumor cells (*arrowheads*) are often associated with necrosis (*asterisk*). (*B*) Coexisting ATC (*right side*, spindled cells) with a well-differentiated papillary thyroid carcinoma (*arrowhead*) showing organized vascular papillae lined by tumor cells. (*C*) Squamous morphology with glassy cells in cohesive nests surrounded by prominent inflammation. (*D*) Variable morphology within the same tumor, including spindled, giant, and epithelioid tumor cells all representing anaplastic carcinoma (hematoxylin-eosin, original magnification ×200).

markers (**Table 1**). In addition, there is a broad differential diagnosis on biopsy, and metastases to the thyroid and thyroid lymphoma must be excluded.

- MTC comprises approximately 1% to 2% of all thyroid cancers in the United States.[2] Despite its rarity, this is a well-characterized neuroendocrine tumor (**Fig. 3**). MTC arises from the parafollicular calcitonin-producing cells in the thyroid (C cells) and can occur sporadically (75%) or in a hereditary (25%) form associated with multiple endocrine neoplasia syndrome (MEN) types 2A and 2B. In patients with a palpable thyroid mass, 70% have cervical lymph node metastases and 10% to 15% have distant metastases. Based on the Surveillance, Epidemiology, and End Results database from 1973 to 2002, the 10-year survival rates for patients with MTC with localized, regional, and distant disease were 96%, 76%, and 40%, respectively.[3]

GENETICS OF THYROID CANCER

In the last decade, molecular diagnostics have improved the care of patients with thyroid cancer. The Ras-Raf-MEK-MAP-ERK (MAPK) kinase signaling pathway plays a key role in development of thyroid cancer. Several studies have reported a high frequency of genetic alterations involved in the MAPK and phosphatidylinositol 3 kinase (PI3K) pathway (**Table 2**):

- *BRAF, RAS, PTEN* mutations in DTC and ATC. Molecular alterations of ATC overlap with DTC and commonly have additional mutations in p53, beta-catenin, and PIK3CA.
- *RET* fusions in DTC.

Table 1
Histologic differential diagnosis and immunophenotype for anaplastic thyroid carcinoma (ATC)

	CKs	Immunohistochemical Analysis			
		TTF1	Thyroglobulin	PAX8	Other
ATC	+ (75%)[d]	+ (5%–18%)	+ (1%–15%) (8%)	+ (30%–70%)	p53 (50%–75%)
Spindled Pattern					
MTC	+	+	−	−	Synaptophysin, chromogranin, calcitonin[c]
True sarcoma (rare)	−	−	−	−	Various but not specific/differentiating
Epithelioid Pattern					
Solid papillary thyroid carcinoma	+	+ (98%)	+ (>90%)	+ (100%)	—
Solid follicular thyroid carcinoma	+	+	+	+	—
PDTC	+	+ Variable	Variable/weak	+	—
Lymphoma	−	−	−	−[a]	CD45, various[b]
Metastasis to thyroid	—	—	—	—	—
Renal, GYN, GU, thymic	+	−	−	+	Various
Lung	+	+	−	−	—
Melanoma	− (Rare +)	−	−	−	Melan A, Tyrosinase, HBME-1
Neuroendocrine carcinoma	+	+ In some sites	−	−	Synaptophysin, chromogranin
Squamoid Pattern					
SCC from adjacent H&N site	+, usually CK5/6[d]	—	—	—	—
Metastatic SCC from another site	+, usually CK5/6[d]	—	—	—	—

Abbreviations: CK, cytokeratin; H&N, head and neck; SCC, squamous cell carcinoma.
[a] Caution: some pax8 antibodies cross react with PAX5, which may be expressed on lymphoma cells.
[b] Immuno pattern varies with type of lymphoma.
[c] Calcitonin is not specific for MTC and occasionally is expressed in neuroendocrine carcinomas from other anatomic sites.
[d] Cytokeratin 5/6 may be expressed in ATC with squamoid differentiation; does not help with differentiating squamoid pattern tumors.

Medullary thyroid carcinoma
2–5% of thyroid carcinomas

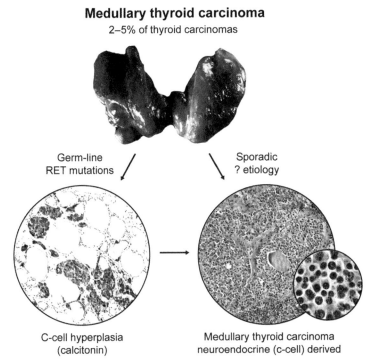

Germ-line   Sporadic
RET mutations   ? etiology

C-cell hyperplasia   Medullary thyroid carcinoma
(calcitonin)   neuroendocrine (c-cell) derived

Fig. 3. Medullary thyroid cancer (MTC) histology. MTCs are neuroendocrine tumors and are derived from the neuroendocrine C cells in the thyroid gland. These tumors may be hereditary (caused by germline RET mutations) or sporadic (Calcitonin, original magnification ×100; hematoxylin-eosin, original magnification ×100 and ×400).

- *TERT* promoter mutations in more aggressive, less-differentiated PTCs.[4]
- Somatic *RET*, *RAS* mutations in MTC.
- Patients with MEN2A and MEN2B have a *RET* germline mutation that serves as the oncogenic basis of their MTC.

Baseline Evaluation

Thyroid cancers are often diagnosed by fine-needle aspiration (FNA) of a thyroid nodule. Accuracy increases with immunohistochemical staining, particularly in MTC with calcitonin, chromogranin-A, or carcinoembryonic antigen (CEA).[5] Suspicious lymph nodes should be sampled in order to plan the best possible curative-intent surgery. Evaluation of patients with suspected ATC often requires a rapid multidisciplinary team with experience with treating ATC. A diagnostic tissue specimen should be obtained without delay. Although FNA or core biopsy is usually sufficient, an open biopsy may be needed if FNA or core biopsy is nondiagnostic. Once the diagnosis is made, a preoperative evaluation should be performed. Recommended testing is listed in **Table 3**.

Primary Treatment

The standard therapy for patients with DTC includes surgery followed by RAI in select patients, and thyroid-stimulating hormone (TSH) suppression (**Fig. 4**). The role of prophylactic central lymph node dissection in PTC is controversial. The paradigms

Table 2
Mutations in thyroid nodule and thyroid cancer

Genes	Molecular Alteration	FA (%)	PTC Conventional (%)	PTC FV (%)	FC (%)	PD (%)	ATC (%)	MTC (%)
BRAF	Mutations; rare fusions	0	71	20	0	15	25	—
RAS[a]	Mutations	30	7	35	45	30	50	—
PAX8/PPARg	Fusion	10	0	2	35	0	0	0
RET/PTC[b]	Fusion	0	0	5	0	0	0	0
RET	Mutations	0	0	0	0	0	0	50[c]
p53	Mutations	0	Rare	0	Rare	30	65	—
b-catenin	Mutations	0	Rare	0	0	25	65	—
EIF1AX	Mutations	Unk	0	Rare	Unk	Unk	Unk	Unk
ETV6-7/NTRK3	Fusion	Unk	0	Rare	Unk	Unk	Unk	Unk
ALK	Fusion	Unk	0	Rare	Unk	Rare	Rare	Unk

Abbreviations: FA, follicular adenoma; FC, follicular carcinoma; FV, follicular variant; PD, poorly differentiated; PTC, papillary thyroid carcinoma; Unk, unknown.
[a] Ras mutation frequency based on The Cancer Genome Atlas: NRAS (Q61R) 65%, HRAS (Q61R>Q61K) 27%, KRAS (EXON 61 and 12) 8%.
[b] The RET gene is fused with multiple different gene partners in papillary thyroid carcinoma, which are termed RET/PTC1, RET/PTC2, and RET/PTC3, although several others exist.
[c] RET mutations are present in all germline MTC and approximately 50% of sporadic cases.

Table 3
Preoperative evaluation in patients with histologic diagnosis of thyroid cancer

	DTC	ATC	MTC
Tumor marker and other laboratory testing	Thyroglobulin (limited value preoperatively), TSH, free T4	No tumor marker Routine laboratory tests	Calcitonin, CEA, genetic test for *RET* germline mutation (due to delays in germline testing results, rule out of pheochromocytoma and primary hyperparathyroidism should be performed before surgery)
Consultation	Surgical	Surgical (preferably an experienced head and neck surgeon)	• Genetic counselor • Surgical (preferably an experienced MTC surgeon)
Radiologic assessment	Ultrasonography examination of neck in all patients If advanced disease is seen on ultrasonography or clinically suspected, perform cross-sectional imaging of the neck (contrast CT neck or MRI) FDG-PET/CT not recommended to detect distant metastases	• Ultrasonography examination of neck • Cross-sectional imaging of neck/chest/abdomen or FDG-PET/CT • MRI brain If distant metastases or surgery unlikely to result in R0 or R1 resection, surgery is of little or no benefit FDG-PET/CT is useful to detect distant metastases	Ultrasonography examination of neck in all patients With any of the following, perform contrast-enhanced CT neck/chest, 3-phase contrast-enhanced CT liver (or contrast-enhanced MRI liver), axial skeleton MRI, and bone scintigraphy: • Extensive neck disease • Signs/symptoms of regional or distant metastases • Calcitonin level >500 pg/mL FDG-PET/CT and F-DOPA-PET/CT not recommended to detect distant metastases
Other assessments	In patients with advanced disease or hoarseness, fiberoptic laryngoscopy	All patients should undergo fiberoptic laryngoscopy before surgery	In patients with advanced disease or hoarseness, fiberoptic laryngoscopy

Abbreviations: CT, computed tomography; FDG, fluorodeoxyglucose; F-DOPA, fluoro-DOPA.

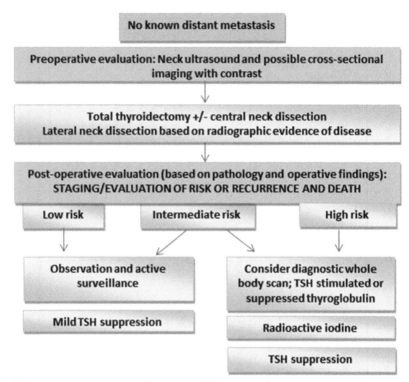

Fig. 4. Management of newly diagnosed differentiated thyroid cancer with no known distant metastases.

of treatment have shifted over the years, with an emphasis on less aggressive approach for selected patients.[6,7]

Although patients with DTC with localized disease have a good prognosis (5-year relative survival rate of 98%), those with distant metastases have a 10-year median survival of only 42% and the prognosis differs based on age, histology, location, and size of the distant disease, as well as whether the disease responds to RAI.[8] Patients with newly diagnosed DTC with known distant metastases (**Fig. 5**) should still be considered for thyroidectomy in order to protect the airway and other regional structures and in order to facilitate administration of RAI. Once the thyroid gland and involved cervical lymph nodes are removed, RAI may be effective to target distant metastatic disease in selected cases (especially if the tumor burden is small). However, if the distant disease is RAI refractory (**Table 4**), monitoring for pace of progression in most cases is warranted. New approaches, such as BRAF and MEK inhibition, are being tested in the hope of increasing RAI incorporation.[9,10]

Patients with ATC should be evaluated for resectability by an experienced head and neck surgeon. If a grossly negative margin can be achieved, surgery should be considered.[11–13] Local therapy is often multimodal. The patient's ability to tolerate aggressive therapy is determined in the treatment plan. After surgery and in patients with unresectable disease, postoperative radiotherapy or concurrent chemoradiotherapy should be considered.[14–16] The presence of distant metastases does not preclude the use of palliative locoregional therapy to treat or prevent symptoms of tracheal or esophageal compromise.[16] **Table 5** lists treatment modalities for patients with ATC.

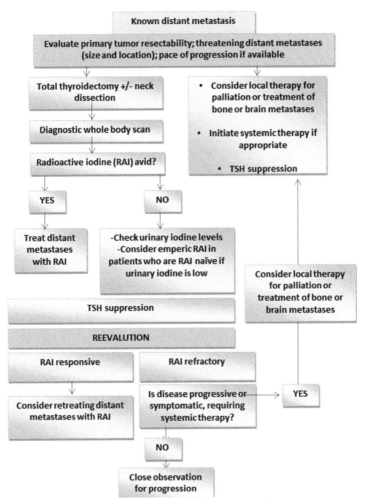

Fig. 5. Management of newly diagnosed differentiated thyroid cancer with known distant metastases.

After the diagnosis of MTC has been established, determination of the cause as either germline or sporadic must be established by germline RET mutation testing. If a germline RET mutation is identified or unknown at the time of surgery, preoperative evaluation for a pheochromocytoma and primary hyperparathyroidism (pHPT) is

Table 4
Definition of RAI–refractory differentiated thyroid cancer
Definition of Radioactive iodine-refractory (any of the following):
The disease does not take up radioactive iodine at known sites of metastatic disease on diagnostic or post-treatment whole body scan
Progression of structural disease over a 16–12 mo period after radioactive iodine therapy despite confirmed uptake
Progression of disease despite a total cumulative dose of radioactive iodine of ≥600 mCi

Table 5
Treatment modalities for anaplastic thyroid carcinoma

Treatment	Indication	Comments
Surgery	Stage IVA (T4a, resectable)	Curative in select (few) patients in combination with postoperative/adjuvant radiation therapy
Tracheotomy	Urgent airway in patients who want treatment	May delay effective therapy because of wound healing
EBRT to neck with radiosensitizing chemotherapy	Stage IVA resected (postoperative): curative intent Stage IVB, IVC: palliative, but often with additional goal of durable local control	IVC and patients with micrometastatic dissemination: distant disease goes untreated
Cytotoxic chemotherapy (full dose)	Treat progressive cervical disease Treat distant metastatic disease	Responses are usually not durable
Targeted therapies/ clinical trials	Treat progressive cervical disease Treat distant metastatic disease	Access to newer agents that may be effective Little evidence of efficacy to date

Abbreviation: EBRT, external beam radiation therapy.

required given that these are potential concomitant diseases associated with MEN2. If a pheochromocytoma is identified, adrenalectomy (cortical sparing if feasible) is performed before treatment of MTC. If pHPT is diagnosed, parathyroidectomy should be performed at the time of the thyroidectomy. Surgery for primary MTC consists of a total thyroidectomy and bilateral central neck dissection, irrespective of absence of radiographic or clinical evidence of central neck disease. More controversial is treatment of the lateral neck fields; we recommend anatomical compartment–defined lateral neck dissection in the presence of radiographically evident disease and do not base this decision on a calcitonin level.

Specific germline *RET* mutations have been associated with certain phenotypic behaviors and guide recommendation for timing of prophylactic thyroidectomy in patients with MEN2 diagnosed on genetic screening. The most recent American Thyroid Association MTC Taskforce has created the groups of highest risk (*RET* codon *M918T* mutation), high risk (*RET* codon *C634* mutations and *A883F* mutation), and moderate risk (including but not limited to *RET* codon *C609*, *C611*, *C618*, *C620*, and *V804* mutations) based on aggressiveness of MTC.[2]

Long-term Surveillance

Long-term surveillance for DTC requires ongoing dynamic risk assessment, which is based on the initial risk assessment and then incorporates new data obtained during the surveillance period. There are 2 initial risk assessments that should be performed:

- Risk of death based on age, tumor size, histology, completeness of surgery, nodal involvement, and distant metastasis[6]
- Risk of recurrence in patients with no distant disease (based on age, tumor size, histology, and nodal involvement).[17]

The level of risk of recurrence or death can change throughout the surveillance period and is based on thyroglobulin (Tg) levels, Tg trends, and imaging (**Fig. 6**).

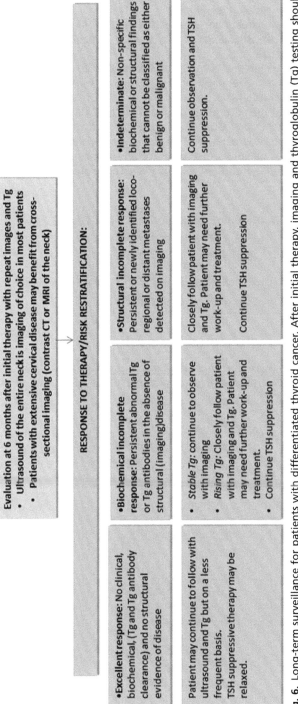

Evaluation at 6 months after initial therapy with repeat images and Tg
- Ultrasound of the entire neck is imaging of choice in most patients
- Patients with extensive cervical disease may benefit from cross-sectional imaging (contrast CT or MRI of the neck)

RESPONSE TO THERAPY/RISK RESTRATIFICATION:

- **Excellent response:** No clinical, biochemical, (Tg and Tg antibody clearance) and no structural evidence of disease

  Patient may continue to follow with ultrasound and Tg but on a less frequent basis.
  TSH suppressive therapy may be relaxed.

- **Biochemical incomplete response:** Persistent abnormal Tg or Tg antibodies in the absence of structural (imaging)disease
  - *Stable Tg:* continue to observe with imaging
  - *Rising Tg:* Closely follow patient with imaging and Tg. Patient may need further work-up and treatment.
  - Continue TSH suppression

- **Structural incomplete response:** Persistent or newly identified loco-regional or distant metastases detected on imaging

  Closely follow patient with imaging and Tg. Patient may need further work-up and treatment.

  Continue TSH suppression

- **Indeterminate:** Non-specific biochemical or structural findings that cannot be classified as either benign or malignant

  Continue observation and TSH suppression.

Fig. 6. Long-term surveillance for patients with differentiated thyroid cancer. After initial therapy, imaging and thyroglobulin (Tg) testing should be performed. Response to therapy and risk restratification is then determined based on new information. Biochemically incomplete refers to TSH-suppressed Tg less than 0.2 ng/mL or TSH-stimulated Tg less than 1 ng/mL.

Patients who have persistent or distant disease after initial therapy require an individualized plan to determine the need for and timing of surgery (for localized disease) and treatment of distant disease (see **Fig. 5**).

Surveillance following treatment in patients with ATC is individualized, but, given the propensity for early relapse, surveillance imaging is generally comprehensive. Serum biomarkers have no role.

In postoperative patients with MTC, calcitonin and CEA should be measured no sooner than 3 months after surgery. **Fig. 7** shows the standard treatment and follow-up for patients with MTC.

In patients with progressive MTC, calcitonin and CEA levels typically increase at similar rates. Calcitonin and CEA doubling times (DTs) correlate with rate of progression, recurrence, and survival.[18] Reliable calculations of DTs require at least 4 time points over a minimum of 2 years of observation. Higher disease-specific survival and recurrence-free survival rates are associated with DTs greater than

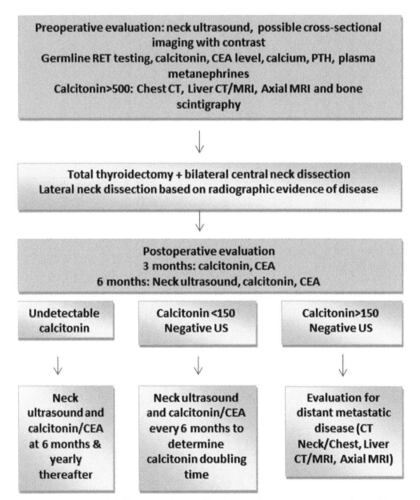

Fig. 7. Management and follow-up of medullary thyroid cancer. PTH, parathyroid hormone; US, ultrasonography.

1 year. CEA DT has a higher predictive value than calcitonin DT. DTs can guide the frequency of imaging studies. Patients with prolonged DTs (>1 year) can have imaging studies every 6 to 12 months, thus reducing cost and radiation exposure.

NONPHARMACOLOGIC THERAPY
External Beam Radiation

The lack of prospective studies to assess the role of external beam radiation therapy (EBRT) in DTC and MTC limits its routine use. Although controversial, postoperative/adjuvant EBRT may improve locoregional control for patients judged to be at highest risk for nonsalvageable (or overly morbid) central compartment recurrence (largely surgeon determined). In general, this represents older patients, pT4 or multiply recurrent disease, and/or aggressive histologic variants.[19,20] At our center, other than for purely palliative situations, EBRT is rarely used to treat gross disease from DTC or MTC in the neck, because EBRT is likely to preclude future neck surgery and radiation doses that can safely be delivered to the low neck and central compartment are limited by the tolerance of the esophagus and brachial plexus. EBRT may delay initiation of systemic therapy and may increase the risk of tracheoesophageal and tracheotumor fistula formation when antiangiogenic kinase inhibitors (KIs) are used.[21]

Localized Therapies

Localized therapies refer to treatments of active disease with nonpharmacologic therapies. **Table 6** shows several choices of localized therapies available to patients with thyroid cancer. Localized therapy is useful for palliating or treating active disease either in conjunction with or without pharmacologic methods.

Table 6
Nonpharmacologic and pharmacologic therapies and their recommended applications for thyroid cancer treatment

Treatment	Application
Nonpharmacologic Therapies	
Surgery	Oligometastases, locoregional disease
EBRT, IMRT, SBRT, gamma knife	Postoperative for locoregional disease (in ATC; controversial in DTC and MTC) or for palliation of soft tissue, bone, lung, liver, brain
Laser treatment	Endobronchial lesions
Thermal ablation (RFA, cryoablation)	Soft tissue, liver
Embolization	Soft tissue, liver
Ethanol ablation	Locoregional disease
Pharmacologic Therapies	
Intravenous bisphosphonates	Bone metastases
RANK ligand inhibitors	Bone metastases
Kinase inhibitors	RAIR, progressive or symptomatic DTC Progressive or symptomatic MTC

Abbreviations: IMRT, intensity-modulated radiation therapy; RAIR, RAI refractory; RANK, receptor activator of nuclear factor kappa-B; RFA, radiofrequency ablation; SBRT, stereotactic body radiation therapy.

Table 7
Kinase inhibitor drugs that are FDA approved for thyroid cancer and their non-FDA-approved uses in thyroid cancer

Drugs	FDA-approved Indication; Trial Phase and Design; Trial Results; (Reference)	Not an FDA-approved Indication; Earlier Phase Trial Completed or Reported; (Reference or NCT#)	Starting Dose (mg)	Frequency	Other Dose Levels (mg)
Sorafenib	RAIR-DTC DECISION trial: phase III, randomized, double blinded, placebo controlled Median PFS sorafenib 10.8 mo vs placebo 5.8 mo; HR = 0.59 (Brose et al,[45] 2014)	MTC (Lam et al,[46] 2010)	400	bid	400 once daily; 200 bid; 200 once daily
Lenvatinib	RAIR-DTC EXAM trial: phase III, randomized, double blinded, placebo controlled Median PFS lenvatinib 18.3 mo vs placebo 3.6 mo; HR = 0.21 (Schlumberger et al,[47] 2015)	MTC (Schlumberger et al,[48] 2012)	24	Once daily	20, 14, and 10 once daily
Vandetanib	Progressive MTC ZETA trial: phase III, randomized, double blinded, placebo controlled Median PFS vandetanib 30.5 mo (estimated) vs placebo 19.3 mo; HR = 0.46 (Wells et al,[49] 2012)	RAIR-DTC (Leboulleux et al,[50] 2012)	300	Once daily	150 once daily
Cabozantinib	Progressive MTC EXAM trial: phase III, randomized, double blinded, placebo controlled Median PFS cabozantinib 11.2 mo vs placebo 4 mo; HR = 0.28 (Schoffski et al,[51] 2012)	RAIR-DTC (Cabanillas et al,[52] 2014, NCT01811212; NCT01896479)	140	Once daily	100, 60, 40 once daily

Abbreviations: bid, twice a day; HR, hazard radio; MTC, medullary thyroid cancer; NCT, National Clinical Trial; PFS, progression-free survival; RAIR-DTC, RAI-refractory DTC.
Data from Refs.[45-52]

PHARMACOLOGIC THERAPIES
Bone-modulating Drugs

Bone is a common site of distant metastases in thyroid cancer and is a poor prognostic factor.[22,23] In DTC, RAI should be considered; however, few patients have complete resolution of their bony metastases.[24] In addition, bone metastases are challenging to treat with the KIs. As with other solid tumors, bone-modulating drugs that inhibit osteoclast activity, such as the intravenous bisphosphonates (zoledronic acid, pamidronate) and the RANK ligand inhibitors (denosumab), are often used alone or in conjunction with localized therapies or KIs for 2 purposes: to control pain and to minimize skeletal-related events. Better strategies for managing bony metastases from thyroid cancer are needed.

Kinase Inhibitors

Several KIs are now US Food and Drug Administration (FDA) approved for metastatic DTC and MTC. **Table 7** lists information regarding the FDA-approved drugs in DTC and MTC. In addition, these drugs and many other KIs have been studied in several trials in other thyroid cancer types (see **Table 7** and **Table 8**). Because most patients with DTC and MTC have indolent disease, understanding the indications for systemic therapy with KIs is critical in order to select appropriate candidates for these drugs. For patients with DTC, it is important to determine whether they are RAI refractory (RAIR; see **Table 3**). **Fig. 8** shows 3 categories of patients with DTC and MTC who meet criteria for systemic therapy, with specific examples. Note that these drugs do not cure the disease, and invariably patients eventually progress. Salvage therapy seems to be a reasonable strategy in patients with DTC who have failed previous KIs.[25]

Systemic therapy may be considered for patients with ATC with distant metastatic disease or progressive locoregional disease after prior surgery and/or radiotherapy. Taxanes, doxorubicin, and platinum chemotherapy have shown low to moderate

Table 8			
Kinase inhibitor drugs studied in thyroid cancer			
Drug	**Type of Thyroid Cancer**	**Study Design**	**References**
Axitinib	ATC, DTC, MTC	II	Cohen et al,[28] 2008
Dabrafenib	DTC	I	Falchook et al,[29] 2014
Everolimus	ATC, DTC, MTC	II	Lorch et al,[30,31] 2013, Lim et al,[32] 2013
Everolimus + sorafenib	DTC, MTC	II	Sherman et al,[33] 2014
Motesanib	DTC, MTC	II	Sherman et al,[34] 2008 and Schlumberger et al,[35] 2009
Pazopanib	ATC, DTC, MTC	II	Bible et al,[36–38] 2012; 2010; 2014
Selumetinib	DTC	II and pilot	Hayes et al,[39] 2012 and Ho et al,[9] 2013
Sunitinib	DTC, MTC	II	Carr et al,[40] 2010, Cohen et al,[41] 2008, De Souza,[42] 2010
Tipifarnib + sorafenib	DTC, MTC	I	Hong et al,[43] 2011
Vemurafenib	DTC	II	Brose et al,[44] 2013

Abbreviations: ATC, anaplastic thyroid cancer; DTC, differentiated thyroid cancer; MTC, medullary thyroid cancer.
Data from Refs.[9,28–44]

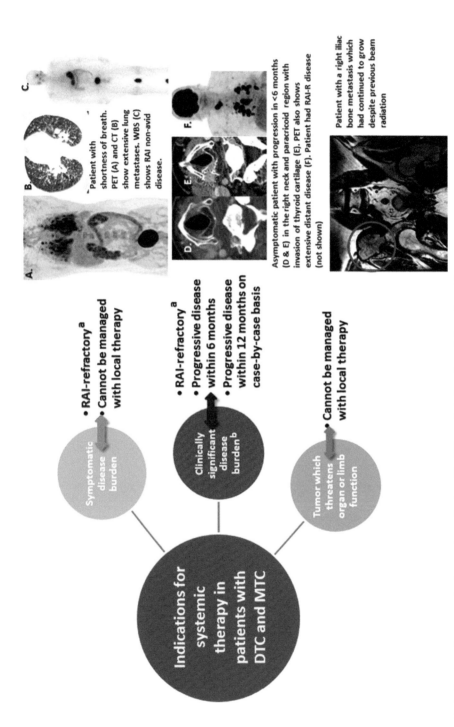

Fig. 8. Indications for systemic therapy in patients with differentiated and medullary thyroid cancer.
[a]Applied only to patients with DTC. [b]Clinically significant disease burden is defined as multiple target lesions, of which one is at least 1.5 cm in diameter, and likely to cause symptomatic disease if left untreated.

Table 9
Completed ATC clinical trials (with >10 participants) and ongoing trials enrolling ATC or ATC cohorts

Targeted Therapy Drug	Number of Patients Participating	Mutation Requirement	Median OS (mo)	Median PFS (mo)	Response Rate: PR/SD/PD, n (%)	Reference and ClinicalTrials.gov Identifier
Trial Results with Results Reported as of 7/8/15						
Sorafenib 400 mg twice per day	20[a]	None	3.9	1.9	2 (10)/ 5 (25)/ 13 (65)	Savvides et al,[53] 2012 NCT00126568
Pazopanib 800 mg once daily	15	None	3.6	2.0 (TTP)	0/ 12 (80)/ 3 (20)	Bible et al,[36] 2012 NCT00625846
Efatutazone + paclitaxel (cohort 1 = 0.15 mg bid; cohort 2 = 0.3 mg bid)	13	None	Cohort 1 = 3.2 Cohort 2 = 4.5	Cohort 1: 1.6 (TTP) Cohort 2 = 2.2 (TTP)	Cohort 1 = 0/ 4 (57)/2 (29)[b] Cohort 2 = 1 (17)/ 3 (50)/ 2 (33)	Smallridge et al,[54] 2013 NCT00603941
Paclitaxel and carboplatin vs carboplatin + fosbretabulin	80[a]	None	4 vs 5.2	3.1 vs 3.3	Not reported	Sosa et al,[55] 2013 NCT01701349
Lenvatinib	11	None	10.6	7.4	3 (27.3)/ 7 (63.6)/ 1 (9.1)	Takahashi et al,[56] 2014 NCT01728623
Ongoing Trials With No Results Reported as of 7/8/15						
Radiation plus either: paclitaxel + pazopanib vs (or) paclitaxel alone	121	None	—	—	—	NCT01236547
Dabrafenib 150 mg twice per day + trametinib 2 mg daily	25 in ATC cohort	BRAF V600E	—	—	—	NCT02034110
MPDL3280A (anti-PD-L1)	10 in ATC cohort	None	—	—	—	NCT02458638
MLN0128 (mTOR inhibitor)	25	None	—	—	—	NCT02244463
Crolibulin + cisplatin vs cisplatin alone (phase II)	70	None	—	—	—	NCT01240590
Efatutazone + paclitaxel vs paclitaxel alone	50	None	—	—	—	NCT02152137
Ceritinib 750 mg daily	10	Alk rearrangements	—	—	—	NCT02289144

Abbreviations: OS, overall survival; PD, progressive disease; PFS, progression-free survival; PR, partial response; SD, stable disease; TTP, time to progression.

[a] Trial did not complete enrollment, thus likely was underpowered.
[b] One patient never restaged; failed because of serious adverse event.

activity in ATC. Because of the low incidence of ATC and frequent presentation with acute symptoms and rapid clinical deterioration, clinical trials have been difficult to complete. In light of the limited efficacy of cytotoxic chemotherapy, enrolling patients with ATC on clinical trials with novel agents is encouraged. **Table 9** lists the targeted therapy trials that have been reported in trials enrolling at least 10 patients and the ongoing trials in ATC. One attractive approach being studied is the use of selective BRAF inhibitors in BRAF-mutated ATC. A recent case report described a dramatic response to vemurafenib, a selective BRAF inhibitor, in a patient with BRAF-mutated ATC[26] and Hyman and colleagues[27] reported on 7 ATC patients on this drug. The overall response rate was 29%. Improvements in systemic therapy for ATC are likely to require the identification of patient subgroups with driver genetic abnormalities in which molecular targeted therapies can be tested.

SUMMARY

In recent decades effective systemic therapies have been discovered for thyroid cancer and 4 antiangiogenic KIs have been approved for DTC and MTC. More chemotherapeutic drugs with different mechanisms of action will be or are currently being tested for these diseases, such as highly selective mTOR inhibitors, second-generation BRAF inhibitors, anti-CTLA4, anti-PD1, and anti-PDL1. Progress in ATC treatments continues to be a challenge. It will require a concerted worldwide effort to further research in ATC. In addition, the future of oncologic endocrine tumors will be affected by the financial toxicity these drugs introduce. A more cost-effective solution to thyroid cancer care needs to be taken into consideration.

REFERENCES

1. Kebebew E, Greenspan FS, Clark OH, et al. Anaplastic thyroid carcinoma. Treatment outcome and prognostic factors. Cancer 2005;103(7):1330–5.
2. Wells SA Jr, Asa SL, Dralle H, et al. Revised American Thyroid Association guidelines for the management of medullary thyroid carcinoma. Thyroid 2015;25(6):567–610.
3. Roman S, Lin R, Sosa JA. Prognosis of medullary thyroid carcinoma: demographic, clinical, and pathologic predictors of survival in 1252 cases. Cancer 2006;107(9):2134–42.
4. Xing M, Liu R, Liu X, et al. BRAF V600E and TERT promoter mutations cooperatively identify the most aggressive papillary thyroid cancer with highest recurrence. J Clin Oncol 2014;32(25):2718–26.
5. Chen H, Sippel RS, O'Dorisio MS, et al. The North American Neuroendocrine Tumor Society consensus guideline for the diagnosis and management of neuroendocrine tumors: pheochromocytoma, paraganglioma, and medullary thyroid cancer. Pancreas 2010;39(6):775–83.
6. Haugen BR, Alexander EK, Bible KC, et al. American Thyroid Association Management Guidelines for Adult Patients with Thyroid Nodules and Differentiated Thyroid Cancer. Thyroid 2015. [Epub ahead of print].
7. Tuttle RM, Haddad R, Ball DW, et al. NCCN clinical practice guidelines in oncology: thyroid carcinoma. J Natl Compr Canc Netw 2014;1:2014.
8. Durante C, Haddy N, Baudin E, et al. Long-term outcome of 444 patients with distant metastases from papillary and follicular thyroid carcinoma: benefits and limits of radioiodine therapy. J Clin Endocrinol Metab 2006;91(8):2892–9.

9. Ho AL, Grewal RK, Leboeuf R, et al. Selumetinib-enhanced radioiodine uptake in advanced thyroid cancer. N Engl J Med 2013;368(7):623–32.

10. Rothenberg SM, McFadden DG, Palmer E, et al. Re-differentiation of radioiodine-refractory *BRAF* V600E-mutant thyroid carcinoma with dabrafenib: a pilot study. J Clin Oncol 2013;31(Suppl):2013 [abstract: 6025].

11. Haigh PI, Ituarte PH, Wu HS, et al. Completely resected anaplastic thyroid carcinoma combined with adjuvant chemotherapy and irradiation is associated with prolonged survival. Cancer 2001;91(12):2335–42.

12. Ito K, Hanamura T, Murayama K, et al. Multimodality therapeutic outcomes in anaplastic thyroid carcinoma: improved survival in subgroups of patients with localized primary tumors. Head Neck 2012;34(2):230–7.

13. Swaak-Kragten AT, de Wilt JH, Schmitz PI, et al. Multimodality treatment for anaplastic thyroid carcinoma–treatment outcome in 75 patients. Radiother Oncol 2009;92(1):100–4.

14. Levendag PC, De Porre PM, van Putten WL. Anaplastic carcinoma of the thyroid gland treated by radiation therapy. Int J Radiat Oncol Biol Phys 1993;26(1): 125–8.

15. Sherman EJ, Lim SH, Ho AL, et al. Concurrent doxorubicin and radiotherapy for anaplastic thyroid cancer: a critical re-evaluation including uniform pathologic review. Radiother Oncol 2011;101(3):425–30.

16. Smallridge RC, Ain KB, Asa SL, et al. American Thyroid Association guidelines for management of patients with anaplastic thyroid cancer. Thyroid 2012;22(11): 1104–39.

17. Tuttle RM, Sabra MM. Selective use of RAI for ablation and adjuvant therapy after total thyroidectomy for differentiated thyroid cancer: a practical approach to clinical decision making. Oral Oncol 2013;49(7):676–83.

18. Meijer JA, le Cessie S, van den Hout WB, et al. Calcitonin and carcinoembryonic antigen doubling times as prognostic factors in medullary thyroid carcinoma: a structured meta-analysis. Clin Endocrinol (Oxf) 2010;72(4):534–42.

19. Su SY, Milas ZL, Bhatt N, et al. Well-differentiated thyroid cancer with aerodigestive tract invasion: long-term control and functional outcomes. Head Neck 2014. [Epub ahead of print].

20. Schwartz DL, Lobo MJ, Ang KK, et al. Postoperative external beam radiotherapy for differentiated thyroid cancer: outcomes and morbidity with conformal treatment. Int J Radiat Oncol Biol Phys 2009;74(4):1083–91.

21. Blevins DP, Dadu R, Hu M, et al. Aerodigestive fistula formation as a rare side effect of antiangiogenic tyrosine kinase inhibitor therapy for thyroid cancer. Thyroid 2014;24(5):918–22.

22. Pittas AG, Adler M, Fazzari M, et al. Bone metastases from thyroid carcinoma: clinical characteristics and prognostic variables in one hundred forty-six patients. Thyroid 2000;10(3):261–8.

23. Sugitani I, Fujimoto Y, Yamamoto N. Papillary thyroid carcinoma with distant metastases: survival predictors and the importance of local control. Surgery 2008;143(1):35–42.

24. Orita Y, Sugitani I, Matsuura M, et al. Prognostic factors and the therapeutic strategy for patients with bone metastasis from differentiated thyroid carcinoma. Surgery 2010;147(3):424–31.

25. Dadu R, Devine C, Hernandez M, et al. Role of salvage targeted therapy in differentiated thyroid cancer patients who failed first-line sorafenib. J Clin Endocrinol Metab 2014;99(6):2086–94.

26. Rosove MH, Peddi PF, Glaspy JA. BRAF V600E inhibition in anaplastic thyroid cancer. N Engl J Med 2013;368(7):684–5.

27. Hyman DM, Puzanov I, Subbiah V, et al. Vemurafenib in multiple nonmelanoma cancers with BRAF V600 mutations. N Engl J Med 2015;373(8):726–36.

28. Cohen EE, Rosen LS, Vokes EE, et al. Axitinib is an active treatment for all histologic subtypes of advanced thyroid cancer: results from a phase II study. J Clin Oncol 2008;26(29):4708–13.

29. Falchook GS, Millward M, Hong D, et al. BRAF inhibitor dabrafenib in patients with metastatic BRAF-Mutant Thyroid Cancer. Thyroid 2014;25(1):71–7.

30. Lorch JH, Busaidy N, Ruan DT, et al. A phase II study of everolimus in patients with aggressive RAI refractory (RAIR) thyroid cancer (TC). J Clin Oncol 2013; 21(Suppl) [abstract: 6023].

31. Wagle N, Grabiner BC, Van Allen EM, et al. Response and acquired resistance to everolimus in anaplastic thyroid cancer. N Engl J Med 2014;371(15):1426–33.

32. Lim SM, Chang H, Yoon MJ, et al. A multicenter, phase II trial of everolimus in locally advanced or metastatic thyroid cancer of all histologic subtypes. Ann Oncol 2013;24(12):3089–94.

33. Sherman E, Ho AL, Fury M, et al. Combination of everolimus and sorafenib in the treatment of thyroid cancer: Update on phase II study. J Clin Oncol 2014; 33(Suppl) [abstract: 6069].

34. Sherman SI, Wirth LJ, Droz JP, et al. Motesanib diphosphate in progressive differentiated thyroid cancer. N Engl J Med 2008;359(1):31–42.

35. Schlumberger MJ, Elisei R, Bastholt L, et al. Phase II study of safety and efficacy of motesanib in patients with progressive or symptomatic, advanced or metastatic medullary thyroid cancer. J Clin Oncol 2009;27(23):3794–801.

36. Bible KC, Suman VJ, Menefee ME, et al. A multiinstitutional phase 2 trial of pazopanib monotherapy in advanced anaplastic thyroid cancer. J Clin Endocrinol Metab 2012;97(9):3179–84.

37. Bible KC, Suman VJ, Molina JR, et al. Efficacy of pazopanib in progressive, radioiodine-refractory, metastatic differentiated thyroid cancers: results of a phase 2 consortium study. Lancet Oncol 2010;11(10):962–72.

38. Bible KC, Suman VJ, Molina JR, et al. A multicenter phase 2 trial of pazopanib in metastatic and progressive medullary thyroid carcinoma: MC057H. J Clin Endocrinol Metab 2014;99(5):1687–93.

39. Hayes DN, Lucas AS, Tanvetyanon T, et al. Phase II efficacy and pharmacogenomic study of selumetinib (AZD6244; ARRY-142886) in iodine-131 refractory papillary thyroid carcinoma with or without follicular elements. Clin Cancer Res 2012;18(7):2056–65.

40. Carr LL, Mankoff DA, Goulart BH, et al. Phase II study of daily sunitinib in FDG-PET-positive, iodine-refractory differentiated thyroid cancer and metastatic medullary carcinoma of the thyroid with functional imaging correlation. Clin Cancer Res 2010;16(21):5260–8.

41. Cohen EE, Needles BM, Cullen KJ, et al. Phase 2 study of sunitinib in refractory thyroid cancer. J Clin Oncol 2008;26(Suppl) [abstract: 6025].

42. De Souza JA, Busaidy N, Zimrin A, et al. Phase II trial of sunitinib in medullary thyroid cancer (MTC). J Clin Orthod 2010;28(Suppl) [abstract: 5504].

43. Hong DS, Cabanillas ME, Wheler J, et al. Inhibition of the Ras/Raf/MEK/ERK and RET kinase pathways with the combination of the multikinase inhibitor sorafenib and the farnesyltransferase inhibitor tipifarnib in medullary and differentiated thyroid malignancies. J Clin Endocrinol Metab 2011;96(4):997–1005.

44. Brose MS, Cabanillas ME, Cohen EE, et al. An open-label, multi-center phase 2 study of the BRAF inhibitor vemurafenib in patients with metastatic or unresectable papillary thyroid cancer positive for the BRAF V600 mutation and resistant to radioactive iodine. Proc European Cancer Congress. Amsterdam, September 27–October 1, 2013. oral abstr 28.

45. Brose MS, Nutting CM, Jarzab B, et al. Sorafenib in radioactive iodine-refractory, locally advanced or metastatic differentiated thyroid cancer: a randomised, double-blind, phase 3 trial. Lancet 2014;384(9940):319–28.

46. Lam ET, Ringel MD, Kloos RT, et al. Phase II clinical trial of sorafenib in metastatic medullary thyroid cancer. J Clin Oncol 2010;28(14):2323–30.

47. Schlumberger M, Tahara M, Wirth LJ, et al. Lenvatinib versus placebo in radioiodine-refractory thyroid cancer. N Engl J Med 2015;372(7):621–30.

48. Schlumberger M, Jarzab B, Cabanillas ME, et al. A phase 2 trial of the multi-targeted tyrosine kinase inhibitor lenvatinib (E7080) in advanced medullary thyroid cancer (MTC). Clin Cancer Res 2015. [Epub ahead of print].

49. Wells SA Jr, Robinson BG, Gagel RF, et al. Vandetanib in patients with locally advanced or metastatic medullary thyroid cancer: a randomized, double-blind phase III trial. J Clin Oncol 2012;30(2):134–41.

50. Leboulleux S, Bastholt L, Krause T, et al. Vandetanib in locally advanced or metastatic differentiated thyroid cancer: a randomised, double-blind, phase 2 trial. Lancet Oncol 2012;13(9):897–905.

51. Schoffski P, Elisei R, Miller S, et al. An international, double-blind, randomized, placebo-controlled phase III trial (EXAM) of cabozantinib (XL184) in medullary thyroid carcinoma (MTC) patients (pts) with documented RECIST progression at baseline. J Clin Oncol 2012;30(Suppl) [abstract: 5508].

52. Cabanillas ME, Brose MS, Holland J, et al. A phase I study of cabozantinib (XL184) in patients with differentiated thyroid cancer. Thyroid 2014;24(10):1508–14.

53. Savvides P, Nagaiah G, Lavertu P, et al. Phase II trial of sorafenib in patients with advanced anaplastic carcinoma of the thyroid. Thyroid 2013;23(5):600–4.

54. Smallridge RC, Copland JA, Brose MS, et al. Efatutazone, an oral PPAR-gamma agonist, in combination with paclitaxel in anaplastic thyroid cancer: results of a multicenter phase 1 trial. J Clin Endocrinol Metab 2013;98(6):2392–400.

55. Sosa JA, Elisei R, Jarzab B, et al. Randomized safety and efficacy study of fosbretabulin with paclitaxel/carboplatin against anaplastic thyroid carcinoma. Thyroid 2013.

56. Takahashi S, Tahara M, Kiyota N, et al. Phase II study of lenvatinib, a multitargeted tyrosine kinase inhibitor, in patients with all histologic subtypes of advanced thyroid cancer (differentiated, medullary, and anaplastic). Ann Oncol 2014;24(suppl 4).

Salivary Gland Malignancies

Cristina P. Rodriguez, MD[a], Upendra Parvathaneni, MBBS, FRANZCR[b],
Eduardo Méndez, MD, MS[c,d], Renato G. Martins, MD, MPH[a,*]

KEYWORDS

- Salivary cancer • Therapy • Review • Management • Systemic

KEY POINTS

- Salivary gland cancers are morphologically and biologically diverse.
- Surgical resection with postoperative radiation is considered a treatment standard for localized disease.
- Systemic therapy can be considered for patients with unresectable or metastatic disease with the goal of palliation of symptoms.

INTRODUCTION

Primary salivary gland malignancies represent less than 5% of all new head and neck cancers, with approximately 3000 new cases diagnosed in the United States annually. These diverse cancers arise from the malignant transformation of the various myoepithelial, ductal, and acinic components of 3 paired major (parotid, submandibular, and sublingual) and minor salivary glands distributed throughout the upper aerodigestive tract. The World Health Organization classifies 24 subtypes[1] characterized by marked biological heterogeneity. For example, high-grade mucoepidermoid carcinomas, salivary duct carcinomas, malignant mixed tumors, and high-grade adenocarcinomas have the most aggressive clinical course, with frequent early spread to regional lymph nodes and distant sites. In contrast, adenoid cystic carcinomas generally display an indolent natural history with a propensity for local or distant recurrence even 10 to 15 years after initial treatment. Knowledge of these unique factors is essential in planning the nuances of therapy.

Conflicts of Interest: The authors have no potential conflicts of interest to disclose.
[a] Division of Medical Oncology, Department of Medicine, University of Washington, 825 Eastlake Avenue East, MS G4940, Seattle, WA 98109, USA; [b] Division of Radiation Oncology, Department of Medicine, University of Washington, 1959 Northeast Pacific Street, Box, Seattle, WA 98195, USA; [c] Department of Otolaryngology, Head and Neck Surgery, University of Washington, 1959 Northeast Pacific Street, Box 356515, Seattle, WA 98195, USA; [d] Clinical Research Division, Fred Hutchinson Cancer Research Center, 1959 Northeast Pacific Street, Box 356515, Seattle, WA 98195, USA
* Corresponding author.
E-mail addresses: rgmart@uw.edu; rgmart@u.washington.edu

Hematol Oncol Clin N Am 29 (2015) 1145–1157
http://dx.doi.org/10.1016/j.hoc.2015.08.002
0889-8588/15/$ – see front matter © 2015 Elsevier Inc. All rights reserved.

INITIAL EVALUATION

The clinical presentation of a salivary gland mass can reveal a great deal about its nature, with certain symptoms and physical findings associated with malignancy. Rapid growth and/or pain (either localized or referred to the temporomandibular joint or the ear), and paresthesias/hypesthesias caused by perineural spread are concerning signs for malignancy.[2,3] Facial nerve dysfunction, firmness and fixation of a mass, the presence of trismus for tumors of the parapharyngeal space, and nodal involvement in the neck are findings that increase suspicion for a malignant process.[4–6]

Computed tomography (CT) and MRI are the two most common imaging modalities used to evaluate salivary gland lesions, with the latter being the method of choice for patients with palpable masses and a strong suspicion for malignancy.[7,8] Contrast enhancement per se cannot distinguish benign versus malignant processes but it can be critical in delineating the extent of the lesion. Irregular margins; bony invasion; presence of metastatic lymph nodes; and perineural spread along cranial nerve VII (stylomastoid foramen), cranial nerve V-3 (foramen ovale), or V-2 (foramen rotundum) can all be concerning signs of malignancy.[6,9] Necrosis can also characterize malignancy, particularly in primary squamous cell carcinomas of the salivary glands (likely caused by squamous metaplasia in patients with chronic inflammation). In addition, PET is now being studied for its utility in evaluating salivary gland tumors. Keyes and colleagues[10] found high sensitivity (100%) but low specificity (30%) in predicting malignancy in a cohort of 26 patients with parotid masses.

Histologic confirmation can be acquired before a definitive surgical procedure and this can be useful in planning the type and extent of definitive therapy. Fine-needle aspiration biopsy (FNAB) is the most widely used method for obtaining diagnostic tissue because of its convenience as an office procedure and its associated high sensitivity and specificity.[11,12] In clinical scenarios in which surgical resection of a growing lesion is planned regardless of the histology, patients may opt to forgo FNAB. With respect to obtaining tissue for surgical preplanning, clinicians should consider the risk of performing unnecessary surgery before knowing the diagnosis based on permanent section evaluation. A frozen section intraoperatively can be useful for a diagnosis but its value compared with FNAB is controversial because its accuracy depends on the experience of the on-call pathologist. Some studies have shown that intraoperative diagnoses can change after permanent section examination.[13,14] Others have shown the sensitivity and specificity of frozen sections to be 77% and 100%.[15] The risk of either test is in performing unnecessary surgery, like a radical resection or a cervical lymphadenectomy, if a diagnosis of an aggressive malignancy is erroneously reported. Thus, the ultimate scope of treatment should be reserved until permanent section analysis is performed.

SURGICAL MANAGEMENT

Surgical excision of a primary salivary gland malignancy can be curative for most cases when the tumor is small, low grade, and easily accessible. Parotid malignancies are most curable with surgery, followed by the submandibular and sublingual glands. Ultimately, prognosis depends on the gland of origin, histology, grade, and extent of disease (ie, American Joint Commission for Cancer stage). Bulkier tumors or those of aggressive histology/grade are best treated with surgery first, followed by adjuvant therapy.

Surgery of the Parotid Gland and Management of the Facial Nerve

Among parotid tumors, avoiding injury to the facial nerve is critical when tumors are not fixed to, or encasing, the nerve. Thus, surgery typically involves removing the superficial lobe of the gland above the plane of the facial nerve or the deep lobe just underneath it. A superficial parotidectomy can be considered the treatment of choice for most tumors in the superficial lobe of the gland. Enucleation of a tumor should be avoided because this has been associated with tumor spillage and higher recurrence rates. However, patients should be consented for total parotidectomy in cases in which there is deep lobe involvement, because preservation of the nerve often requires removing the superficial lobe to then dissect any deep lobe component from the nerve.

The decision on whether or not the facial nerve should be sacrificed is complex and should be considered on a case-by-case basis. When dealing with a malignant tumor, some general guidelines can be followed, such as preservation of the nerve when the tumor is not involving it. In contrast, sacrifice may be necessary if preservation would lead to grossly positive margins or tumor spillage.[16–18] This decision can also be influenced by the options available postoperatively. For example, clinicians may err on the side of nerve sacrifice in cases of recurrent disease in which surgical salvage is considered after failed radiation therapy (RT). In cases in which the tumor is noted to abut the mastoid bone or the stylomastoid foramen, the patient should be consented for a mastoidectomy to identify the nerve trunk more proximally. This procedure would expose a portion of uninvolved nerve for grafting if sacrifice is required at the level of the stylomastoid foramen. Besides nerve grafting when the nerve is not working preoperatively or must be sacrificed, the surgeon should be prepared for facial reanimation procedures, such as a gold-weight eyelid implant and/or oral commissure facial sling suspension, to prevent corneal damage and preserve oral competence. This outcome can be accomplished either at the time of tumor resection or later, as an elective procedure. Larger tumors involving the ear canal or middle ear require a temporal bone resection. Patients should be counseled with respect to hearing loss if the ear canal is involved and requires obliteration.

Surgery of the Submandibular and Sublingual Glands

Surgery for tumors of the submandibular and sublingual glands also has its own set of special considerations. When submandibular malignancy is known *a priori*, clinicians must avoid shelling out the gland, and instead dissection should incorporate the adjacent lymph nodes of a level I cervical lymphadenectomy. Surgical management of a sublingual gland malignancy can be approached transorally. Obtaining negative margins for the sublingual gland can be more challenging because it is not encapsulated by the cervical fascia as is the submandibular gland, because of its location abutting the lingual cortex of the mandible, and its close relationship to the lingual nerve and Wharton duct of the submandibular gland. Often reposition of this duct is necessary to avoid chronic obstruction and inflammation of the submandibular gland.

Surgical considerations for minor salivary glands vary depending on their location. In general, the goal is to perform a wide local excision with clear margins confirmed intraoperatively with frozen sections. The procedure is determined by the location and extent of disease. Given the most common locations where tumors present, mainly the palate and base of tongue, surgical defects can have a significant impact on speech, swallowing, and velopharyngeal competence. Because of the low risk of occult metastatic spread, a prophylactic neck dissection is often not warranted. Smaller tumors of the parapharyngeal space may be approached transorally, whereas larger ones require a transcervical/transparotid approach with or without a mandibulotomy.[19]

Management of the Neck

The overall incidence of cervical lymph metastases is low for patients with malignant salivary cancer, with about 16% of parotid carcinomas and 8% of submandibular/sublingual malignancies presenting with lymphadenopathy. Surgical management of cervical lymph nodes is usually performed in the presence of adenopathy or high-grade histology. Because of the low risk of occult disease, a prophylactic neck dissection is not often performed in other circumstances. Often the final diagnosis of the tumor depends on permanent pathologic analysis after tumor resection. Thus, treatment of the lymph nodes would be considered after the initial surgery. When the risk of occult disease is higher because of aggressive histology or high-grade features (such as advanced T and N descriptors, positive resection margins, perineural invasion) and the need for adjuvant treatment to the resected bed is indicated, management of the N0 neck can be accomplished effectively in this setting.[20,21]

RADIATION THERAPY

Unresectable locally advanced tumors with involvement of the skull base or encasing of the carotid vessels, and patients who decline surgery because of the requirement of sacrifice of an intact facial nerve or who are otherwise challenged with medical comorbidities, could be treated with primary RT.[22,23] Mendenhall and colleagues[24] reported on 160 patients who were treated with surgery and RT and compared outcomes with 64 patients treated with RT alone. The 10-year local control rate was 42% for RT alone versus 90% for surgery plus RT. There are obvious selection biases favoring combined modality treatment in these patients, because the patients receiving RT alone tend to have more medical comorbidities that often preclude effective control of the cancer by diminishing tolerance to treatment.

Small, well-localized, low-grade tumors excised with clear margins are best treated with surgery alone.[25–28] High-grade, advanced stage (T3/4), and inadequately excised tumors treated with surgery alone have a poor prognosis compared with those treated with adjuvant RT, with an overall local regional control rate of 82% compared with 59% for the group treated with surgery alone in several nonrandomized studies.[24–27,29–37] High tumor grade, advanced stage (T3/4), close or positive margins, and nodal involvement[24–28,32] are the pathologic factors most commonly associated with a high risk of locoregional failure (30%–60%) after surgery. These patients are the ones most likely to benefit from the addition of postoperative radiotherapy.

A recurring theme with most high-grade salivary gland cancers is that, despite adequate long-term locoregional control rates of 80% to 90%, with surgery and RT, the overall rate of distant failures is in the order of 30% to 50%. Effective systemic therapy agents are likely to dramatically affect the survival outcome in these patients, and several novel agents are being studied.

Evaluation of response following primary RT to indolent varieties of salivary gland cancers, including adenoid cystic carcinomas, poses a problem. Radiological responses in these tumors are gradual, and often barely perceptible when annual interval images are compared. In addition, histologic appearances of posttreatment biopsy-detected residual tumor can be confusing, and do not necessarily represent active malignancy. Hence, patient management should take into consideration the presence of symptoms suggesting disease recurrence/progression in these situations.

Neutron Radiotherapy

Fast neutrons are a form of radiation with high linear energy transfer (LET) that directly damages DNA, independent of the presence of molecular oxygen. In comparison, low-LET radiation (X rays, electrons, protons) causes mostly indirect DNA damage, mediated by an oxygen-dependent pathway. In addition, high-LET RT has significantly higher relative biological effectiveness (RBE) for slowly cycling tumors.[38] The RBE for neutron radiotherapy (NRT) versus fractionated RT was 8.0, compared with 3 to 3.5 for most late-responding normal tissues, with a therapeutic gain factor of 2 to 2.5. Damage by NRT is not readily repairable and there is less variation of sensitivity through the cell cycle.[38] Therefore, NRT has a clear theoretic advantage compared with low-LET radiation in tumor models that have 1 or more of the mechanisms discussed earlier contributing to radioresistance to low-LET radiotherapy.

A prospective Radiation Therapy Oncology Group (RTOG)/Medical Research Council (MRC) randomized controlled study[39] compared low-LET radiotherapy (X rays and electrons) with NRT for unresectable primary and recurrent salivary gland tumors. This study could only enroll 32 patients over a 6-year period, which indicates the rarity of the disease and the difficulty in conducting a prospective multicenter randomized study. An interim analysis at 2 years on 25 eligible patients showed that the NRT group achieved significantly better local control both at the primary site and in the lymph nodes (67% vs 17%; $P<.005$) and there was a trend toward improved survival (62% vs 25%; $P = .1$). Hence, the data monitoring committee deemed it unethical to offer any treatment other than NRT for salivary gland cancers. With longer follow-up the survival curves merged and patterns of failure analysis showed that delayed distant metastases accounted for most of the failures in the NRT arm, and local/regional failures predominated in the low-LET arm. The toxicity was worse with NRT in this study, with 9 patients having at least 1 severe or greater complication compared with 4 patients on the low-LET arm. There were no fatal events in either arm. In our experience at the University of Washington, using modern RT techniques, severe toxicity is rare. A retrospective study of 148 patients reported by Douglas and colleagues[40] showed only 6% of patients developing grade 3 or 4 complications using the RTOG/European Organisation for Research and Treatment of Cancer grading system. To date, NRT is currently available only at our center, the University of Washington, creating an issue with access and logistics.

Using conventional RT, selected institutional outcomes seem favorable. For example, Pohar and colleagues[29] reported a local control rate of 85% with primary RT, and Wang and Goodman[41] reported a 5-year actuarial local control of 100% for 9 unresectable parotid gland tumors treated with RT. However, comparison between studies is hampered by methodological problems.

In the postoperative setting, multiple investigators[24–27,42] showed good local control rates of approximately 80% to 85% for patients treated with conventional RT. There are also a few recently reported good outcomes with proton beam therapy[43]; however, longer follow-up will be important to interpret the results in the context of the natural history of salivary gland malignancies.

SYSTEMIC THERAPY

The use of systemic agents in salivary gland cancers is often considered among patients with recurrent/metastatic disease who are not deemed candidates for curative intent therapy. The different histologic subtypes and the heterogeneous natural history within these groups make the determination of the standard of care for systemic therapy challenging. **Table 1** outlines the most common of these histologic subtypes. Several issues complicate the interpretation of the data:

1. Metastatic salivary tumors are rare. Consequently, it is difficult to conduct randomized studies.

Table 1	
Relative frequencies of most common salivary gland carcinoma histologies	
Histology	Frequency (%)
Mucoepidermoid carcinoma	34
Adenoid cystic carcinoma	21
Adenocarcinoma	21
Acinic cell carcinoma	7
Other subtypes	13

Data from Spiro RH. Management of malignant tumors of the salivary glands. Oncology (Williston Park) 1998;12(5):672.

2. Single or multi-institutional phase II trials almost always include all histologies, even though they may have different biological behaviors and responses to therapy. The small number of patients included in each histology may lead to misinterpretation of drug activity.[44,45]
3. Subsets of salivary gland cancers, such as adenoid cystic and acinic cell carcinomas, frequently have an indolent growth pattern. The development of asymptomatic, slowly growing pulmonary metastasis can be observed years after the initial diagnosis, which makes it difficult to interpret the time to progression and stable disease rates described in the studies, particularly considering the lack of randomization.
4. As a consequence of the neurotropism of some of these histologies, particularly adenoid cystic carcinomas, patients may be very symptomatic (nerve palsies/paralysis). However, they may have disease that it is not easily measurable, particularly in the setting of prior surgeries and radiotherapy, and consequently may be excluded from clinical trials.

The Role of Conventional Chemotherapy

Several conventional chemotherapy agents have some activity in advanced salivary gland tumors. These agents include cisplatin, paclitaxel, vinorelbine, epirubicin, mitoxantrone, and methotrexate.[46]

In the mid-1990s investigators from Italy conducted a randomized phase II trial comparing single-agent vinorelbine with the combination of vinorelbine and cisplatin.[47] Exemplifying the difficulties discussed earlier, this study randomized only 36 patients between both arms. Multiple histologies were included but most patients had adenoid cystic carcinoma (n = 22) or adenocarcinoma (n = 9). Patients treated with the combination had a higher response rate (45% vs 19%). More patients were alive at 12 months with the combination (6 vs 1). The investigators concluded that the combination of cisplatin and vinorelbine was superior to single-agent vinorelbine.

Investigators of the National Cancer Institute Clinical Trials Group conducted a phase II study investigating the use of gemcitabine in combination with cisplatin (carboplatin was used when cisplatin was contraindicated).[48] A total of 32 patients were treated. Multiple histologies were included, with a predominance of adenoid cystic carcinoma (n = 10) and adenocarcinoma (n = 8). The initial doublet included cisplatin in 27 cases. Toxicities observed were those expected with these combinations. Prespecified criteria required 13 responses to declare the combination as active; however, only 8 (24%) responses were observed.

Gilbert and colleagues[44] published results from a phase II trial of single-agent paclitaxel in salivary gland cancers conducted through the Eastern Cooperative Oncology

Group (ECOG). Fifty patients with salivary gland cancer were enrolled in this study, with adenocarcinomas, mucoepidermoid carcinomas, and adenoid cystic carcinomas representing the most common histologies. Note that patients were not required to have evidence of disease progression to participate. There were 8 partial responses to paclitaxel. None of the 14 patients with adenoid cystic carcinoma showed an objective response to systemic therapy, and the median overall survival of the cohort of patients was 12.5 months.

Studies of Target Agents

The use of drugs directed to specific molecular abnormalities (target therapies) has transformed the therapy for many malignancies. Because these agents are approved for use in common tumors they have been tested in salivary gland tumors. Most of this work has not been based in the characterization of activating mutations and many remain in abstract format.

Overexpression of c-kit was identified in a high proportion of patients with adenoid cystic carcinoma.[49] Small case series suggested possible activity of imatinib,[50] a drug approved for the therapy for gastrointestinal stromal tumors because of its inhibition of c-kit. Based on this observation, investigators from Canada conducted a phase II trial of imatinib in patients with unresectable or metastatic adenoid cystic carcinoma expressing c-kit.[51] Sixteen patients were included and no responses were observed. This lack of activity was confirmed by investigators from Israel.[52] These disappointing results are likely explained by the fact that c-kit activating mutations, not expression, are the biomarkers that predict response, and are rarely present in adenoid cystic carcinoma.[53]

Epidermal growth factor receptor (EGFR) is strongly expressed by immunohistochemistry (IHC) in 24% of adenoid cystic carcinomas and 52% of mucoepidermoid carcinomas.[54] However, activating mutations are rarely present. Based on the IHC data and the activity in other tumor types, several EGFR targeting agents were tested in salivary gland malignancies. However, gefitinib[55] and cetuximab[56] were not associated with any objective responses. As an example of the challenges in the conduct and interpretation of trials in this disease, the investigators of the cetuximab article were encouraged by the proportion of patients achieving stable disease (80%) and recommended further investigation of EGFR targeting.

HER2 overexpression by IHC and even amplification detected by fluorescence in situ hybridization (FISH) can be found in a few cases of salivary malignancies. Salivary duct carcinomas (SDCs) have the highest rates of both 3+ IHC and FISH high polysomy or amplification.[57] Investigators from Boston, Massachusetts, treated 13 patients with SDC and HER2 expression by IHC[58] with a combination of paclitaxel, carboplatin, and trastuzumab. Eight patients received adjuvant therapy, which makes analysis of efficacy challenging. Among the 5 patients who received palliative therapy, all had 3+ IHC and amplification by FISH. One patient had a complete response, 2 patients had a partial response, and 2 others had progressive disease. The investigators also described that 2 of the patients treated for metastatic disease had received prior trastuzumab as a single agent with prolonged disease control. The frequent finding of HER2 amplification suggests that this may be a viable target in SDC.

Carcinoma ex pleomorphic adenomas, adenocarcinomas, and SDCs have been observed to overexpress estrogen, progesterone, and androgen receptors, making hormonal therapy an intriguing avenue for targeted therapeutics. However, data on the success of this approach are limited to case reports.[59–62]

Based on 2 observed responses in patients with adenoid cystic carcinoma in a phase I study of vorinostat, investigators from Detroit, Michigan, led a multicenter phase II trial.[63] Thirty patients with locally advanced or metastatic disease were enrolled. The treatment was well tolerated. Only 2 patients had confirmed partial responses, both documented late during treatment, after 8 and 10 cycles. Twenty-six patients had stable disease and 45% of those lasted 12 months. Overall, the median progression-free survival was 11.4 months.

ONGOING RESEARCH AND FUTURE DIRECTIONS

Scientific inquiry and prospective clinical investigation among salivary gland malignancies are challenging because of this disease's infrequency and underlying heterogeneity in both histology and biological behavior. Notwithstanding, thoughtful clinical trial design coupled with improvements in molecular profiling technology holds promise in being able to answer relevant clinical questions in the management of this disease, and may ultimately lead to improvements in therapeutic outcomes.

Locally Advanced Disease

Among salivary gland carcinomas treated with curative intent, the observed survival improvement over the past 3 decades is widely attributed to the adoption of postoperative RT.[27,42,64] RT is now considered a treatment standard despite the absence of prospective clinical data supporting its use. In this population, patients with high-risk features such as advanced T and N stages, and positive margins of resection, continue to have suboptimal outcomes and represent a population in need of better treatment options.

In resected squamous cell carcinomas of the head and neck with extracapsular nodal extension and positive margins, benefit from the addition of systemic platinum-based chemotherapy to postoperative radiation has been shown by 2 large clinical trials jointly published in 2004.[65,66] This intensified treatment strategy is intuitively attractive among high-risk resected salivary gland malignancies. Single-institution data with small numbers have reported encouraging results of platinum-based chemoradiation in the postoperative setting.

The NRG/RTOG has recently completed a randomized phase II clinical trial (RTOG 1008 NCT01220583) comparing postoperative RT alone with postoperative cisplatin concurrent with radiation. Note that the design of this study limited enrollment to the most commonly occurring, highest risk resected salivary gland subtypes in an effort to limit the biological heterogeneity inherent in this disease.

Also noteworthy is that RTOG 1008 was an unprecedented attempt to study this rare malignancy in the cooperative group setting. Feasibility was one of its primary end points, which was met with accrual exceeding projected rates. This adjuvant trial also mandated tumor tissue submission and successfully established a prospectively collected salivary gland cancer tissue repository to be used for correlative studies. The success of its completion supports the cooperative groups as a viable setting for the conduct of large clinical trials with the potential to answer critical management questions in rare diseases.

Recurrent/Metastatic Disease

There is currently no standard of care for the management of salivary gland malignancies that are not amenable to curative intent treatment. As previously described, the low incidence and heterogeneity of histologic and clinical behavior pose significant challenges for clinical investigation.

In order to arrive at relevant and interpretable results, the design of clinical trials in the metastatic setting has to accommodate these unique disease features. Modifying the study design to include patients with demonstrated progression of measurable disease, or more aggressive disease subtypes, may enrich the patient population for those in which drug activity may be more objectively determined.

Molecular profiling technology is evolving at a rapid pace and represents a tool with tremendous potential to identify drug targets in this disease. Because of the absence of US Food and Drug Administration–approved targeted drugs for this indication, the role of the routine use of this technology in the clinical setting is unclear. Single-institution reports using genomic profiling are emerging and suggest that these could lead to appropriate drug selection and resultant clinical benefit to patients.[67] Further study of these techniques and their validation in predicting responses to novel agents and/or identifying driver mutations are needed in order to facilitate rational drug selection for clinical investigation.

In addition, therapeutic approaches targeting immune evasion by malignant tumors are gaining relevance in both solid and hematologic malignancies.[68] Immunotherapy and immune checkpoint inhibitors are currently unexplored in salivary gland malignancies. There are provocative preclinical and clinical data suggesting that histone deacetylate inhibitors alter the biology of intratumoral regulatory T cells and may increase tumor PD-L1 expression, and lead to improved responses to PD-1 checkpoint inhibitors in other epithelial malignancies.[69–72] Vorinostat is a histone deacetylase inhibitor that has been studied in adenoid cystic carcinomas.[63] Our group is about to embark on a clinical trial examining the combination of vorinostat and pembrolizumab (a PD-1 inhibitor) in patients with recurrent metastatic salivary gland carcinomas, with the aim of defining the activity and toxicity profiles of these agents in this disease.

REFERENCES

1. Seifert G, Sobin LH. Histological typing of salivary gland tumors. WHO international histological classification of tumors. 2nd edition. Berlin (Germany); New York; Heidelberg (Germany): Springer-Verlag; 1991.
2. Speight PM, Barrett AW. Salivary gland tumors. Oral Dis 2002;8(5):229–40 [Review].
3. Theriault C, Fitzpatrick PJ. Malignant parotid tumors. Prognostic factors and optimum treatment. Am J Clin Oncol 1986;9(6):510–6.
4. Witten J, Hybert F, Hansen HS. Treatment of malignant tumors in the parotid glands. Cancer 1990;65(11):2515–20.
5. Pedersen D, Overgaard J, Søgaard H, et al. Malignant parotid tumors in 110 consecutive patients: treatment results and prognosis. Laryngoscope 1992; 102(9):1064–9.
6. Zbären P, Schüpbach J, Nuyens M, et al. Carcinoma of the parotid gland. Am J Surg 2003;186(1):57–62.
7. Thoeny HC. Imaging of salivary gland tumours. Cancer Imaging 2007;7:52–62 [Review].
8. Yousem DM, Kraut MA, Chalian AA. Major salivary gland imaging. Radiology 2000;216(1):19–29 [Review].
9. Som PM, Curtin HD. 3rd edition. Head and neck imaging, vol. 2. St Louis (MO): Mosby; 1996. p. 877–912.
10. Keyes JW Jr, Harkness BA, Greven KM, et al. Salivary gland tumors: pretherapy evaluation with PET. Radiology 1994;192(1):99–102.
11. Zurrida S, Alasio L, Tradati N, et al. Fine-needle aspiration of parotid masses. Cancer 1993;72(8):2306–11.

12. Wong DS, Li GK. The role of fine-needle aspiration cytology in the management of parotid tumors: a critical clinical appraisal. Head Neck 2000;22(5):469–73.

13. Hillel AD, Fee WE Jr. Evaluation of frozen section in parotid gland surgery. Arch Otolaryngol 1983;109(4):230–2.

14. Wheelis RF, Yarington CT Jr. Tumors of the salivary glands. Comparison of frozen-section diagnosis with final pathologic diagnosis. Arch Otolaryngol 1984;110(2): 76–7.

15. Seethala RR, LiVolsi VA, Baloch ZW. Relative accuracy of fine-needle aspiration and frozen section in the diagnosis of lesions of the parotid gland. Head Neck 2005;27(3):217–23.

16. Scianna JM, Petruzzelli GJ. Contemporary management of tumors of the salivary glands. Curr Oncol Rep 2007;9:134–8.

17. Day TA, Deveikis J, Gillespie MB, et al. Salivary gland neoplasms. Curr Treat Options Oncol 2004;5:11–26.

18. Bell RB, Dierks EJ, Homer L, et al. Management and outcome of patients with malignant salivary gland tumors. J Oral Maxillofac Surg 2005;63(7):917–28.

19. Olsen KD. Tumors and surgery of the parapharyngeal space. Laryngoscope 1994;104(5 Pt 2 Suppl 63):1–28 [Review].

20. Bhattacharyya N, Fried MP. Nodal metastasis in major salivary gland cancer: predictive factors and effects on survival. Arch Otolaryngol Head Neck Surg 2002; 128(8):904–8.

21. Stennert E, Kisner D, Jungehuelsing M, et al. High incidence of lymph node metastasis in major salivary gland cancer. Arch Otolaryngol Head Neck Surg 2003;129(7):720–3.

22. Conley J, Baker DG. "Cancer of the salivary glands." Cancer of the head and neck. New York: Churchill Livingstone; 1981. p. 524–56.

23. Vikram B, Strong EW, Shah JP, et al. Radiation therapy in adenoid cystic carcinoma. Int J Radiat Oncol Biol Phys 1984;10:221–3.

24. Mendenhall WM, Morris CG, Amdur RJ, et al. Radiotherapy alone or combined with surgery for salivary gland carcinoma. Cancer 2005;103:2544–50.

25. Terhaard CHJ, Lubsen H, Rasch CRN, et al. The role of radiotherapy in the treatment of malignant salivary gland tumors. Int J Radiat Oncol Biol Phys 2005;61: 103–11.

26. Chen AM, Granchi PJ, Garcia J, et al. Local-regional recurrence after surgery without post-operative irradiation for carcinomas of the major salivary glands: implications for adjuvant therapy. Int J Radiat Oncol Biol Phys 2007;67:982–7.

27. Armstrong JG, Harrison LB, Spiro RH, et al. Malignant tumors of major salivary gland origin. A matched-pair analysis of the role of combined surgery and postoperative radiotherapy. Arch Otolaryngol Head Neck Surg 1990;116(3):290–3.

28. Kokemueller H, Swennen G, Brueggemann N, et al. Epithelial malignancies of the salivary glands: clinical experience of a single institution—a review. Int J Oral Maxillofac Surg 2004;33:423–32.

29. Pohar S, Gay H, Rosenbaum P, et al. Malignant parotid tumors: presentation, clinical/pathologic prognostic factors, and treatment outcomes. Int J Radiat Oncol Biol Phys 2005;61:112–8.

30. Frankenthaler RA, Luna MA, Lee SS, et al. Prognostic variables in parotid gland cancer. Arch Otolaryngol Head Neck Surg 1991;117:1251–6.

31. Miglianico L, Eschwege F, Marandas P, et al. Cervico-facial adenoid cystic carcinoma: study of 102 cases. Influence of radiation therapy. Int J Radiat Oncol Biol Phys 1987;13:673–8.

32. Renehan AG, Gleave EN, Slevin NJ, et al. Clinico-pathological and treatment-related factors influencing survival in parotid cancer. Br J Cancer 1999;80: 1296–300.

33. Chen AM, Bucci MK, Weinberg V, et al. Adenoid cystic carcinoma of the head and neck treated by surgery with or without postoperative radiation therapy: prognostic features of recurrence. Int J Radiat Oncol Biol Phys 2006;66:152–9.

34. North CA, Lee DJ, Piantadosi S, et al. Carcinoma of the major salivary glands treated by surgery or surgery plus postoperative radiotherapy. Int J Radiat Oncol Biol Phys 1990;18:1319–26.

35. Tran L, Sadeghi A, Hanson D, et al. Major salivary gland tumors: treatment results and prognostic factors. Laryngoscope 1986;96:1139–44.

36. Reddy SP, Marks JE. Treatment of locally advanced, high-grade, malignant tumors of major salivary glands. Laryngoscope 1988;98:450–4.

37. Bissett R, Fitzpatrick P. Malignant submandibular gland tumors. A review of 91 patients. Am J Clin Oncol 1988;11:46–51.

38. Hall EJ, Giaccia AJ. Radiobiology for the radiologist. 6th edition. Philadelphia: Lippincott Wilkins & Williams; 2006.

39. Laramore GE, Krall JM, Griffin TW, et al. Neutron versus photon irradiation for unresectable salivary gland tumors: final report of an RTOG-MRC randomized trial. Int J Radiat Oncol Biol Phys 1993;27:235–40.

40. Douglas JD, Silbergeld DL, Laramore GE. Gamma knife stereotactic radiosurgical boost for patients treated primarily with neutron radiotherapy for salivary gland neoplasms. Stereotact Funct Neurosurg 2004;82:84–9.

41. Wang CC, Goodman M. Photon irradiation of unresectable carcinomas of salivary glands. Int J Radiat Oncol Biol Phys 1991;21:569–76.

42. Garden AS, el-Naggar AK, Morrison WH, et al. Postoperative radiotherapy for malignant tumors of the parotid gland. Int J Radiat Oncol Biol Phys 1997;37(1): 79–85.

43. Frank SJ, Cox JD, Gillin M, et al. Multifield optimization intensity modulated proton therapy for head and neck tumors: a translation to practice. Int J Radiat Oncol Biol Phys 2014;89(4):846–53.

44. Gilbert J, Li Y, Pinto HA, et al. Phase II trial of Taxol in salivary gland malignancies (E1394): a trial of the Eastern Cooperative Oncology Group. Head Neck 2006;28: 197–204.

45. Till BG, Martins RG. Response to paclitaxel in adenoid cystic carcinoma of the salivary glands. Head Neck 2008;30:810–4.

46. Laurie SA, Licitra L. Systemic therapy in the palliative management of advanced salivary gland cancers. J Clin Oncol 2008;24:2673–8.

47. Airoldi M, Pedani F, Succo G, et al. Phase II randomized trial comparing vinorelbine versus vinorelbine plus cisplatin in patients with recurrent salivary gland malignancies. Cancer 2001;91:541–7.

48. Laurie SA, Siu LL, Winquist E, et al. A phase II study of platinum and gemcitabine in patients with advanced salivary gland cancer. Cancer 2010;116:362–8.

49. Jeng YM, Lin CY, Hsu HC. Expression of c-kit is associated with certain subtypes of salivary gland carcinoma. Cancer Lett 2000;154:107111.

50. Alcebo JC, Fabrega JM, Arosena JR, et al. Imatinib mesylate as treatment for adenoid cystic carcinoma of the salivary glands; report of two successfully treated cases. Head Neck 2004;26:829–31.

51. Hotte SJ, Winquist EW, Lamont E, et al. Imatinib mesylate in patients with adenoid cystic cancers of the salivary gland expressing c-kit: a Princess Margaret Hospital phase II consortium study. J Clin Oncol 2005;23:585–90.

52. Pfeffer MR, Talmi Y, Catane R, et al. Phase II study of imatinib for advanced adenoid cystic carcinoma of the head and neck salivary glands. Oral Oncol 2007;43:33–6.

53. Wetterskog D, Wilkerson PM, Rodrigues DN, et al. Mutation profiling of adenoid cystic carcinomas from multiple anatomical sites identifies mutations in the RAS pathway, but no KIT mutations. Histopathology 2013;62:543–50.

54. Clauditz TS, Gontarewicz A, Lebok P, et al. Epidermal growth factor receptor (EGFR) in salivary gland carcinomas: potential as therapeutic target. Oral Oncol 2012;48:991–6.

55. Jakob JA, Kies MS, Glisson BS, et al. Phase II study of gefitinib in patients with advanced salivary gland cancers. Head Neck 2015;37(5):644–9.

56. Locati LD, Bossi P, Perrone F, et al. Cetuximab in recurrent and/or metastatic salivary gland carcinoma: a phase II study. Oral Oncol 2009;45:574–8.

57. Etti T, Stiegler C, Zeitler K, et al. EGFR, HER2, surviving, and loss of pSTAT3 characterize high-grade malignancy in salivary gland cancer with impact on prognosis. Hum Pathol 2012;43:921–31.

58. Limaye SA, Posner MR, Krane JF. Trastuzumab for the treatment of salivary duct carcinoma. Oncologist 2013;18:294–300.

59. Nasser SM, Faquin WC, Dayal Y. Expression of androgen, estrogen, and progesterone receptors in salivary gland tumors. Frequent expression of androgen receptor in a subset of malignant salivary gland tumors. Am J Clin Pathol 2003; 119(6):801–6.

60. Jaspers HC, Verbist BM, Schoffelen R, et al. Androgen receptor-positive salivary duct carcinoma: a disease entity with promising new treatment options. J Clin Oncol 2011;29(16):e473–6.

61. Campos-Gómez S, Flores-Arredondo JH, Dorantes-Heredia R, et al. Case report: anti-hormonal therapy in the treatment of ductal carcinoma of the parotid gland. BMC Cancer 2014;14:701.

62. Elkin AD, Jacobs CD. Tamoxifen for salivary gland adenoid cystic carcinoma: report of two cases. J Cancer Res Clin Oncol 2008;134(10):1151–3.

63. Goncalves PH, Kummar S, Siu LL, et al. A phase II study of suberoylanilide hydroxamic acid (SAHA) in subjects with locally advanced, recurrent, or metastatic adenoid cystic carcinoma. J Clin Oncol 2013;31, 203(suppl):[abstr: 6045].

64. Terhaard CH, Lubsen H, Van der Tweel I, et al. Salivary gland carcinoma: independent prognostic factors for locoregional control, distant metastases, and overall survival: results of the Dutch Head and Neck Oncology Cooperative Group. Head Neck 2004;26(8):681–92 [discussion: 692–3].

65. Bernier J, Domenge C, Ozsahin M, et al. Postoperative irradiation with or without concomitant chemotherapy for locally advanced head and neck cancer. N Engl J Med 2004;350(19):1945–52.

66. Cooper JS, Pajak TF, Forastiere AA, et al. Postoperative concurrent radiotherapy and chemotherapy for high-risk squamous-cell carcinoma of the head and neck. N Engl J Med 2004;350(19):1937–44.

67. Chintakuntlawar AV, Okuno SH, Andress Rowe Price K. Genomic testing may offer therapeutic opportunity in salivary gland cancers. J Clin Oncol 2015; 33(Suppl) [abstr: e17053].

68. Disis ML. Immune regulation of cancer. J Clin Oncol 2010;28(29):4531–8.

69. Christiansen AJ, West A, Banks KM, et al. Eradication of solid tumors using histone deacetylase inhibitors combined with immune-stimulating antibodies. Proc Natl Acad Sci U S A 2011;108(10):4141–6.

70. Shen L, Ciesielski M, Ramakrishnan S, et al. Class I histone deacetylase inhibitor entinostat suppresses regulatory T cells and enhances immunotherapies in renal and prostate cancer models. PLoS One 2012;7(1):e30815.
71. Wrangle J, Wang W, Koch A, et al. Alterations of immune response of non-small cell lung cancer with azacytidine. Oncotarget 2013;4(11):2067–79.
72. Yang H, Bueso-Ramos C, DiNardo C, et al. Expression of PD-L1, PD-L2, PD-1 and CTLA4 in myelodysplastic syndromes is enhanced by treatment with hypomethylating agents. Leukemia 2014;28(6):1280–8.

Supportive Care and Survivorship Strategies in Management of Squamous Cell Carcinoma of the Head and Neck

Aru Panwar, MD[a,b], Veronique Wan Fook Cheung, MD[a], William M. Lydiatt, MD[a,b],*

KEYWORDS

- Head and neck • Squamous cell carcinoma • Supportive care • Survivorship
- Cancer treatment • Depression

KEY POINTS

- Management of head and neck squamous cell carcinoma (HNSCC) can result in significant short- and long-term physical and psychosocial impact.
- Patients with HNSCC have unique needs for follow-up, surveillance, and management of acute and delayed toxicity from treatment, which can result in significant adverse functional, cosmetic, and behavioral health outcomes.
- Effective supportive care and survivorship strategies require collaborative and multidisciplinary efforts.

INTRODUCTION

Head and neck cancer contributes significantly to the global burden of cancer-related disease and is ranked fifth worldwide in overall incidence.[1] Squamous cell carcinoma may arise in the mucous membranes of the oral cavity, oropharynx, larynx, paranasal sinuses, nasopharynx, skin, and, infrequently, in the salivary glandular tissue. Management of such malignancies involves use of surgery and irradiation, alone or in combination with chemotherapy. Each therapy has significant potential for treatment-related adverse effects. When management involves a combination of therapeutic choices, treatment-related side effects are exacerbated.[2]

Patients who receive treatment of HNSCC often experience significant acute toxicities as well as a plethora of long-term sequelae. The unique combination of challenges posed by cosmetic disfigurement, physical and functional impairment, and

The authors have no relevant financial disclosures.

[a] Division of Head and Neck Surgical Oncology, University of Nebraska Medical Center, 981225 Nebraska Medical Center, Omaha, NE 68198-1225, USA; [b] Head and Neck Surgical Oncology, Nebraska Methodist Hospital, 8303 Dodge St., Omaha, NE 68154, USA

* Corresponding author. 981225 Nebraska Medical Center, Omaha, NE 68198-1225.

E-mail address: wmlydiatt@cox.net

Hematol Oncol Clin N Am 29 (2015) 1159–1168

http://dx.doi.org/10.1016/j.hoc.2015.07.010

psychosocial stress resulting from the disease and its treatment requires dedicated and multidisciplinary collaborative efforts for effective management.

Improved diagnostic tools, more effective and diverse therapeutic choices, and the changing demographics of the population with head and neck cancer have led to significantly improved survival rates.[3,4] A longer posttreatment survival is, however, accompanied by additional long-term morbidities resulting from therapy. These complications of therapy may not become manifest for 5 or 10 years, but the younger patient population and improved survival makes these considerations all the more germane. As a result, identification of strategies aimed at minimizing treatment-related complications and optimizing their long-term management are increasingly critical.

Institutions and head and neck cancer teams devoted to the multidisciplinary care of patients with HNSCC should incorporate a robust plan for addressing survivorship. The goals for ongoing care should include not only early identification and management of locoregional or distant failure and second primary malignancies but also effective management of treatment-related complications such as xerostomia, dental disease, osteoradionecrosis (ORN), hypothyroidism, speech, and swallowing disturbances. Other areas critical to healthy survivorship that require specialized attention to diagnose and treat include nutritional deficiency, substance abuse, and behavioral health. Although an in-depth examination of available evidence for individual management strategies for these diverse but related issues is beyond the scope of this article, it outlines recommended management strategies, provides consensus guidelines, and identifies areas where controversy and knowledge gaps exist.

SURVIVORSHIP CARE PLANS

Care of the patient with head and neck cancer is complex and, in addition to engagement of the patients and their families, requires involvement of multiple health care teams, including surgeons, medical and radiation oncologists, dental providers, speech and language pathology professionals, social workers, nurse managers, psychologists, and the patients' primary care providers. Efficient and cost-effective care patterns require superior interdisciplinary coordination and safe and effective transitions of care to community physicians when considered appropriate. Survivorship care plans (SCPs) may serve as important tools in helping achieve these goals.

The Institute of Medicine (IOM) recommendations stress the importance of measures geared toward improving awareness about unique needs of a cancer survivor and the significance of a comprehensive care summary describing follow-up plans and ongoing management for patients on completion of primary therapy.[5] The IOM recommendations are rooted in the 2 key observations that many cancer survivors are lost to follow-up and that important opportunities for intervention are missed during transitions of care.[5]

However, adoption of SCP has been far from universal. Among the National Cancer Institute–designated cancer centers, only about half of the patients who underwent therapy for breast or colorectal malignancies received SCPs.[6,7] Although SCPs may lead to increased sense of comfort for primary care providers entrusted with caring for cancer survivors and reduction in anxiety related to care transitions for the patients, several barriers continue to limit the use of such tools.[6] These barriers include the additional demands relating to time, personnel, and resources that may be needed for generating and communicating effective SCPs to the intended audience, in a cost-sensitive health care environment, with no additional reimbursements for such efforts.[6,8]

Concerns about the ability of patients and providers to integrate SCPs into ongoing clinical care exist, and the additional documentation can easily be lost within the large volume of documentation encountered through the process of cancer care. Studies indicate that a large number of patients and many physicians failed to remember if they received an SCP document, and most patients could not locate the document 3 years after therapy completion. In addition, scientifically accurate verbiage in such a document may hold little or no value to patients, and hence a single static document may not effectively serve the needs of a community physician and the patient during care transitions.[9]

Regardless of the medium used, effective communication between health care providers and the patient is critical to reduce errors, improve efficiencies, ensure timely interventions, and avoid duplicity of efforts and investigations. Such communication should include clear summation of the disease process, administered therapy, ongoing interventions, and future plans for follow-up, investigations, and interventions. Whenever possible, the rational for future interventions and investigations should be included.

Although consensus guidelines specific to the care of HNSCC survivors are not readily available, physicians may use standardized guidelines and resources from a global cancer care perspective to help manage patients, including clinical practice guidelines from the IOM and cancer survivorship guidelines from the National Comprehensive Cancer Network (NCCN).[5,10] Other guidelines addressing chemotherapy-related neuropathy, fatigue, and anxiety and depression have been made available by the American Society of Clinical Oncology.[11]

CANCER TREATMENT–RELATED PHYSICAL EFFECTS

Head and neck cancer therapy can be associated with debilitating physical effects. Although acute toxicity related to irradiation and chemotherapeutic or targeted agents may subside soon after therapy cessation, some, including mucositis, may persist for a significant duration. Other side effects may persist for a long time, be permanent, or may appear after a delay. These treatment sequelae contribute toward long-term toxicity and the associated compromise in quality of life, including issues such as xerostomia, hypothyroidism, radiation-related accelerated vascular disease, ORN, and associated symptoms such as dysphagia, pain, chronic aspiration, and decline in nutrition and general well-being. Other long-term sequelae, such as lymphedema, soft-tissue fibrosis, decreased range of motion, trismus, and speech and swallowing disturbances, require continued participation of physical therapists and speech and language pathology specialists in survivor care.[12]

A variety of regimens and agents have been tried for the management of mucositis with variable benefit. Poor quality of available evidence limits interpretation of value of individual agents used in the management of oral mucositis. Recently published consensus guidelines indicate that relief of pain associated with mucositis, using 2% morphine oral rinse and tricyclic antidepressants such as doxepin may be of value. The role of antifungals and topical anesthetic agents remains unclear. Evidence suggests that routine use of oral antibiotics, chlorhexidine mouthwashes, and coating agents such as sucralfate did not improve outcomes, and use of these agents is generally not recommended.[13,14] Small-scale studies and a randomized control trial investigating the role of low-level laser therapy to affected mucosa has shown some promise.[13,15,16]

Radiation-induced xerostomia contributes to life-long morbidity with associated symptoms that include burning sensation, pain, altered taste, poor dentition, and malnutrition. Strategies for management include maintenance of oral hygiene, salivary substitutes (including lysozyme-containing gels, lactoferrin, and peroxidase), sialogogues such as pilocarpine, xylitol chewing gums, sorbitol lozenges, hydration, fluoride-rich agents, and antimicrobials.[12,17,18] However, data regarding individual efficacy of these agents are difficult to interpret. Early and continued involvement of an experienced dental provider may help to mitigate and manage risks related to xerostomia-related dental caries and ORN.[17,19] Finally, the role of acupuncture has been investigated in a randomized controlled trial, and there seems to be increased salivary flow and symptomatic relief.[20]

Nearly half of the patients treated for HNSCC with irradiation to the neck develop hypothyroidism months or years after completion of therapy. Symptoms of hypothyroidism can be innocuous, and diagnosis may be suspected in a patient with vague features such as fatigue, depression, and poor energy levels.[21,22] A high index of suspicion and appropriate screening with serum measurements of thyroid stimulating hormone every 6 to 12 months is recommended, and thyroid hormone replacement should be instituted as appropriate when hypothyroidism is identified.[12,23]

Investigators report a high incidence of accelerated atherosclerotic cardiovascular disease and related mortality risk in HNSCC survivors with advanced age.[24] Higher incidence of carotid stenosis and cerebrovascular events in patients following radiation therapy to head and neck may contribute to a substantial number of deaths in HNSCC survivors.[21,24,25] Although evidence-based guidelines for prevention and management of radiation-associated vasculopathy are scarce, patients should be evaluated based on individual risks, suspicious examination findings such as vascular bruits, and symptoms related to cerebral ischemia.[26] Screening tools such as vascular duplex ultrasound imaging, may be used and lifestyle modifications may be indicated in patients, because many patients share common risk factors for vascular disease (such as tobacco and alcohol use).[27] In these patients, risk reduction strategies such as use of statins or antiplatelet therapy should be based on their overall cardiovascular risk.

Perhaps the most significant long-term complication occurs because of fibrosis of the muscles of swallowing. The slow but relentless loss of ability to elevate the larynx, invert the epiglottis, and protect from aspiration is one of the mechanisms for all-cause survival being reduced in survivors of health and neck cancer. Coupled with cranial neuropathies that reduce the ability of the tongue and vocal cords to perform their function, chronic aspiration is a slow but relentless enemy of survival and quality of life. The combination of irradiation and chemotherapy increase this risk. Prevention and strengthening exercises may mitigate this risk to some degree and, although not definitively proven to decrease long-term swallowing and cranial neuropathies, they at least enhance awareness.[28]

CANCER-RELATED PSYCHOLOGICAL DISTRESS

Fear of cancer recurrence, treatment-related anxiety, and depression are often underrecognized in HNSCC survivors.[29] Although most patients experience a modest fear of cancer recurrence, such fear is more strongly felt among patients with lower education levels and lack of optimism and among patients who identify as Hispanic or white.[30] Such fear affects quality of survivorship experience, psychosocial well-being, and risk for continued tobacco abuse.[31,32] A high index of suspicion, appropriate screening, and evaluation by trained behavioral health professionals are often required, along with behavioral therapy, when indicated for management of patient symptoms.[31,33] Additional sources of psychosocial stress may stem from treatment-related disfigurement, altered social interactions, loss of professional position, and perceived compromise to humanity in the setting of impaired breathing, speech, eating, and challenges with physical intimacy.[34,35] One-half of HNSCC survivors report quality-of-life issues relating to food intake, whereas 1 in every 5 patients has long-term pain issues and one-third of the patients report significant long-term psychological distress.[35,36]

Development of depression is common in HNSCC survivors, and 13% to 44% of patients reported symptoms of depression. These statistics are comparable with other cohorts of patients with cancer.[34,35,37–39] Patients who experience depression during the treatment of HNSCC are 1.5 times more likely to inflict self-harm and commit suicide.[40] Management strategies depend on early identification of at-risk patients, use of screening tools, involvement of social contacts and/or family, psychotherapy, counseling, and antidepressants.[36]

There is randomized, placebo-controlled evidence to support the role of prophylactic antidepressants in patients who undergo therapy for HNSCC. In a randomized controlled trial published by the authors' group, prophylactic use of escitalopram led to a 50% reduction in the rate of depression in patients being treated for HNSCC. In addition, prophylactic pharmacotherapy resulted in improved quality of life for up to 3 months after cessation of therapy.[40]

SUBSTANCE ABUSE AND SURVIVORSHIP

Many patients with HNSCC have a shared history of exposure to tobacco, alcohol, and potentially other substances. Patients should be asked about ongoing or previous history of substance use. Data suggest that patients who continue to smoke on diagnosis and through therapy are at higher risk for death and progression of disease.[41] Continued smoking is associated with a 5-fold elevated risk for second primary malignancies.[42–45] Counseling and dedicated smoking cessation programs with use of pharmacologic adjuncts may be useful when isolated use of smoking cessation aids proves ineffective.[44]

The role of electronic cigarettes in smoking cessation remains under scrutiny, because concerns exist about potential for increased nicotine dependence.[46] In other studies, use of electronic cigarettes was associated with reduction in the number of cigarettes smoked, comparable with transdermal nicotine patch use.[47,48] Similarly, continued alcohol dependence may be associated with 2- to 3-fold increased incidence of second primary malignancy, and appropriate counseling and assistance for its cessation are advisable.[43,49]

ONCOLOGIC SURVEILLANCE AND DETECTION OF SECOND PRIMARY MALIGNANCIES

Surveillance strategies are tailored for potential early detection of locoregional recurrences, thus affording potential opportunities for intervention and salvage. However, the value of intense surveillance strategies in improving overall survival and outcomes remains controversial, especially in patients with HNSCC with advanced-stage tumors and those who require irradiation as part of their primary therapy. However, surveillance visits offer additional opportunities for reassurance, psychosocial support, nutritional management, and management of long-term treatment-related toxicities.

Most recurrences are detected within the initial 2 to 3 years after therapy completion. HNSCC survivors experience a 25% higher risk for long-term mortality than age- and gender-matched counterparts in the general population, and nearly 1 in 3 deaths observed in the initial decade after primary therapy relate to recurrence or metachronous malignancies.[50,51]

Current recommendations from NCCN suggest complete head and neck examination, using in-office fiberoptic examination, when applicable, as an extension of clinical examination, every 1 to 3 months for year 1, every 2 to 4 months for year 2, every 4 to 6 months for years 3 to 5, and annually thereafter.[12]

Posttreatment imaging should be obtained for establishing a new baseline for the primary site and nodal basins usually within 3 to 6 months after completion of primary therapy. Routine imaging is not advisable as part of follow-up and should be used in the setting of new or concerning symptoms or signs on clinical examination.[12]

Second primary malignancies account for nearly 25% of HNSCC survivor deaths. With an annual incidence of 3% to 7%, detection of these tumors is an important goal of ongoing survivorship. More than half of these arise in lung parenchyma or bronchi, whereas esophageal and colorectal malignancies contribute to 10% and 5% of these tumors.[22] The clustering of these malignancies in patients with HNSCC may occur in the setting of shared exposure to tobacco, alcohol, and other causative agents resulting in field cancerization of the upper aerodigestive tract.[52–54] However, the incidence of second primary malignancies is estimated to be lower in patients with p16-associated oropharyngeal squamous cell carcinoma.[55] Overall, routine screening for malignant neoplasms should be tailored to individual patient characteristics, including age, heredity, and personal history of at-risk behavior, in light of existing disease-specific screening guidelines.

Screening for lung masses has largely been addressed by way of annual chest radiography in many centers because of ease of access, limited radiation exposure, and health care economics. However, chest radiography is a poor screening tool and may fail to detect clinically relevant pulmonary lesions in up to 65% of cases. As a result, the NCCN and American Cancer Society recommend against the use of chest radiography for lung cancer screening.[56,57] Low-dose computerized tomography (LDCT) is superior to chest radiography in detecting lung malignancy in high-risk population with history of tobacco smoking and may reduce lung cancer–specific mortality by 20%. However, meta-analyses reveal that LDCT may not affect all-cause mortality and may result in higher false-positive rates.[56,58,59] HNSCC survivors between ages 55 and 74 years, with 30 or more pack-year history of smoking, are eligible for annual lung cancer screening using LDCT.[60,61] Patients should be counseled about the risk of false-positive results and the failure to reduce all-cause mortality while opting for LDCT screening while considering costs and false-positive rates.[60,62]

SUMMARY

Supportive care and survivorship strategies in the management of HNSCC revolve around continued collaborative efforts aimed at early identification of and intervention for locoregional disease recurrence, second primary malignancy, management of treatment-related side effects, and provision for psychosocial support. Development of evidence-based guidelines and optimization of these strategies is increasingly important in the setting of improved survival of patients with HNSCC owing to a variety of diagnostic and therapeutic advances and evolving demographics of HNSCC patient population, specifically p16-associated oropharyngeal squamous cell carcinoma.

REFERENCES

1. Goon PK, Stanley MA, Ebmeyer J, et al. HPV & head and neck cancer: a descriptive update. Head Neck Oncol 2009;1:36.

2. Trotti A, Bellm LA, Epstein JB, et al. Mucositis incidence, severity and associated out-comes in patients with head and neck cancer receiving radiotherapy with or without chemotherapy: a systematic literature review. Radiother Oncol 2003;66(3):253–62.

3. Survival, epidemiology and end results program website. http://seer.cancer.gov/faststats/selections.php?#Output. Accessed July, 2015.

4. Pulte D, Brenner H. Changes in survival in head and neck cancers in the late 20th and early 21st century: a period analysis. Oncologist 2010;15(9):994–1001.

5. National Research Council. Cancer patient to cancer survivor: lost in transition. Washington, DC: The National Academies Press; 2005.

6. Salz T, Oeffinger KC, McCabe MS, et al. Survivorship care plans in research and practice. CA Cancer J Clin 2012;62(2):101–17.

7. Stricker CT, Jacobs LA, Risendal B, et al. Survivorship care planning after the Institute of Medicine recommendations: how are we faring? J Cancer Surviv 2011;5(4):358–70.

8. Hewitt ME, Bamundo A, Day R, et al. Perspectives on post-treatment cancer care: qualitative research with survivors, nurses, and physicians. J Clin Oncol 2007; 25(16):2270–3.

9. Campbell BH, Massey BL, Myers KB. Survivorship care plans for patients with head and neck cancer. Arch Otolaryngol Head Neck Surg 2012;138(12):1116–9.

10. National Comprehensive Cancer Network clinical practice guidelines in oncology - survivorship. http://www.nccn.org/professionals/physician_gls/pdf/survivorship.pdf. Accessed July, 2015.

11. Practice guidelines: ASCO Institute for Quality. http://www.instituteforquality.org/practice-guidelines. Accessed July, 2015.

12. National Comprehensive Cancer Network clinical practice guidelines in oncology - head and neck cancer. http://www.nccn.org/professionals/physician_gls/pdf/head-and-neck.pdf. Accessed July 2015.

13. Mallick S, Benson R, Rath GK. Radiation induced oral mucositis: a review of cur-rent literature on prevention and management. Eur Arch Otorhinolaryngol 2015. [Epub ahead of print].

14. Saunders DP, Epstein JB, Elad S, et al. Systematic review of antimicrobials, mucosal coating agents, anesthetics, and analgesics for the management of oral mucositis in cancer patients. Support Care Cancer 2013;21(11):3191–207.

15. Oton-Leite AF, Silva GB, Morais MO, et al. Effect of low-level laser therapy on chemoradiotherapy-induced oral mucositis and salivary inflammatory mediators in head and neck cancer patients. Lasers Surg Med 2015;47(4):296–305.

16. Gautam AP, Fernandes DJ, Vidyasagar MS, et al. Effect of low-level laser therapy on patient reported measures of oral mucositis and quality of life in head and neck cancer patients receiving chemoradiotherapy–a randomized controlled trial. Support Care Cancer 2013;21(5):1421–8.

17. Epstein JB, Guneri P, Barasch A. Appropriate and necessary oral care for people with cancer: guidance to obtain the right oral and dental care at the right time. Support Care Cancer 2014;22(7):1981–8.

18. Hutchinson CT, Suntharalingam M, Strome SE. What are the best management stra-tegies for radiation-induced xerostomia? Laryngoscope 2014;124(2):359–60.

19. Ruggiero S, Gralow J, Marx RE, et al. Practical guidelines for the prevention, diagnosis, and treatment of osteonecrosis of the jaw in patients with cancer. J Oncol Pract 2006;2(1):7–14.

20. Meng Z, Garcia MK, Hu C, et al. Randomized controlled trial of acupuncture for prevention of radiation-induced xerostomia among patients with nasopharyngeal carcinoma. Cancer 2012;118(13):3337–44.

21. Choi M, Craft B, Geraci SA. Surveillance and monitoring of adult cancer survivors. Am J Med 2011;124(7):598–601.
22. Zohar Y, Tovim RB, Laurian N, et al. Thyroid function following radiation and surgical therapy in head and neck malignancy. Head Neck Surg 1984;6(5):948–52.
23. Garcia-Serra A, Amdur RJ, Morris CG, et al. Thyroid function should be monitored following radiotherapy to the low neck. Am J Clin Oncol 2005;28(3):255–8.
24. Baxi SS, Pinheiro LC, Patil SM, et al. Causes of death in long-term survivors of head and neck cancer. Cancer 2014;120(10):1507–13.
25. Bashar K, Healy D, Clarke-Moloney M, et al. Effects of neck radiation therapy on extra-cranial carotid arteries atherosclerosis disease prevalence: systematic review and a meta-analysis. PLoS One 2014;9(10):e110389.
26. Plummer C, Henderson RD, O'Sullivan JD, et al. Ischemic stroke and transient ischemic attack after head and neck radiotherapy: a review. Stroke 2011;42(9):2410–8.
27. Xu J, Cao Y. Radiation-induced carotid artery stenosis: a comprehensive review of the literature. Interv Neurol 2014;2(4):183–92.
28. Hutcheson KA, Lewin JS, Barringer DA, et al. Late dysphagia after radiotherapy-based treatment of head and neck cancer. Cancer 2012;118(23):5793–9.
29. Boyajian RN, Grose A, Grenon N, et al. Desired elements and timing of cancer survivorship care: one approach may not fit all. J Oncol Pract 2014;10(5):e293–8.
30. Koch L, Jansen L, Brenner H, et al. Fear of recurrence and disease progression in long-term (>/= 5 years) cancer survivors–a systematic review of quantitative studies. Psychooncology 2013;22(1):1–11.
31. Thewes B, Brebach R, Dzidowska M, et al. Current approaches to managing fear of cancer recurrence; a descriptive survey of psychosocial and clinical health professionals. Psychooncology 2014;23(4):390–6.
32. Van Liew JR, Christensen AJ, Howren MB, et al. Fear of recurrence impacts health-related quality of life and continued tobacco use in head and neck cancer survivors. Health Psychol 2014;33(4):373–81.
33. Ghazali N, Cadwallader E, Lowe D, et al. Fear of recurrence among head and neck cancer survivors: longitudinal trends. Psychooncology 2013;22(4):807–13.
34. Chen AM, Daly ME, Vazquez E, et al. Depression among long-term survivors of head and neck cancer treated with radiation therapy. JAMA Otolaryngol Head Neck Surg 2013;139(9):885–9.
35. Funk GF, Karnell LH, Christensen AJ. Long-term health-related quality of life in survivors of head and neck cancer. Arch Otolaryngol Head Neck Surg 2012;138(2):123–33.
36. Bjordal K, Kaasa S. Psychological distress in head and neck cancer patients 7-11 years after curative treatment. Br J Cancer 1995;71(3):592–7.
37. Zabora J, BrintzenhofeSzoc K, Curbow B, et al. The prevalence of psychological distress by cancer site. Psychooncology 2001;10(1):19–28.
38. Katz MR, Kopek N, Waldron J, et al. Screening for depression in head and neck cancer. Psychooncology 2004;13(4):269–80.
39. Moubayed SP, Sampalis JS, Ayad T, et al. Predicting depression and quality of life among long-term head and neck cancer survivors. Otolaryngol Head Neck Surg 2015;152(1):91–7.
40. Lydiatt WM, Bessette D, Schmid KK, et al. Prevention of depression with escitalopram in patients undergoing treatment for head and neck cancer: randomized, double-blind, placebo-controlled clinical trial. JAMA Otolaryngol Head Neck Surg 2013;139(7):678–86.

41. Gillison ML, Zhang Q, Jordan R, et al. Tobacco smoking and increased risk of death and progression for patients with p16-positive and p16-negative oropharyngeal cancer. J Clin Oncol 2012;30(17):2102–11.

42. Khuri FR, Kim ES, Lee JJ, et al. The impact of smoking status, disease stage, and index tumor site on second primary tumor incidence and tumor recurrence in the head and neck retinoid chemoprevention trial. Cancer Epidemiol Biomarkers Prev 2001;10(8):823–9.

43. Lin K, Patel SG, Chu PY, et al. Second primary malignancy of the aerodigestive tract in patients treated for cancer of the oral cavity and larynx. Head Neck 2005;27(12):1042–8.

44. Vander Ark W, DiNardo LJ, Oliver DS. Factors affecting smoking cessation in patients with head and neck cancer. Laryngoscope 1997;107(7):888–92.

45. de Bruin-Visser JC, Ackerstaff AH, Rehorst H, et al. Integration of a smoking cessation program in the treatment protocol for patients with head and neck and lung cancer. Eur Arch Otorhinolaryngol 2012;269(2):659–65.

46. Borderud SP, Li Y, Burkhalter JE, et al. Electronic cigarette use among patients with cancer: characteristics of electronic cigarette users and their smoking cessation outcomes. Cancer 2014;120(22):3527–35.

47. Bullen C, Howe C, Laugesen M, et al. Electronic cigarettes for smoking cessation: a randomised controlled trial. Lancet 2013;382(9905):1629–37.

48. Franck C, Budlovsky T, Windle SB, et al. Electronic cigarettes in North America: history, use, and implications for smoking cessation. Circulation 2014;129(19):1945–52.

49. Druesne-Pecollo N, Keita Y, Touvier M, et al. Alcohol drinking and second primary cancer risk in patients with upper aerodigestive tract cancers: a systematic review and meta-analysis of observational studies. Cancer Epidemiol Biomarkers Prev 2014;23(2):324–31.

50. Fuller CD, Wang SJ, Thomas CR Jr, et al. Conditional survival in head and neck squamous cell carcinoma: results from the SEER dataset 1973-1998. Cancer 2007;109(7):1331–43.

51. van der Schroeff MP, van de Schans SA, Piccirillo JF, et al. Conditional relative survival in head and neck squamous cell carcinoma: permanent excess mortality risk for long-term survivors. Head Neck 2010;32(12):1613–8.

52. Cognetti DM, Weber RS, Lai SY. Head and neck cancer: an evolving treatment paradigm. Cancer 2008;113(7 Suppl):1911–32.

53. Pelucchi C, Tramacere I, Boffetta P, et al. Alcohol consumption and cancer risk. Nutr Cancer 2011;63(7):983–90.

54. Slaughter DP, Southwick HW, Smejkal W. Field cancerization in oral stratified squamous epithelium; clinical implications of multicentric origin. Cancer 1953; 6(5):963–8.

55. Ang KK, Harris J, Wheeler R, et al. Human papillomavirus and survival of patients with oropharyngeal cancer. N Engl J Med 2010;363(1):24–35.

56. Manser R, Lethaby A, Irving LB, et al. Screening for lung cancer. Cochrane Database Syst Rev 2013;(6):CD001991.

57. Shah SI, Applebaum EL. Lung cancer after head and neck cancer: role of chest radiography. Laryngoscope 2000;110(12):2033–6.

58. Fu C, Liu Z, Zhu F, et al. A meta-analysis: is low-dose computed tomography a superior method for risky lung cancers screening population? Clin Respir J 2014. [Epub ahead of print].

59. National Lung Screening Trial Research Team, Aberle DR, Adams AM, et al. Reduced lung-cancer mortality with low-dose computed tomographic screening. N Engl J Med 2011;365(5):395–409.

60. National Comprehensive Cancer Network clinical practice guidelines in oncology - lung cancer screening. http://www.nccn.org/professionals/physician_gls/pdf/lung_screening.pdf. Accessed July 2015

61. Wood DE, Eapen GA, Ettinger DS, et al. Lung cancer screening. J Natl Compr Canc Netw 2012;10(2):240–65.

62. Wender R, Fontham ET, Barrera E Jr, et al. American Cancer Society lung cancer screening guidelines. CA Cancer J Clin 2013;63(2):107–17.

Index

Note: Page numbers of article titles are in **boldface** type.

Hematol Oncol Clin N Am 29 (2015) 1169–1177
http://dx.doi.org/10.1016/S0889-8588(15)00166-5
0889-8588/15/$ – see front matter © 2015 Elsevier Inc. All rights reserved.

Moving?

Make sure your subscription moves with you!

To notify us of your new address, find your **Clinics Account Number** (located on your mailing label above your name), and contact customer service at:

Email: journalscustomerservice-usa@elsevier.com

800-654-2452 (subscribers in the U.S. & Canada)
314-447-8871 (subscribers outside of the U.S. & Canada)

Fax number: 314-447-8029

**Elsevier Health Sciences Division
Subscription Customer Service
3251 Riverport Lane
Maryland Heights, MO 63043**

*To ensure uninterrupted delivery of your subscription, please notify us at least 4 weeks in advance of move.

Printed and bound by CPI Group (UK) Ltd, Croydon, CR0 4YY

03/10/2024

01040497-0002